Handbook of Psychosocial Interventions with Older Adults

In the past decade, evidence based practice (EBP) has emerged as one of the most important movements to improve the effectiveness of clinical care. As the number of older adults continues to grow, it is essential that practitioners have knowledge of effective strategies to improve both the medical and the psychosocial aspects of older persons' lives. The purpose of this work is to present systematic reviews of research-based psychosocial interventions for older adults and their caregivers.

The interventions presented focus on a variety of critical issues facing older adults today including medical illnesses (cardiac disease, diabetes, arthritis/pain, cancer, and HIV/AIDS), mental health/cognitive disorders (depression/anxiety, dementia, substance abuse), and social functioning (developmental disabilities, end-of-life, dementia caregivers, grandparent caregivers). For each of these areas the prevalence of the problem, the demographics of those affected, and the nature and consequences of the problem are discussed. The empirical literature is then reviewed. A treatment summary highlights the type and nature of research supporting the interventions reviewed and is followed by a conclusion section that summarizes the status of intervention research for the specified issue. A Treatment Resource Appendix for each area is included. These appendices highlight manuals, books, articles and web resources that detail the treatment approaches and methodologies discussed.

This book was previously published as a special issue of the *Journal of Gerontological Social Work.*

Sherry M. Cummings is Associate Dean and Associate Professor in the College of Social Work at the University of Tennessee. She is the current president of the Association for Gerontological Education in Social Work (AGE-SW) and a Hartford Geriatric Social Work Scholar (2001-2003).

Nancy P. Kropf is Professor and Director of the School of Social Work at Georgia State University. She is a former president of AGESW and a Hartford Geriatric Social Work Scholar (2000-2002). Her area of research and scholarship is lat*e lif*e caregiving relationships, with the focus specifically c

D0149122

Handbook of Psychosocial Interventions with Older Adults

Evidence-based approaches

Edited by Sherry M. Cummings and
Nancy P. Kropf

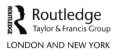
Routledge
Taylor & Francis Group

LONDON AND NEW YORK

First published 2009 by Routledge
2 Park Square, Milton Park, Abingdon, Oxon, OX14 4RN

Simultaneously published in the USA and Canada
by Routledge
711 Third Avenue, New York, NY 10017
Reprinted 2009

Routledge is an imprint of the Taylor & Francis Group, an informa business

Typeset in Times by Value Chain, India

British Library Cataloguing in Publication Data
A catalogue record for this book is available from the British Library

ISBN13: 978-0-415-48185-4 (h/b)
ISBN13: 978-0-415-48186-1 (p/b)

CONTENTS

Over the past decade, there has been tremendous growth in the movement to enhance the delivery of quality services through the use of evidence-based interventions. While a growing number of reviews have examined the effectiveness of pharmacological interventions for older adults, few have examined the status of psychosocial interventions for the older population. The purpose of this special volume is to increase researchers' and practitioners' knowledge of evidencebased treatments for older adults and their family members. To this end, a thorough review of the extant research on psychosocial interventions available to address the varied health, mental health/cognitive, and social role challenges faced by older adults and family caregivers is provided.

KEYWORDS. Evidence-based treatment, psychosocial intervention, older adult, caregivers

EVIDENCE-BASED INTERVENTIONS FOR HEALTH CONDITIONS

Cardiovascular disease (CVD) is the leading cause of death in the US. The growth of the older population in coming decades will inevitably increase the incidence of age-related cardiac disease. Increasing evidence has shown the prevalence of co-morbid mental health conditions in CVD patients. Specifically, depression and anxiety have been linked with CVD mortality. Due to the risk of psychosocial conditions with cardiac patients, mental health practitioners in health and gerontology need to be well-informed about CVD-related mental health co-morbidity and current research developments. Accordingly, this article provides a systematic review of the clinical evidence about the efficacy, cost-effectiveness, and any potential risk *of psychosocial intervention with cardiac patients.*

KEYWORDS. Cardiovascular disease, coronary heart disease, psychosocial interventions

Cancer is of particular importance to gerontology due to the changing nature of the disease. Survival rates are at all time highs as a result of technological advances in early detection and treatment of cancer. Some less aggressive or invasive forms of cancer are now seen as chronic illnesses rather than acute, terminal diseases. As a result, demand is increasing for evidence-based psychosocial interventions designed to improve the health and well-being of people living with cancer. This article reviews evidence-based psychosocial interventions designed to address the needs of persons with cancer and their family members. Traditional and technology-enhanced interventions are discussed as are complementary and alternative therapies designed to augment traditional interventions.

KEYWORDS. Cancer, breast cancer, prostate cancer, psychosocial interventions

Arthritic pain is a common and disabling problem for many older adults. There is widespread evidence that despite its prevalence and debilitating effects on the physical, emotional and cognitive status of older adults, arthritic pain remains under-treated in those age 65 and older. This condition significantly and negatively impacts older adults' quality of life and is a critical problem that requires the attention of gerontological social work. This chapter provides a brief summary of arthritic pain in older adults. It also discusses the treatment efficacy of cognitive-behavioral therapy and psycho-educational programs for older adults with this type of pain.

KEYWORDS. Arthritis, pain, cognitive-behavioral therapy, psycho-educational therapy

With the aging of the population, physical inactivity, and growing rates of obesity, there has been a dramatic rise in the incidence of diabetes. Diabetes and its treatment is a holistic and dynamic experience, shaping many aspects of a person's life and well-being. Despite the biopsychosocial nature of this chronic disease, medications tend to be the principal intervention among medical professionals. Over the past fifteen years, however, diabetes researchers and clinicians have begun to develop interventions addressing the psychosocial aspects of diabetes. The majority of these interventions fall within the knowledge base and clinical abilities of social work practitioners. This paper systematically reviews psychosocial intervention studies with older adults, identifying and summarizing treatment protocols.

KEYWORDS. Diabetes mellitus, type I diabetes, type II diabetes, individual interventions, group interventions

Charles A. Emlet, MSW, PhD
R. Andrew Shippy, MA

Although fewer people are being diagnosed with AIDS in the U.S. and deaths continue to decline, the number of adults age 50 and older who are living with HIV/AIDS is larger than ever. It is likely that older people will continue to comprise an increasingly larger proportion of individuals diagnosed with HIV/AIDS, reflecting both the ineffective prevention efforts targeting older adults and the highly effective antiretroviral therapies that allow many people to live for significantly longer periods of time. These recent trends have created two distinct populations of older persons with HIV/AIDS: those who were infected later in life and those infected earlier and now aging with HIV disease. Aging with HIV/AIDS presents unique psychosocial challenges that may be exacerbated by the aging process. HIV-related stigma, social support and coping issues and evidence-based psychosocial interventions for older adults with HIV/AIDS are reviewed in this paper and suggestions for future research are discussed.

KEYWORDS. HIV/AIDS, stigma, social support, coping, psychosocial intervention studies

EVIDENCE-BASED INTERVENTIONS FOR COGNITIVE AND MENTAL HEALTH ISSUES

Margaret E. Adamek, PhD
Greta Yoder Slater, PhD

Depression and anxiety are the most common psychiatric conditions in late life. Despite their prevalence, we know relatively little about their unique manifestation in older adults. And, although the most common intervention for late-life depression and anxiety continues to be medication, research on psychosocial interventions for late-life depression and anxiety has burgeoned in the past several years. Unfortunately, this growing body of intervention research has yet to be widely translated into improved systems of care for late-life depression. This article is one step toward synthesizing the knowledge in this growing area of research. The review of literature presents the conclusions of several meta-analyses that have reviewed psychosocial interventions for late-life depression and anxiety. In addition, intervention studies concerning the effectiveness of cognitive behavioral therapy, interpersonal therapy, reminiscence therapy, and alternative therapies with depressed and/or anxious older adults are reviewed. A brief description of various approaches to psychosocial intervention with anxious and/or depressed older adults is also presented.

KEYWORDS. Depression, anxiety, cognitive behavioral therapy, reminiscence therapy, interpersonal therapy

Sara Sanders, PhD
Carmen Morano, PhD

The number of individuals with Alzheimer's disease or a related dementia is growing at a staggering rate. Thus, it is essential that social workers in geriatric settings are knowledgeable about this disorder and the appropriate interventions to use at all stages of the disease. The purpose of this article is to examine the types of non-pharmacological, psychosocial treatments that are used to manage the behavioral manifestations and changes in the mood of individuals with Alzheimer's disease or a related dementia. While great strides have been made in pharmacological treatments of Alzheimer's disease, less attention has been given to the types of psychosocial interventions that are readily employed in community-based and long-term care settings to assist in the care of these individuals. This article provides an overview of psychosocial interventions, as well as identifies the direction for future evidence-based treatment studies, for individuals with Alzheimer's disease and related dementia.

KEYWORDS. Alzheimer's disease, dementia

Alcohol abuse poses special risks for increased morbidity and mortality among older adults, contributing to the heightened use of medical resources and the related increase in medical costs. Although the prevalance of alcohol use disorders in the older adults is generally less than that found in younger groups, it is expected to increase with the aging of the "baby-boom" generation. In spite of this, little attention has focused on developing, and evaluating the efficacy of, treatment programs for older adults with alcohol-related disorders. This article discusses the availability of effective treatment strategies for older alcohol abusers and reviews the epidemiological and outcomes research literatures related to alcohol abuse and older adults. The few empirical studies that examine outcomes associated with the treatment of older substance abusers reveal positive outcomes, especially when "age-specific," cognitive-behavioral, and less confrontational treatment approaches are employed.

KEYWORDS. Alcohol, substance abuse, aging-specific treatment, psychosocial interventions

EVIDENCE-BASED INTERVENTIONS FOR SOCIAL FUNCTIONING

Adults with Developmental Disabilities (DD) are experiencing increased longevity and the projected number of older persons with DD is expected to double by 2020. As a result, concerns have been raised that agencies and professional staff are illprepared to address the increased needs of an older population with lifelong disabilities. The caregiving life of families of persons with DD now spans multiple decades and is increasingly a feature of advanced age for *parents and grandparents, and of old age for siblings. Problem behaviors, onset or poor management of mental health concerns and inadequate planning for their aging years are the biggest barriers to successful aging for persons with developmental disabilities. However, psychosocial interventions have the potential to alleviate these barriers and promote positive aging for older persons with developmental disabilities. The evidence for the effectiveness of such interventions will be examined within this article.*

KEYWORDS. Developmental disabilities, intellectual disabilities, caregiving, futures planning

Deborah P. Waldrop, MSW, PhD

End-of-life care has gained recognition as an important interdisciplinary clinical domain during the past three decades largely because scientific and medical advances have changed the nature of dying in the US. Advances in the treatment of lifelimiting illness have typically focused on medical issues and on treating the physical symptoms that accompany the final stage of a terminal illness. However, because the lengthening life span has made more choices available at the end of life, there is also greater need for evidence-based psychosocial treatment to diminish some of the prolonged emotional, psychological social, and spiritual distress that accompanies dying. Both terminally ill older adults and their caregivers can be helped by interventions that address the need for information, education, preparation, communication, emotional support, and advocacy. This paper presents a review of evidence-based psychosocial treatments at the end of life for both older adults and their caregivers.

KEYWORDS. End-of-life care, terminal illness, grief, bereavement, psychosocial intervention

Kimberly McClure Cassie, MSSW, MA
Sara Sanders, PhD

Caregivers of older adults face many obstacles as they balance family, career, and caregiving demands. Caregivers are at an increased risk for burden, stress, depression, and a variety of other mental and physical health complications. It is not uncommon for caregivers to receive some form of pharmacological therapy to treat the physical and mental health changes that may occur throughout their caregiving career. However, while pharmacological forms of treatment are invaluable, medications only may not be sufficient to treat the needs of caregivers. As such, geriatric professionals also have a responsibility to intervene with caregivers through psychosocial interventions. This paper provides an overview of caring, a summary of evidence-based psychosocial interventions for family caregivers of older adults, and recommendations for future interventions.

KEYWORDS. Caregivers, older adults, dementia, interventions, evidence-based treatments

Although grandparent caregiving is not a new phenomenon in the United States, there has been a dramatic increase in grandparent-headed households in the last two decades. Many of these care providers are older and feel somewhat unprepared to raise a new generation of children. As a result, grandparent caregivers are at risk for multiple physical, mental, and emotional problems due to the stresses and strains of care provision. This article summarizes characteristics of grandparent caregivers in our society, the challenges that they face, and how organizations are attempting to assist these older adults with their care provision responsibilities. Recommendations for future research and intervention design will also be discussed.

KEYWORDS. Granparent caregivers, grandparents as parents, skipped generation households

Taken collectively, the articles in this volume provide a method to assess psychosocial outcome research in aging. Although the outcome literature on effective interventions with older adults is uneven across condition and treatment approaches, there are some particular intervention methods that have received consistent research support. This article condenses the rich analyses presented by the volume authors and summarizes the interventions for which some evidence base exists by life issue/condition (health, mental health/cognitive and social roles) and outcomes achieved.

KEYWORDS. Evidence-based treatment, psychosocial intervention, older adult, caregivers

Preface

At one time social work practice with older adults was perceived as limited to the domain of social workers in geriatric sites. This perception has now changed as increasingly the major foci of social work practice in health and mental health settings, such as hospitals and community-based services, are older adults and their families. Social work now must address intersecting practice issues in aging and health care.

It is well-known that there are significant health and mental health illnesses and conditions which challenge the quality of life of older persons and their caregivers. Therefore, the goal of health care is not only to provide excellent medical and nursing care but also to help older people and their caregivers manage their health with quality of life. Thus, excellent social work practice is needed. Older people with chronic illness and activity limitations represent an increasing percentage of all persons helped by social workers who have important roles in helping patients and caregivers deal with the challenge of complex treatments, their side effects and the uncertainty of the future. Careful assessment and intervention by social workers can lead to reduced emotional disability and enhanced quality of life. In addition, social workers bring unique perspectives to health and mental health treatments, such as attention to the differential impact and response to treatments of older patients from different racial and ethnic backgrounds. And, social workers do not overlook the needs of caregivers because their needs, if not addressed, may cause physical and psychological stress and negatively impact patient outcomes. Concomitant with this critical counseling role, social workers assume an important function in identifying needed community support services and resources, and in enabling patients and caregivers to access these services.

Evidence is mounting that regardless of the particular condition, attention to the psychological consequences of aging related disease and disability is a critical component of overall care (Horowitz, 2006). Experts in all fields of health care express the need for more well-designed controlled intervention studies that test service models targeted to improving the care and quality of life of older adults. For social work practice to achieve excellence, psychosocial treatment options must be put to the test of effectiveness. At this time in our profession's history we are beginning to develop an evidence-based practice repertoire. As Sherry Cummings and Nancy Kropf note, the adoption of interventions in which effectiveness has been demonstrated can serve to enhance the quality of service delivery. With this as their mantra, the two editors have selected specific health and mental health areas in which social workers are heavily engaged in practice. They have asked gerontological social work experts in each arena to review the extant research on the effectiveness of various psychosocial interventions. Five chapters deal with health conditions (cardiovascular disease, cancer, arthritis, diabetes, and HIV/AIDS) and three chapters deal with mental health/cognitive disorders (depression and anxiety, Alzheimer's disease and related dementias, and substance abuse). In addition, four chapters are included which relate to later life transitions that necessitate a demand for the older adult or family member to engage in challenging shifts in role and social functioning . The various topics that address these social changes include the adjustment to a terminal diagnosis, caring for the changing needs of an adult child with developmental disabilities, raising grandchildren, and providing care for older adults with dementia and other related dementia.

Cummings and Kropf have delineated five levels of review criteria to be used in determining whether a treatment is evidence-based when subjected to systematic review. Randomized controlled studies are their gold standard with the lowest acceptable level of evidence being consensus review which represents the opinions of authorities. They have asked their chapter authors to address their specific arena's evidence-based practices. For example, Maramaldi, Dungan and Poorvu in their chapter conduct a systematic review of psychosocial interventions with cancer patients. More than 1.4 million people are diagnosed with cancer annually, with an estimate that 9.8 million people are survivors of cancer. While cancer was once viewed as an acute illness, which was inevitably terminal, there are some cancers which can now be viewed as chronic diseases. As Emlet and Shippy describe in their chapter, HIV/AIDS was once seen as a death sentence, but currently an increasing number of individuals are living many years and aging with this virus. With so many individuals living with serious chronic conditions, the social worker's role in helping older patients manage their lives with quality of life has become a major sphere of practice.

Many chapter authors note that while true rigorous controlled trials are sparse, there are a growing number of empirically tested psychosocial interventions for older patients and their caregivers for which outcomes are measurable. In any systematic review of psychosocial treatments it is important to be specific as to the type and subtype of diseases or conditions that older adults are facing, as each has different trajectories and psychosocial impacts. And, to complicate such a review even more, within some diseases such as cancer, there are different stages of disease and different treatments necessary. Maramaldi and colleagues, in their review of cancer intervention studies, separate the studies by type of cancer, such as breast or prostate cancer, and further examine the studies by stages of disease. To provide easier access to the information discussed, all chapters in this volume include a table summarizing the studies reviewed. Of great significance for those of us who wish to utilize practices proven to be effective, is that this type of table can help us make informed decisions as to which interventions might be beneficial for specific treatment groups (e.g., Supportive-expressive group therapy [SET] with metastatic breast cancer patients).

Health conditions affect more than the patient. Independent relationships can be suddenly changed when family members must assume new responsibilities for caregiving and this can create new psychosocial stressors. There is a need for well-designed, controlled intervention studies that test service models which aim to enhance the lives of older adults and their caregivers. This book reflects our profession's determination to treat with effective proven interventions.

Barbara Berkman, MSW, PhD
Helen Rehr/Ruth Fizdale Professor, Health and Mental Health
Columbia University
PI and National Director
Hartford Geriatric Social Work Faculty Scholars Program

REFERENCES

Horowitz, Amy. "Overview," *Handbook of Social Work in Health and Aging*, ed: B. Berkman, Oxford University Press (2006), 5-6.

Maramaldi, P. and Lee, J. "Older Adults with Cancer," *Handbook of Social Work in Health and Aging*, ed: B. Berkman, Oxford University Press (2006), 7.

Chapter 1

Overview of Evidence-Based Practice with Older Adults and Their Families

Sherry M. Cummings, PhD
Nancy P. Kropf, PhD

Currently, there are about 37 million persons 65 years of age and over in the United States. By the year 2030, the number of older adults will more than double to about 80 million, with the greatest increase occurring among those aged 85 years and older (Census Bureau, 2004). Later life often ushers in a variety of challenges for older individuals such as acute medical illnesses, chronic conditions, functional impairment, loss of family and friends, and cognitive changes. These challenges represent risks to older adults for decreased quality of life and for increased morbidity and mortality.

In the past decade, there has been a tremendous growth in research for interventions for older adults. Unfortunately, however, interventions supported by research are not routinely offered in many practice settings. Although older adults are responsive to mental health treatment, for example, those with mental health disorders are more likely to receive inadequate or no treatment as compared to younger adults (Bartles, Dums, Oxamn, Schneider, Arean, Alexopoulos, & Jeste, 2002). In addition, while many conditions experienced by older adults are treated medically, the emotional, psychological, and social aspects of their illnesses or conditions often remain unaddressed. The neglect of such critical dimensions of an older client's life may result in non-compliance with medical regimens, increased stress, delayed recovery from medical conditions, and increased impairment. As the number of older adults continues to grow, it is essential that practitioners have knowledge of effective strategies to improve both the medical and the psychosocial aspects of older persons' lives.

Over the past decade, there has been tremendous growth in the movement to enhance the delivery of quality services through the use of evidence-based interventions. It is now widely agreed that in order to ensure the delivery of the best services to meet clients' needs, practitioners' decisions must go beyond clinical judgment and expertise to include knowledge of evidence-based practices (Gambril, 1999, 2001; Gilgun, 2005). The adoption of interventions whose effectiveness have been demonstrated by clinical and social services research can serve to enhance the quality of service delivery and, thereby, improve the lives of many individuals.

For this reason, in the last decade evidence-based practice (EBP) has emerged as one of the most important movements to improve the effectiveness of clinical care. EBP can be understood as the conscientious, explicit and judicious use of current best evidence in making decisions about the care of individuals (Sackett, Richardson, Rosenberg, & Haynes, 1997). Begun in the field of medicine in the early 1990s, the emphasis on EBP has now spread to a variety of fields including nursing (Sackett, Rosenberg, Muir Gray, Haynes, & Richardson, 1996), psychology (Gatz, Fiske, Fox, Kaskie, Kasl-Godley, McCallum, & Wetherhall, 1998), psychiatry (Bartles et al., 2002), and social work (Gambrill, 2001, 1999, 2005; Gilgun, 2005).

Although there is a body of evidence supporting the effectiveness of certain interventions for older adults, a substantial gap remains between this growing body of knowledge and treatments routinely used in practice settings (Torrey, Drake, Dixon, Burns, Flynn, Rush, Clark, & Klatzker, 2001). Recognizing that access to relevant research findings is critical to fostering awareness and usage of evidence-based interventions, there have been increased calls for greater availability of rigorous research reviews in recent years (Gambril, 1999; Gilgun, 2005). While a growing number of reviews have examined the effectiveness of pharmacological interventions for older adults, few have examined that status of psychosocial interventions for the older population. The purpose of this current work is to address this gap by presenting systematic reviews of research-based psychosocial interventions for older adults and their caregivers.

The interventions presented within the following articles focus on a variety of critical issues facing older adults today including medical illnesses (cardiac disease, diabetes, arthritis/pain, cancer, and HIV/AIDS), mental health/cognitive disorders (depression/anxiety, dementia, substance abuse), and social roles (developmental disabilities, end-of-life, dementia caregivers, grandparent caregivers). Each article discusses the prevalence of the problem, the demographics of those affected, and the nature and consequences of the problem. The empirical literature is then reviewed using specific parameters. The following criteria for evidence-based treatment were utilized:

> *Level 1*–evidence is obtained from a meta-analysis of all relevant randomized controlled studies (RCS) or from a systematic review of RCS
>
> *Level 2*–evidence is obtained from at least one properly designed RCS
>
> *Level 3*–evidence is obtained from well-designed controlled studies without randomization
>
> *Level 4a*–evidence is obtained from non-controlled studies
>
> *Level 4b*–evidence consists of consensus reviews that represent the opinions of respected authorities based on clinical experience or reports of expert committees.

Studies of individual, family, and group interventions as well as com-

munity and institution-based interventions were considered for each review. Only those research studies whose participants consisted of older
adults were included; however, no one established definition of older
adult was provided. Rather, older adult is defined within the context of
each specified illness/condition. For each review, information concerning the databases searched, search terms used, and time period considered is clearly provided. A treatment summary highlights the nature and
type of evidence-based interventions reviewed and is followed by a
conclusion section that summarizes the status of intervention research
for the specified issue, identifies gaps in knowledge, and suggests directions for future research. Each article concludes with a *Treatment Resource Appendix* that highlights manuals, books, articles and web
resources that describe treatment approaches and methodologies.

ORGANIZATION OF VOLUME

Health Conditions

The article by Peck and Ai addresses the status of psychosocial interventions designed to enhance the well-being of older adults with cardiovascular disease (CVD), the leading cause of death in the US. The
impact of psychosocial issues on CVD morbidity and mortality is well-
documented. Co-morbid mental health disorders, for instance, are common in CVD patients and are linked with CVD mortality and poor quality of life. Poor social support has also been identified as a predictor of
CVD mortality while stress is a major risk factor for the development of
CVD. Over the past 20 years psychosocial interventions for persons
with CVD have been offered to improve the psychological and physical
well-being of CVD patients through the modification of thoughts, behaviors and mood. Common intervention approaches to accomplish this
goal include health education, stress management, relaxation therapy,
cognitive behavioral therapy (CBT), and group support. The review of
two decades of research affirms the efficacy of psychosocial interventions to enhance the mental health and quality of life of older persons
with CVD. This same research, however, calls into question the utility
of such interventions as methods for reducing mortality in this population.

Maramaldi, Dungan, and Poorvu discuss issues confronting older individuals diagnosed with cancer and the status of interventions that seek to improve their psychosocial and physical functioning. A wide variety of psychosocial treatments for older persons with cancer have been developed and tested. The majority of these utilized group formats and incorporate education, support, psychotherapy, and/or relaxation techniques in order to improve mood, increase knowledge, enhance coping, and decrease stress. Some interventions have also targeted spouses of cancer patients and employed group formats to enhance spousal coping and marital satisfaction. Although the emotional, psychological and social impact of living with cancer is well-recognized and a variety of psychosocial treatments have been tested, information concerning empirically validated psychosocial interventions with cancer patients is limited when compared with the extensive medical intervention literature in this field.

The article by Yoon and Doherty focuses on psychosocial interventions for one of the most prevalent chronic health problems and the leading cause of disability among older Americans, arthritis and arthritic pain. Because the importance of psychological and social factors in the management of chronic pain is well-recognized, a range of psychosocial treatments exists. Among these, cognitive behavioral therapy and psychoeducational interventions have received the greatest empirical support. Meta-analyses and randomized controlled studies have documented the benefits of interventions incorporating these approaches. Some of the interventions utilizing these techniques have also been replicated with Spanish-speaking elders and with older adults living in foreign countries. However, the authors note that since many of the psychosocial treatments studied were multi-modal and integrated a variety of psychosocial approaches, it is difficult to determine which particular components or combinations of components have the greatest treatment efficacy.

In the fifth chapter, Vaughn DeCoster discusses diabetes, a leading cause of disability and death in older adults. Close to 20% of persons 60 years of age and older have diabetes while another 20% are at heightened risk of developing this disease. Proper diabetes management involves significant life-style changes including adherence to a medication regime, dietary control, and exercise. Non-compliance with the prescribed routine of care can result in blindness, amputations, kidney disease and death. In response, psychosocial interventions have been developed to increase compliance with care regimens through modification of health and life-style behaviors, and to improve quality of life through enhanced psychological and social well-being. Currently, much of the psychosocial intervention research in this area concentrates on exploratory research and pilot testing of intervention protocols. Psychosocial interventions in this area utilize a variety of group and individual approaches that incorporate social support, education, problem-solving, case management, exercise, and computer assisted diabetes care. The studies reviewed suggest that such interventions are efficacious in helping older persons with diabetes to increase their knowledge and self-care behaviors, and to improve their diet, quality of life and blood sugar levels.

Emlet and Shippy provide an overview of the unique challenges faced by older persons living with HIV/AIDS in chapter six. These challenges represent the convergence of physical, psychosocial, spiritual and service issues faced by a hidden group of older adults. Although AIDS cases among Americans over 50 have quintupled since 1990 and older adults now represent approximately 20% of all persons living with HIV, little attention has focused on the needs of this population. The number of older adults with HIV/AIDS, however, is expected to grow rapidly due to highly effective therapies that allow many people to live for significantly longer periods of time, and to ineffective HIV/AIDS prevention efforts targeting older adults. Research on psychosocial interventions for persons with HIV/AIDS is in the nascent stage and even within this arena studies focused on older adults are rare. However, within the past five years a few such studies have taken place. These studies represent emerging efforts to conceptualize and test psychosocial HIV/AIDS interventions and, through such efforts, lay the beginning groundwork for future development and exploration of treatments to promote the functioning and well-being of older adults living with HIV/AIDS.

COGNITIVE AND MENTAL HEALTH ISSUES

Turning to later-life mental health/cognitive disorders, Adamek and Slater, in chapter seven, review the multiple studies and meta-analyses that have examined the efficacy of psychosocial interventions to treat depression and anxiety in older adults. These studies provide strong evidence that a range of psychosocial interventions, such as CBT, Reminiscence Therapy, and Problem-Solving Therapy, provide significant benefit over and above placebos for improving the mental health status of depressed older adults. Although not as many studies have been conducted on psychosocial treatments for late life anxiety as have been for depression, a substantial number of studies do exist that support the usefulness of CBT, offered in either individual or group format, for reducing anxiety among older adults.

Due to the devastating and costly nature of Alzheimer's Disease for older adults, their families, and society as a whole, much research has been focused on determining strategies to slow or stop the progression of this disease. However, much less attention has been paid to developing and testing psychosocial treatments to reduce problematic behaviors and negative mood states among those afflicted. Sanders and Morano examine the small but varied body of research in this area. They report that while interventions for individuals with dementia have had mixed results, evidence does suggest that psychosocial treatments can reduce depression, anxiety, and agitation and improve social interactions, awareness, and recognition among those with dementia.

Cummings, Bride, Cassie, and Rawlins-Shaw discuss the nature of and treatment for substance abuse among older adults in chapter nine. Research in this area is complicated by definitional ambiguity. No agreement exists as to what constitutes an older person in addictions research and persons defined as older in the studies examined ranged in age from 45 years and over to 60 and above. Likewise, definitions of conditions such as alcohol abuse also vary significantly. However, the available research does reveal positive outcomes for older substance abusers including abstinence, reduction in use, and improved general health. The research also suggests that older substance abusers achieve the best results when a cognitive-behavioral approach is utilized, and have better treatment compliance and outcome when treated in an older adult specific program.

SOCIAL FUNCTIONING

Articles nine through twelve turn our attention to interventions designed to promote social role functioning among older adults and their caregivers. In chapter ten, McCallion and Nickle review psychosocial treatment studies focused on older adults with developmental disabilities (DD) and their family members. Research in this area is in the beginning stages and, thus far, has focused on promoting life skills among older adults with DD and on strategies to enhance caregivers' future planning ability. These studies suggest that futures planning interventions can enhance caregivers' knowledge and awareness of planning resources and their competence, confidence, and progress in future planning for their aging son or daughter. In addition, research on social role functioning of adults with DD themselves is included in this article. Examples of particular issues and conditions include dealing with residential concerns and leisure-based options, and assisting the person with DD deal with grief and loss situations. While many studies in this area suffer from small sample size and lack of control/comparison groups, they do lay the groundwork for future research on interventions to promote the quality of life and care for this growing and vulnerable population of older adults.

Scientific and medical advances have changed the nature of dying in the US and have highlighted the need for comprehensive approaches to end-of-life care. In chapter eleven, Deborah Waldrop underscores the essential interrelationship between the patient experience, caregiver experience, and advanced care planning in end-of-life treatment. While a myriad of intervention studies exist that examine the medical aspects of end-of-life care, those exploring the psychosocial aspects are less common. Thus far, the psychosocial intervention studies that have been conducted, focus on enhancing end-of-life care for terminally ill older adults and on promoting healthy grief experiences for surviving caregivers. In particular, these studies examine the impact of psychosocial treatments on dying individuals' quality of life, end-of-life preferences, satisfaction, and emotional and cognitive functioning, while bereavement studies target family members' grief, coping, and mood. Results of research studies in this emerging field affirm the promise of psychosocial treatments to promote enhanced care at end-of-life, and highlight the need for further development in the area of bereavement intervention.

In chapter twelve, Cassie and Sanders explore the results of psychosocial interventions designed to enhance the functioning of family members providing care to older relatives in the well-developed field of caregiver research. Results of meta-analyses and research studies on individual and group caregiver interventions, as well as multi-modal and technology-based interventions for caregivers are reviewed. Results of these studies provide strong evidence supporting the utility of psychosocial interventions for reducing negative mental and physical consequences of providing care and for enhancing caregivers' coping and quality of life.

In the final chapter on social roles, Stacey Kolomer examines developments in the much more recent field of intervention research for grandparent caregivers. As the expected life span increases and the average size of families declines, an increasing number of older adults are called upon to carry out child rearing duties. Grandparents are often unprepared to deal with the emotional, legal, financial, educational, and social challenges related to providing care for younger family members. A small but varied group of innovative interventions using group formats and/or interdisciplinary case management models to assist this population of caregivers has been developed and tested. Thus far, the majority of intervention studies report the results of small pilot programs. This handful of studies, however, provides support for the effectiveness of such interventions in improving the mental health, coping, social support, and access to needed services among grandparent caregivers.

These articles provide a thorough review of the extant research on psychosocial interventions available to address the varied health, mental health/cognitive, and social role challenges faced by older adults and family caregivers. It is hoped that such a review will help increase practitioners' knowledge of evidence-based treatments and, thereby, facilitate the usage of such interventions in practice settings. The information provided in these articles also points to gaps in the knowledge base and suggests areas in which future psychosocial intervention research for older adults is urgently needed. It is critical that careful investigation of such interventions continues and expands. Only through such efforts can we extend our knowledge and use of the best available methods for improving the lives of current and future older adults.

REFERENCES

Bartels, S. J. et al. (2002). Evidence-based practives in geriatric mental health care. *Psychiatric Services, 53*, 1419-1431.

Gambrill, E. (2001). Social work: An authority-based profession. *Research on Social Work Practice, 11*, 166-175.

Gambrill, E. (1999). Evidence-based practice: An alternative to authority-based practice. *Families in Society, 80*, 341-349.

Gatz, M., Fiske, A., Fox, L., Kaskie, B., Kasl-Godley, J. E., McCallum, T. J., & Wetherhall, J. L. (1998). Empirically validated psychological treatments for older adults. *Journal of Mental Health and Aging, 4*, 9-45.

Gilgun, J. F. (2005). The four cornerstones of evidence-based practice in social work. *Research on Social Work Practice, 15*, 52-59.

Sackett, D. L., Richardson, W. S., Rosenberg, W., & Haynes, R. B. (1997). *Evidence-based medicine: How to practice and teach EBM.* New York: Churchill Livingstone.

Sackett, D., Rosenberg, W., Muir Gray, J., Haynes, B., & Richardson, W. S. (1996). Evidence-based medicine: What it is and what isn't. *British Medical Journal, 312,* 71-72.

Torrey, W. C., Drake, R. E., Dixon, L., Burns, B. J., Flynn, L., Rush, A. J., Clark, R. E., & Klatzker, D. (2001). Implementing evidence-based practices for persons with severe mental illnesses. *Psychiatric Services, 52,* 45-50.

US Census Bureau. http://www.census.gov/prod/2004pubs/04statab/pop.pdf

EVIDENCE-BASED INTERVENTIONS FOR HEALTH CONDITIONS

As the body ages, the onset of a chronic or acute health condition can impact the older adult in significant ways. Within this section, intervention approaches to treat five disease categories commonly found within the older population are highlighted: cardiovascular conditions, cancer, arthritis, diabetes, and HIV/AIDS. With medical treatment advances, these conditions no longer foretell a life of dependence and frailty. Greater numbers of older adults are living their lives managing one of these conditions. Clearly, there is a role for social workers to play in promoting the health and wellness of older adults and in keeping these adults as healthy and functional as possible after the onset of a serious illness.

Due to differences in the nature and characteristics of the health conditions discussed in these chapters, the intervention approaches presented focus on various treatment outcomes. Certain educational interventions, for example, enhance older adults' knowledge related to their diagnosis or disease process. Other educational treatments seek to increase older adults' understanding of nutrition and diet management, while yet others teach new approaches to living with arthritis-related pain. Such interventions have been found to positively impact older adults' and family members' knowledge of particular health conditions and their ability to incorporate new behaviors and life-style changes. As a result, the negative components of a particular disease process on older adults are reduced.

Other interventions are employed to alleviate the emotional and social impacts of health conditions. All of the chapters in this section discuss some studies that are focused upon relieving co-morbid mental health issues, such as depression and/or anxiety, that often accompany health problems. Intervention approaches that have some level of efficacy include the use of journals, cognitive behavior therapy, and support and educational groups. Supportive group approaches, which provide a forum for patients to increase their social support and decrease feelings of isolation in dealing with their health crisis, have also been used.

The interventions that are included in the following chapters are found in various health and community-based contexts. Some hospitals have a comprehensive approach to health and wellness, and offer follow-up services as part of the aftercare treatment. Social workers and other health professionals also offer programs within the community, such as nutritional information for cardiovascular or diabetes management. Such topics can easily be incorporated into senior center programs. Support groups, which have been used with several of the client populations in this section, can be based in a variety of settings, including hospitals, senior centers, churches and synagogues. While activity and exercise programs should always be undertaken under the advice of the patient's physician, these interventions also are found in numerous contexts within the community.

With age, a major issue that older adults and their families face is change in health status. Due to technological and medical advances, many of the conditions that previously caused death or incapacitation are now managed through various regimes and programs. Social workers are often involved in treatment with older adults who are dealing with a cardiovascular, cancer, diabetes, or arthritis diagnosis. In addition, some social workers are involved with a growing subgroup of the older populations–those who have a HIV diagnosis. The social work profession offers an important perspective by looking beyond particular disease conditions to the psychosocial impacts that such diseases have on older adults and their families. The following five chapters provide an important overview of the treatment approaches that have demonstrated efficacy in improving the functioning and well-being of older adults with common, yet threatening, health conditions.

Chapter 2

Cardiac Conditions

Michel D. Peck, PhD
Amy L. Ai, PhD

The Census Bureau (2004) projected that in 2005, about 37 million Americans would be aged 65 years and older. By the year 2040, the population of older adults in the United States (U.S.) will more than double to about 80 million, with the greatest rate of increase in those aged 85 years and older. This aging trend will inevitably increase the incidence of age-related cardiovascular disease (CVD), the leading cause of death in the U.S. (American Heart Association or AHA, 2005). CVD mainly includes coronary heart disease (CHD), rheumatic heart disease, cardiomyopathy, pulmonary heart disease, congestive heart failure (CHF), ischemic attack in the brain (stroke), myocardial infarction (MI or heart attack), irregular heartbeat (arrhythmia), hypertension (high blood pressure), congenital cardiovascular defects, valvular heart disease, bacterial endocarditis, diseases of the arteries, and thromboembolism. Within this article, CVD will be addressed in general but specific types of CVD, especially CHD, will be highlighted in particular. In this way, the most important information about efficacy, as well as cost-effectiveness and risk, of interventions for cardiac conditions will be presented.

Increasing evidence has shown the prevalence of comorbid mental health conditions in CVD patients (Hemingway, Malik, & Marmot, 2001; Pignay-Demaria, Lesperance, Demaria, Frasure-Smith, & Perrault, 2003; Rozanski, Blumenthal, & Kaplan, 1999). Specifically, depression and anxiety have been linked with CVD mortality (Barth, Schumacher, & Herrmann-Lingen, 2004; van Melle et al., 2004). Due to the risk of psychosocial conditions with cardiac patients, mental health practitioners in health and gerontology need to be well-informed about CVD-related mental health comorbidity and current research developments. Accordingly, this article provides a systematic review of the clinical evidence about the *efficacy, cost-effectiveness, and any potential risk* of psychosocial intervention with cardiac patients. In particular, we attempt to examine which types of therapies may be effective on two types of outcomes based on the available evidence. Primary outcomes include mortality and major cardiac events (e.g., non-fatal MI) and secondary outcomes include cardiovascular measures (e.g., blood pressure, heart rate), risk behavior factors (e.g., smoking, diet), and mental health (e.g., depression, anxiety). To be informative, we begin with some basic information about CVDs.

DEMOGRAPHICS AND PREVALENCE

Of individuals who are aged 65 years and older, an estimated 70% (27 million) have at least one form of CVD (AHA, 2005). In men, the average annual rate for first major CVD increases from seven per 1,000 for those aged 35-44 years to 68 per 1,000 for those aged 85-94 years. In women, comparable rates occur 10 years later. For those older than 75 years, however, the prevalence of CVD is greater in women than that of men. In the U.S., one in four men (AHA, 2006b) and one in three women (AHA, 2006d) suffer from CVD. The development of CVD, stroke, hypertension, arrhythmia, and CHF is related to aging; and, in women the development of these conditions is also related to menopause (AHA, 2005).

For Americans in all racial and ethnic backgrounds, more die of CVD than of the next five leading causes of death combined (cancer, chronic lower respiratory diseases, accidents, diabetes mellitus, and Alzheimer's disease). At birth, the probability of eventually dying from a major CVD is 47%, while the probability of dying from cancer is 22%. Of CVD-related deaths, approximately 84% occur in people 65 years of age and older (AHA, 2005). CVD is a major reason for costly medical expenses; in 2002 there were 6,024,000 outpatient department visits with a primary diagnosis of CVD (AHA, 2005).

Among all types of CVDs, CHD imposes the highest impact on the U.S. population, especially among the elderly. More than 83% of Americans who die from CHD are age 65 years and older (AHA, 2005). After 40 years of age, nearly one in two men and one in three women will have the lifetime risk of CHD. In fact, CHD is the leading reason for short-stay hospitalization (AHA, 2005). In addition, CHD can create additional cardiac problems, such as angina pectoris (chest pain), MI (heart attack), and sudden cardiac arrest.

The Center for Disease Control (CDC) estimates that each year 400,000 to 460,000 people die of heart disease in an emergency department or before reaching a hospital, which accounts for over 60% of all cardiac deaths (AHA, 2005). One of CHD-related emergent conditions is MI (stroke), for which the average age of an American experiencing a first episode is about 66 years for men and 70 years for women. After suffering an MI, one in four men and about two in five women will die within one year. Stroke is a leading cause of serious, long-term disability in the U.S., and rates of stroke increase with age. Nearly 90% of stroke deaths occur in people 65 years of age and older (AHA, 2003).

Taken together, cardiac problems are one of the major health issues confronted by older adults. The significant percentage of baby boomers with CVDs, 36% of all U.S. men and women (AHA, 2006c), signifies that CVD will remain a major health issue for many years. By the year 2020, heart disease and stroke will become the leading cause of both death and disability worldwide (AHA, 2006a). CVD-related fatalities are projected to increase to more than 20 million a year and, by the year 2030, to more than 24 million a year (AHA, 2006a). Cardiovascular disease alone will kill five times as many people as HIV/AIDS worldwide (AHA, 2006a). By 2020, CVD, injury and mental illnesses will be responsible for about one-half of all deaths and one-half of all healthy life years lost, worldwide (AHA, 2006a).

NATURE OF CARDIAC DISEASE

Growing evidence shows that cardiac conditions are associated with psychosocial issues for many people. One of the major mental health comorbid conditions for cardiac patients is depression. People with CHD, for example, are more likely to suffer from depression than are otherwise healthy persons (Nemeroff, Musselman, & Evans, 1998). Carney and colleagues (1999) found that one in five (20%) CHD patients has major depression. Others reported the prevalence of major depression with CHD to range from 16-23%, with clinically significant depressive symptoms ranging from 31.5-60% (Musselman, Evans, & Nemeroff, 1998).

Over the past two decades, community-based and clinical studies have illuminated the connection between CHD and lower social support-related measures (Krantz et al., 2000; Rozanski et al., 1999). Being unmarried or without a confidant, living alone, and having a small social network have been identified as risk factors in CHD and MI-related morbidity and mortality (Krantz et al., 2000; The ENRICHD Investigators, 2001). Higher levels of social support, however, buffer the impact of depression on post-MI mortality (Frasure-Smith et al., 1999). Perceptions of low emotional support predicted increased risk for future cardiac events (Rozanski et al., 1999) and post-MI mortality (The ENRICHD Investigators, 2001).

Clearly, the consequences of CVD are severe. For those living with CVD, needed lifestyle modifications can range from minor changes in diet to significant physical stamina and activity limitations and pain. The psychological and financial impacts on individual patients, their families, and on society are astounding. In the U.S., the total direct and indirect cost for CVD is expected to be $393.5 billion, which includes the following: $109.9 billion in hospital costs, $39.3 billion in nursing home costs, $6.0 billion in professional medical provider costs, $45.9 billion in drugs and medical durables, $10.9 billion in home health care, and $151.6 billion in lost productivity (AHA, 2005). With regard to the individual, CVD-related medical costs are exorbitant, with an average cost of $17,763 for diagnostic cardiac catheterization, $40,852 for a pacemaker, and $60,853 for coronary artery bypass graft (CABG) (AHA, 2005).

Taken collectively, CVD and CVD-related deaths involve staggering costs, and increased risk with advanced age. Therefore, interventions to reduce harm related to CVDs have become an important task for all health and mental health professionals, and are especially critical in gerontology. Given the scope of the impact of CVD, even a modest modification in outcomes will encompass both public health and social significance. This evidence-based review is both timely and critical. Thus, in our review we detail the types of psychosocial interventions traditionally used with CVD, overview their effectiveness and provide recommendations as to best evidence-based practices that social workers can use with clients with CVD.

EMPIRICAL LITERATURE

In general, psychosocial treatments refer to interventions designed to improve psychological and physical well-being by modifying behavior, emotions, and thoughts (Miller & Cohen, 2001). Particular for CHD-related interventions, clinical research has targeted several types of psychosocial modalities including *health education* (HE), *stress-management* (SM), *psychosocial nursing intervention* (PNI), *relaxation training* (RT), *group emotional support* (GES), *individual cognitive-behavioral therapy* (CBT) and *group-mediated cognitive behavioral therapy* (GMCB) (Focht et al., 2004; Krantz et al., 2000). In the literature, many clinical studies on psychosocial treatments involved combined interventions or nonspecified techniques. Among the most frequently specified psychosocial treatments are SM, HE, and CBT. These techniques have also received the most research attention.

The concepts and components of these major interventions are summarized below. Health education (HE) consists of instructional activities organized in a systematic way, including personal contacts between a health professional and patients to facilitate positive changes in risk factors for CHD and associated unhealthy behaviors (Dusseldorp et al., 1999). Stress management (SM) possesses four components: illness education, cognitive restructuring, coping skills training, and psychological support (Dusseldorp et al., 1999; Miller & Cohen, 2001). In addition, relaxation training (RT) involves specified training in various practices such as meditation, relaxation response, progressive muscle relaxation, and biofeedback-assisted relaxation (Miller & Cohen, 2001). PNI tends to be a component of a multidisciplinary intervention involving cardiologists, nurses, dieticians, social workers, and patient decision support systems. It involves repeated evaluation of, and intervention related to, cardiac status, psychosocial difficulties and needs. Additionally, individualized components such as emotional support, reassurance, education, practical advice, and referral to physicians and other health resources are included. Finally, the most noteworthy treatment modality is CBT, which is offered in both individual and group intervention formats. CBT is based on a social learning approach and has been extensively utilized for the treatment of depression and low social support.

To identify empirical-based treatment literature, a systematic computer search was conducted in four primary databases: CINAHL (cumulative index to nursing and allied health literature), Medline, PsycInfo, and PubMed. To be comprehensive, we used the following procedure. First, we identified eight CVD items: (1) CVD, (2) CHD, (3) CHF, (4) MI, (5) ischemic attack, (6) stroke, (7) arrhythmia, and (8) hypertension. Second, in conjunction with each of these eight terms, we repeated searches for keywords concerning psychosocial interventions, i.e., counseling, therapy, psychotherapy, cognitive behavioral interventions or therapy, stress management, support groups, self-help, peer support, and relaxation therapy. Third, we searched combinations of the eight keywords with anxiety, depression, and distress, frequently noted in articles that we identified through the previous searches. These keywords yielded results; the use of keywords concerning other types of psychosocial interventions, such as narrative therapy, failed to produce additional citations.

After identifying a citation, we then followed any hyperlinks to related articles. Next, in reviewing articles, we also examined bibliographies for any additional articles that we had not yet found. To get an initial sense of the breadth of relevant literature, we searched all years and found articles, especially in years from 1980 to present. We reviewed a few articles from the 1970s and noted that, in general, they lacked substantial empirical evidence to support psychosocial interventions with older adults and CVD. Thus, we had confidence that focusing on articles and research from the 1980s and later would provide a meaningfully relevant and systematic review.

Utilizing our search procedures and the protocol for evidence criteria established for this text, we found three meta-analyses (Table 1) completed between the years 1992 and 1999 (Dusseldorp et al., 1999; Linden, Stossel, & Maurice, 1996; Mullen, Mains, & Velez, 1992) and 11 recent randomized controlled trials (RCTs). Table 2 displays an overview of these trials organized alphabetically by name of investigators; we also indicate the country where the study occurred. In the table, the results section details outcomes that we have described as both primary (mortality, major cardiac events) and secondary (cardiovascular measures, risk behaviors, mental health). In addition, we note assessment tools, such as the Geriatric Depression Scale (GDS) and the Symptom Checklist-90-Revised (SCL-90-R). Because this is not a text about assessment tools, we limit our discussion about these measures, although we do make some comments about trial findings relative to the use of measures. For more information about the various measures, we direct readers to the studies cited and texts about health-related assessment.

It should also be emphasized that the surging interest in psychosocial interventions and CHD has led to several large-sample randomized controlled trials (RCTs) currently sponsored by the National Institute of Health (NIH), which set a high standard for new clinical evaluation of psychosocial intervention. In particular, the newly published multi-center "ENRICHD" trial involving thousands of post-MI patients from a variety of backgrounds has drawn national attention (The ENRICHD

TABLE 1. Meta-Analyses with Description and Findings Listed Alphabetically by Author

Authors, Pub. Year, Location	Description	Intervention Types Sample (tx/ctrl)	Findings
Dusseldorp, Elderen, Maes, Meulman, & Kraaij (1999) USA.	37 studies of HE and SM published between 1974 and 1997.	HE, SM, and combined programs	34% reduction in cardiac mortality, 29% reduction in nonfatal MI recurrence, and improvements in systolic blood pressure, cholesterol, body weight, smoking behavior, physical exercise, and eating habits. Programs more successful on secondary outcomes also more effective on primary outcomes.
Linden, Stossel, & Maurice (1996) USA.	23 controlled trials published between 1975 and 1995.	Psychosocial interventions and counseling (tx types poorly specified).	Approximately 41% reduction in cardiac all-cause mortality and 46% reduction in nonfatal MI recurrence at short-term f/u. Improvements in systolic blood pressure, heart rate, cholesterol, Type A behavior, depression, and anxiety. Length of treatment associated with greater reduction in mortality.
Mullen, Mains, & Velez (1992) USA.	28 controlled trials published between 1974 and 1987.	HE	19% improvement in mortality, and improvements in systolic blood pressure, exercise, and diet. Outcome measures were positively influenced by certain moderating programs factors including individualization, feedback, facilitation, relevance, and reinforcement.

ctr l= Control, f/u = Follow-Up, HE = Health Education, SM = Stress Management, tx = Treatment

TABLE 2. RCTs with Intervention Protocol and Outcomes Listed Alphabetically by Author

Authors, Pub. Year, Location	Tx Type 1°/2°	CVD Type, Age, Sample Size (male/female), Group Assignment, Assessment	Intervention Protocol	Outcomes
Black, J.L. et al. (1998). USA.	CBT/ SM, HE	CAD, unstable angina, MI, PTCA, and CABG, all with depressive symptoms. 60.2±10.7y; 53/7 (m/f). Random assignment. Baseline, 3- 6- 9- and 21-month assessments.	G1 (n = 30): Psychiatric eval., issue-focused counseling (1-7x), one or more of BRR, CBT, CI, RT, and SM to reduce distress. G2 (n = 30): Usual care.	G1 (vs G2): Decreased re-hospitalization (35% G1, 48% G2), reduction in general distress (SCL-90-R) (ns), and reduction in symptom-related distress (GSI, p <.034).
Blumenthal et al. (1997, 2002). USA.	SM/ CBT	CAD with MIS, 58.5±8.4y, 94/13 (m/f). Random assign. to G1 and G2, those unable to attend 3x/wk assigned to G3. Baseline, end of treatment, and annual assessments for 5 years.	G1 (n = 33): 1.5-hr/wk group SM, for 16 wks, based on Duke SM Model of CB-SL, focused on interaction between personality and social environment. G2 (n = 34): Aerobic exercise 3x/wk for 16 wks G3 (n = 40): Usual care.	G1 had fewer CAD events than G3 at 1-year (p = .020) and 2-yr (p =.013), and overall 5-yr (p = .037). G1 had trend for fewer CAD events than G2 (ns). G1 had lower 5-yr total costs than G3 (p = .009) but not less than G2 (p = .157).
Campbell, N.C. et al. (1998a), (1998b). Scotland.	PNI/HE	CHD, 66±8 y, 685/488 (m/f). Random assignment stratified by age, sex, and medical practice (28 clinics randomly selected in NE Scotland). Baseline and 1-year assessments.	G1 (n = 593): Clinic staff promoted medical and lifestyle aspects of secondary prevention. Nurse-led protocol of symptom management including contracting for lower pt risk behaviors. G2 (n = 580): Usual care from treating practitioner.	G1 (vs. G2): Fewer hospital admissions; improvements in SF-36 function, pain, and general health scales; improvements in role limits due to physical health; and had fewer reports of worsening chest pain. No sig. effects on anxiety, depression, or general practitioner consultation rates. G1 (vs. G2): Sig. improvements in secondary prevention including aspirin, blood pressure, lipid management, and physical activity.

TABLE 2 (continued)

Authors, Pub. Year, Location	Tx Type 1°/2°	CVD Type, Age, Sample Size (male/female), Group Assignment, Assessment	Intervention Protocol	Outcomes
Cowan, M.J. et al. (2001). (1997). USA.	PNI/HE	Survivors of out-of-hospital ventricular fibrillation or asystole, 60 yrs, 97/36 (m/f). Random assignment to intervention. Baseline and 2-year assessments.	G1 (n = 67): Eleven 90-min (2x/wk) nurse-led individual therapy sessions including RT and biofeedback, CBT, and 90-min health education. G2 (n = 66): Usual care, plus 90-min health education.	Intervention significantly reduced risk for cardiovascular death by 86% and all-cause mortality. G1: 3 deaths, G2: 8 deaths. Controlling for other factors including functional ability, health perception and baseline levels of psychosocial distress, depression significantly lowered (by 62%).
ENRICHD Investigators (2004), (2004), (2003). USA.	CBT	MI patients, 61 yrs (SD = 12.5 yrs) 1397/1084 (m/f), with depression. Intervention occurred in 73 hospitals. Stratified by clinical center, random assignment to intervention. Assessments at baseline, 6-month post intervention, and annually thereafter.	G1 (n = 1238): CBT median of 11 sessions during 6 mo., group therapy when feasible, SSRIs for patients scoring higher than 24 on the HRSD or having a less than 50% reduction in BDI scores after 5 weeks. G2 (n = 1243): Usual care.	The intervention failed to increase survival rates or reduce recurrent MIs. The intervention improved depression and social isolation, although control group also showed improvements in these dimensions.
Focht, B.C. et al. (2004),, Rejeski, W.J. et al. (2003). USA.	GMCB	MI, AP, CHF, 77/70 (m/f), 64.8 yrs (SD = 6.94). Random assignment stratified by sex. Assessment at baseline and 3- and 12-month follow-ups.	G1 (n = 73): GMCB for 20-25 minutes for 3 months following CRP exercise sessions that were consistent with AACVPR guidelines. G2 (n = 74): CRP exercise sessions only.	G1: Significant improvements in MET level, self-efficacy and long-term adherence to exercise. Men (G1 & G2) and women in (G1 only) had significant HRQOL improvements as measured by SF-36.

Authors, Pub. Year, Location	Tx Type 1°/2°	CVD Type, Age, Sample Size (male/female), Group Assignment, Assessment	Intervention Protocol	Outcomes
Kohn, C.S. et al. (2000). USA.	CBT/HE	AR and eligible for ICD implant, 65±10y, 32/17 (m/f). Random assign. Assessment at baseline and 9-month post-ICD implant follow-up.	G1 (n = 25): CBT with HE, pre-implant, pre-d/c, and at seven routine f/u visits (1x/wk first 4 wks, and 1-, 3-, and 5-month f/u's). G2 (n = 24): Usual care.	No difference between groups. G1 less distress than G2 for PAIS in overall adjustment (p = .009), healthcare posture (p = .010), sex fx / relationships (p = .002) and distress (p = .015). G1 vs. G2 less sexual function difficulties at f/u (p = .010), better BDI score (p = .037). Symptoms of major depress in 33% G1 and 11% G2 (ns.) Lower STAI in G1 v. G2 (p = .013). For pts who received 1 or more shocks, G1 showed better outcomes than G2.
Lincoln N.B., Flannaghan, T. (2003). UK.	PNI/CBT	MI pts with depression, 66.1y; 63/60 (m/f). Three groups random assignment. Assessment at baseline, and 3- and 6-month follow-ups.	G1 (n = 39): 1-hr weekly CPN-led CBT (10 wks); included education, task assignment, activity scheduling, and modification of thoughts and beliefs. G2 (n = 43): an attention placebo–visit from a community psychiatric nurse with no CBT. G3 (n = 41): Usual care	There were no significant differences between the groups in patients' mood, independence in instrumental activities of daily living, handicap, or satisfaction with care. CBT in the treatment of depression following stroke was found to be ineffective in this study.
Luskin, F. et al. (2002). USA.	SM	CHF, 66±9y, 13/20 (m/f). Incomplete randomization (location barrier to total random assignment). Assessments 1-2 wk pre-tx and 1-2 weeks post-tx (approx 3 mo.).	G1 (n = 14): Psychotherapist-led 75-min SM group training (8 weekly sessions); didactic with practice assignments and time for personal sharing. G2 (n = 15): Wait-list control.	G1: Improvement in 6 min walk (p < .02) [175ft further than G2], in GDS (p < .02), in PSS (p < .001), and on MOS question #9 (p < .02) [emotional coping].

TABLE 2 (continued)

Authors, Pub. Year, Location	Tx Type 1°/2°	CVD Type, Age, Sample Size (male/female), Group Assignment, Assessment	Intervention Protocol	Outcomes
Rich, M.W., Beckham, V., Wittenburg, C. et al. (1995). USA.	PNI/HE	CHF, 79±6y, 99/183 (m/f). Random assign. Baseline assessment, and 90-days post-d/c.	G1 (n = 140): HE materials to patient and family, prescribed diet, consultation with a social service agent, review of medications, plan for discharge, and intensive follow-up for 90 days. G2 (n = 142): Usual care.	Restricting analysis to survivors of first hospitalization, there were more 90-day survivors in G1 (67%) than G2 (54%, p = .04). Intervention increased QOL, assessed by CHFQ, in G1 vs. G2 (p = .001). Fewer hospital re-admissions in G1 (41 pts) than G2 (59 pts, p = .03). Hospital readmit costs lower in G1 ($3,236/pt) than G2 ($2,178/pt, p = .03).

1° = Primary, 2° = Secondary, AACVPR = American Association of Cardiopulmonary and Pulmonary Rehabilitation, AR = Arrhythmia, BDI = Beck Depression Inventory, BRR = Behavioral Risk Reduction, CB-SL = Cognitive Behavioral Social Learning, CHFQ = Chronic Heart Failure Questionnaire, CPN = Community Psychiatric Nurse, d/c = Discharge, f/u = Follow-Up, GSI = General Severity Index subscale, GDS = Geriatric Depression Scale, GMCB = Group-mediated Cognitive-Behavioral Therapy, HADS = Hospital Anxiety and Depression Scale, HRQOL = Health Related Quality of Life, ICD = Implantable Cardioverter Defibrillator, MET = Maximal Graded Exercise Test (used to assess peak oxygen uptake), MIS = Myocardial Ischemia, MOS = Medical Outcome Survey, ns = non-significant, PSS = Perceived Stress Scale, pt = Patient, pts = patients, RT = Relaxation Therapy, SCL-90-R = Symptom Checklist-90-Revised, SF-36 = Short Form-36, SM = Stress Management, STAI = State Trait Anxiety Inventory, Tx = treatment

Investigators, 2001, 2003). Therefore, our discussion of findings emphasizes these large trials more than that of the smaller trials. However, we begin with details from the three meta-analyses.

Meta-Analysis of Psychosocial Interventions

Three meta-analyses have dealt with psychosocial treatment efficacy in CVD. Of the three somewhat overlapping meta-analyses (Dusseldorp et al., 1999; Linden et al., 1996; Mullen et al., 1992), Mullen and colleagues (1992) reviewed 28 controlled trials, including 47 interventions, related to patient education programs. All studies were published between 1974 and 1987. In the second meta-analysis, Linden et al. (1996) evaluated 23 controlled trials (2024 subjects undergoing treatment vs. 1156 control subjects) that used psychosocial interventions and counseling. All of these studies were published between 1975 and 1995 and some tested psychosocial interventions without clear definitions. The third meta-analysis (Dusseldorp et al., 1999) evaluated 37 studies that explicitly examined HE and SM and were published between 1974 and 1997. These studies included measures of mortality and cardiac events.

In the first meta-analysis (Mullen et al., 1992), the most prominent effect was found in the broadly defined category of "patient education" for both primary outcomes (i.e., 19% improvement in mortality) and secondary outcomes (i.e., systolic blood pressure, exercise, and diet). This analysis also determined that the outcome measures were positively influenced by certain moderating factors concerning program quality (i.e., individualization, feedback, facilitation, relevance, and reinforcement). Other factors, however (i.e., length of intervention, length of measurement period, intervention emphasis, and channel of intervention), were not.

The second meta-analysis (Linden et al., 1996) reported on unspecified psychosocial interventions and counseling. In this analysis, efficacy of interventions was determined for both primary outcomes (i.e., roughly a 41% reduction of cardiac all-cause mortality and 46% reduction in nonfatal MI recurrence for short-term follow-up) and secondary outcomes (i.e., systolic blood pressure, heart rate, cholesterol, Type A behavior, depression, and anxiety). Unlike Mullen et al. (1992), this meta-analysis did not address moderating factors. Rather, it associated the length of treatment, but not the timing of intervention, with greater reduction in mortality.

The third meta-analysis (Dusseldorp et al., 1999) highlighted socio-demographic risks and provided an operational definition of the psychosocial interventions investigated, including HE, SM, and combined programs. This research revealed several noteworthy findings. Primarily, the interventions evaluated had positive influences on both primary outcomes (i.e., a 34% reduction in cardiac mortality and a 29% reduction in nonfatal MI recurrence) and certain secondary outcomes (i.e., systolic blood pressure, cholesterol, body weight, smoking behavior, physical exercise, and eating habits). However, evidence was not reported for changes in reduction of depression and anxiety. The findings of this meta-analysis indicated that cardiac rehabilitation programs that were more successful on proximate targets (e.g., reduced Type A behavior, or other measures of secondary outcomes) were also more effective on distal targets (i.e., primary outcomes). No effect was found concerning other factors such as random assignment, program factors (e.g., type of evaluation, setting and length of the program, profession of the program provider, individual or group treatment, participation of partners), or subject characteristics (e.g., mean age, percentage of gender, type of cardiac event).

Randomized Controlled Trials

Eleven studies that were not included in the three meta-analyses were found. The earliest of these studies was published in 1995; the most recent publications were in 2004. Table 2 indicates that six of the studies focused on CBT interventions. One study focused on CBT as a stress management (SM) intervention. Another specifically examined group-mediated CBT (GMCB), and two others, which were considered PNI studies, reviewed the impact of nursing delivered CBT. Three studies focused on stress management; as mentioned, two of these used CBT as primary or secondary intervention components. There were a total of five new PNI studies identified. Health education (HE) was a secondary component in multiple studies, in particular three PNI, one CBT, and one SM trials. Some study reports refer to HE as psychoeducation. Since education, by definition, is psychological, we utilize the term HE.

The next section provides more details about the interventions. To help elucidate effective intervention protocols, we organize these findings by primary treatment types in the order that follows: stress management (SM), cognitive behavioral therapy (CBT), group-mediated CBT (GMCB), and psychosocial nursing intervention (PNI). To provide readers a format to easily compare intervention protocols and findings, we summarize treatment protocols for the group of studies, followed by a summary of findings.

Stress Management. The SM trial of Blumenthal and colleagues (1997) was reported in a study that included the full sample ($n = 107$, aged 58.5 yrs, $SD = 8.4$), and a sub-study (Blumenthal et al., 2002) of only men ($n = 94$, aged 60 yrs, $SD = 8$). Patients in the initial study exhibited myocardial ischemia (MIS) either via mental stress testing or halter monitoring. They were randomly assigned to an exercise group ($n = 33$) or a stress management program ($n = 34$). Those unable geographically to attend three times per week were assigned to the control group (usual care, $n = 40$). Follow-up assessment occurred at the end of treatment and annually, thereafter, for 5 years.

For the first group, aerobic exercise conditioning occurred three times weekly for 16 weeks. The sessions consisted of a 10-minute warm-up of stretching and pedaling on a stationary bicycle at a heart rate of 50% to 70% of the heart rate reserve. Then 35 minutes of walking and jogging at a target intensity of 70% to 85% of heart rate reserve occurred. Throughout, patients recorded their heart rates and perceived exertion at 10-minute intervals. The second group followed the Duke Stress Management Program, which is based on a cognitive social learning model of behavior-focused interactions between the social environment and personality traits predisposing individuals to respond to situations in particular ways. For 16 weeks, groups of eight patients attended 1.5-hour weekly sessions. Initial sessions were educational; the later sessions involved instruction in specific skills to reduce the affective, behavioral, cognitive, and physiologic components of stress. Therapeutic techniques included: graded task assignments, monitoring irrational automatic thoughts, and generating alternative interpretations of situations. Progressive muscle relaxation techniques were taught, and each patient also had two individual sessions of electromyographic biofeedback training. Patients in the usual care group were monitored on a monthly basis to ensure that they had not joined any exercise or stress management training program. Patients continued their regular medical regimens and visited their local cardiologists as needed; no attempt to alter care plans were made (Blumenthal et al., 2002).

The researchers found that the SM treatment group showed improved health outcomes compared to the control group. In the assessed frequency of cardiac events, the treatment group had significantly fewer cardiac events at 1-year (p = .020), 2-year (p = .013), and overall 5-year (p = .037) follow-up assessments. Although not statistically significant, the SM treatment group had a trend toward fewer cardiac events than did the exercise only group. Further, Blumenthal and colleagues found that the SM intervention had lower 5-year total costs than that of the control group (p = .009) but not less than that of the exercise only group (p = .157).

Luskin and colleagues (2002) performed a clinical trial providing licensed psychotherapist-led stress management training, with cognitive behavioral components. A total of 29 participants diagnosed with CHF were included within the research (average age = 66, *SD* = 9). Because the location of the intervention was a barrier for some participants, this trial used incomplete randomization into treatment (*n* = 14) and wait-list control (*n* = 15) groups with conditions assigned based upon ability to participate in the intervention protocol. Baseline measurement occurred 1-2 weeks prior to the intervention; follow-up assessment occurred 1-2 weeks post-intervention.

For 8 weeks, the intervention group received 75-minute group trainings (10 hours total), with time for practice assignments and personal sharing. Training was didactic, with an emphasis on guided practice of techniques. The intervention group was trained in stress management (SM) techniques including Freeze-Frame, Heart Lock-in, Appreciation, and Care versus Overcare. Freeze-Frame is a stress management technique and starts with the conscious shifting of attention from a stressful experience to the area around one's heart. Then, one takes a few slow and deep breaths into that same area, and one's attention is drawn to a visualization or memory of a positive emotion, such as care or love. The feeling generated by that positive emotion is held in the area around the heart. Heart Lock-in is an extended Freeze-Frame. Further, *care* is distinguished from *overcare* which is defined as the tendency to want something or someone so much that the extra effort and anxiety obscures the positive experience of care and leads to distress. At the completion of the intervention, control group members were invited to attend a 1-day training. The researchers found that those in the treatment group had significant improvements in a 6 minute walk (p < .02), including the ability to walk a greater distance. Additionally, they found significant improvements in treatment versus control group on the geriatric depression scale (GDS; p < .02), the perceived stress scale (PSS; p < .001), and emotional coping–question number 9 on the Medical Outcome Survey (p < .02).

Cognitive Behavioral Treatment. Three trials were classified as CBT (Black et al., 1998; the ENRICHD Investigators, 2003, 2001; Kohn et al., 2000) and one trial as a Group Mediated Cognitive Behavioral (GMCB) treatment approach (Focht et al., 2004; Rejeski et al., 2003).

First, Black and colleagues (1998) studied CAD, in 53 men and seven women, age 60.2±10.7 years. The sample was of consecutive patients referred for cardiac rehabilitation who had depressive symptoms according to the SCL-90-R. Random assignments were made to treatment (n = 30) and control (usual care, n = 30) groups. Data collection occurred at program entry, program exit, 3-, 6-, 9-, and 21-month follow-up visits. In addition to the cardiac rehabilitation protocol (usual care), members of the treatment group were first evaluated by a psychiatrist to assess the source of their distress and the need for psychoactive medications, which were prescribed if considered essential. Eight patients received psychiatric medications. In addition, patients received 1-7 visits with a psychiatrist to do one or more of the following interventions to treat identified sources of distress, such as anxiety, depression, and hostility: (A) relaxation training, (B) stress management, (C) efforts to reduce behavioral risk factors, (D) efforts to improve compliance with medical, dietary, and exercise regimens, and (E) cognitive behavioral. Excluding the initial assessment, the number of additional sessions per patient ranged from 0 to seven sessions.

Usual care included 8 weeks of cardiac rehabilitation involving monitored exercise, according to the American Association of Cardiovascular and Pulmonary Rehabilitation Guidelines, administered 1-3 times per week based. Patients were offered a series of educational lectures which included information about Type A behavior and stress management, a two-part support group for patients and spouses or significant others, and individual dietary counseling. Insofar as physical health-related outcomes, Black and colleagues found that the intervention decreased hospitalizations by 35% for the treatment group versus 48% for the control. The researchers found that the intervention group had statistically non-significant reduction in general psychological distress, measured by the SCL-90-R. However, there was statistically significant improvement in symptom-related psychological distress for the treatment group.

The major multi-site trial in this review is that conducted by The ENRICHD Investigators (2004a, 2004b, 2003). The ENRICHD trial set a higher standard for CHD-related RCTs and has provided the most solid and comprehensive evidence of treatment efficacy related to primary and secondary outcomes (The ENRICHD Investigators, 2001). This trial included a diverse sample that filled a sociodemographic gap found in most previous studies. Counselors who were involved were culturally competent, and trained in the life-styles, values, and customs of diverse groups. In this study, 73 hospitals affiliated with eight clinical centers enrolled 1397 men and 1084 women, with a mean age of 61 years (SD = 12.5 yrs), each with a diagnosis of MI. Stratified by clinical center, participants were randomized into treatment (n = 1238) and control (n = 1243) groups. Follow-up occurred 6 months after randomization, and annually thereafter.

The treatment group received 11 sessions (median) of CBT during a 6-month period, and group therapy when feasible. In addition, patients with clinically significant depression scores were prescribed anti-depressant medications (ENRICHD Investigators, 2004a, 2004b, 2003). In the ENRICHD (2001) trial, licensed mental health professionals, including social workers who received training and certification from the Beck Institute, provided up to 6 months of individual sessions to depressed patients. Consistent with CBT protocols, these sessions included rapport and relationship building, reflection about previous sessions, and a focus on the week's experiences and current goals (The ENRICHD Investigators, 2001). Several components were part of the protocols including reinforcement, the use of homework, and participation in group therapy. The 12-topic group curriculum consisted of: "(1) Role behavior, emotion and thoughts in CHD; (2) Emotions: Identifying and evaluating them; (3) Cognitions; (4) Feeling connected with others; (5) Communicating effectively; (6) Relapse prevention training; (7) Anger management; (8) Assertiveness in communication; (9) Problem solving, relapse prevention, and life project; (10) Personal values and goals; (11) Future plans; and, (12) Holding on to progress and staying well" (The ENRICHD Investigators, 2001, p. 750).

Twelve weekly, 2-hour group sessions complemented individual sessions by providing a venue to rehearse new skills, foster social support, and normalize experiences. A participant could be enrolled into a group any time after three individual sessions had been completed, but no later than 6 months after enrollment. The groups included five to eight participants with depression, lack of perceived social support (LPSS), or both. The intervention helped participants develop an ability to: (1) identify the problem situations and associated cognitions that promote depressed moods; (2) apply cognitive and behavioral skills as needed in their daily life; (3) appraise their thoughts and beliefs about current problematic situations or issues; and (4) apply newly learned skills to problematic situations in the future.

The primary goal of treatment for LPSS was to alter the participant's perception of his or her social support by modifying the environmental, behavioral and/or cognitive factors that lead to LPSS. Treatment was individually tailored on the basis of a multimodal assessment that included both qualitative and quantitative strategies. Modular intervention components were closely linked to this assessment and addressed (1) behavioral/social skill deficits, (2) cognitive factors contributing to the perception or maintenance of unsatisfying levels of social support, and (3) social outreach and network development. Inasmuch as a host of factors provide an individual with a sense of support, most cases of LPSS required an integration of these three treatment modules. Unlike positive findings in the smaller trial by Black, the ENRICHD intervention failed to increase survival rates or to reduce recurrent MIs. While the ENRICHD intervention improved psychosocial outcomes within the treatment group, including improving depression and reducing social isolation, control group members also showed improvements in these dimensions.

Studying patients with arrhythmia (irregular heart beat), Kohn and colleagues (2000) were concerned with the effects of CBT on depression, specifically in patients with arrhythmia who are eligible for implantable cardioverter defibrillators (ICDs). In two teaching hospitals, 32 men and 17 women, aged 65 years (*SD* 10) were randomly assigned to the CBT treatment (*n* = 25) or no therapy control group (*n* = 24). Assessment occurred at baseline and 9-month post-ICD implant follow-up. A doctoral level psychology student administered individual CBT sessions at pre-implant, pre-discharge, once per week for the first 4 weeks, and at 1- 3- and 5-month follow-up visits to the outpatient clinic. Pre-implant and pre-discharge sessions lasted 30-60 minutes, while follow-up sessions lasted 15-30 minutes. CBT addressed "anxiety and apprehensions, avoidance behavior, fear of shocks, stress management, ability to resume work and social activities, and distorted cognitions (e.g., about the safety of the ICD)" (Kohn et al., p. 451). The control group received no therapy, but patients also had follow-up ICD clinic visits at 1-, 3-, 5-, and 9-months. The researchers found no difference in the number of cardiac events between treatment and control groups. However, compared to the control group, treatment participants had less distress, improved overall adjustment, better health care posture, less sexual functioning and relationship difficulties, and better scores on the both Beck Depression Inventory (BDI) and the State Trait Anxiety Inventory (STAI). There was also a statistically non-significant reduction in symptoms of major depression for the treatment group.

Focht et al. (2004) and Rejeski et al. (2003) reported the effects of a group mediated CBT (GMCB) intervention on physical activity and life style behavior change. For this trial, participants aged 50 years and older with CVD were recruited via mass mailings, media advertisements and physician requests. The final sample included 77 men and 70 women (age 65 years, $SD = 7$) diagnosed with MI, AP, or CHF. These 147 subjects were randomized into two groups, both receiving traditional cardiac rehabilitation program (CRP), one also receiving GMCB treatment and CRP ($n = 73$), and the other CRP only ($n = 74$). Data was collected at baseline and 3- and 12-month follow-ups.

The CRP exercise sessions were consistent with American Association of Cardiopulmonary and Pulmonary Rehabilitation (AACVPR) guidelines. The exercise routine included warm-up (5 min.), aerobic stimulus (30-35 min.), upper extremity strength training (15-20 min.), and cool down with stretching (5 min.). Exercise leaders, who were trained in both aspects of the intervention and supervised by the study team, led participants in center-based exercise three times weekly for 3 months. During the third month, members of the GMCB treatment group only received one day of center-based exercise and had personal responsibility for two additional days of self-planned home exercise. As for the GMCB intervention, CBT-based counseling occurred for 20-25 minutes following the first 3 months of exercise. The first month focused on learning and using self-regulatory tools, the second month focused on becoming an "independent exerciser," and the third month focused on self-perception–particularly viewing oneself as an active person. In months 4-9, contact with the treatment group was less intensive and included booster exercise sessions, and contact via telephone and mail–including submission of activity reports. In months 9-12, there was no contact between treatment group and staff. At the end of the GMCB protocol, patients participated again in 30-minute monthly follow-up counseling sessions and bi-weekly telephone contact.

The primary health outcome in the study was the Maximal Graded Exercise Test (MET), which is used to assess peak oxygen uptake. The researchers found that the intervention group performed better on this measure. Further, at the 12-month follow-up, there was evidence for gender $\times$ baseline $\times$ treatment interaction (Focht et al., 2004). Men in both GMCB and standard exercise therapy, and women in GMCB, had desirable improvement in self-reported mental health and vitality. Older persons with lower baseline health status reported the greatest improvements. In addition, the treatment group showed greater improvement in physical activity, fitness, and self-efficacy (Rejeski et al., 2003). Regardless of treatment group, men's outcome scores were better than women in either group.

Psychosocial Nursing Interventions (PNIs). The remaining trials to be discussed are the new trials categorized as psychosocial nursing interventions (PNIs). Campbell and colleagues (1998a, 1998b) targeted 28 different medical practices in NE Scotland. Their sample included 685 men and 488 women with CHD, aged 66±8 years. Using random assignment stratified by age (less or more than 65 years of age), sex, and medical practice, patients were assigned to either treatment (*n* = 593) or control groups (*n* = 580). The clinics ran for 1 year, and all patients were invited for a first visit during the first 3 months of the study. Follow up was encouraged, with timing determined by clinical circumstances, but usually every 2-6 months. Data were colleted at baseline and at 1-year.

The intervention consisted of nurse-run clinics within a general practice. The intervention had four stages. First, symptom review occurred, and appropriate referrals made for poorly controlled symptoms. Second, drug treatment was reviewed, aspirin use–if not contraindicated–was encouraged, and possible drug side effects were identified. Third, using British Hypertension Society guidelines and local lipid management guidelines, blood pressure and lipids were assessed and referral to a medical doctor made if drug treatment was indicated. Finally, behavior risk factors were assessed and needed changes negotiated. Each visit ended with feedback and goal planning, followed by the writing of an action plan in cooperation with the patient. The control group patients received usual care from their treating practitioner during the year-long study (Campbell et al., 1998a, 1998b).

The researchers found that the intervention reduced the number of hospital admissions. In addition, members of the treatment group showed improvements in the health measure (SF-36) and reported declines in role limitations due to physical health, including fewer reports of worsening chest pain. Fewer patients in the treatment group reported worsening chest pain than those in the control group. While intervention effected no statistically significant change in the Hospital Anxiety and Depression Scale (HADS), the treatment group showed improvements in role limitations attributed to physical problems. Finally, the treatment failed to reduce the rates of practitioner consultation, although members of the treatment group had significant improvements in secondary prevention efforts, including the use of aspirin, blood pressure and lipid management, and physical activity.

Cowan and colleagues (2001, 1997) studied psychosocial interventions in survivors of out-of-hospital ventricular fibrillation or asystole. Their sample included 97 men and 36 women, with a mean age of 60 years, who were assigned randomly to either a treatment group of individual therapy sessions ($n = 67$) or a control group ($n = 66$). Two-year follow up data was obtained for 129 of the 133 participants. The treatment group psychosocial therapy intervention consisted of 11 individual sessions, optimally given twice a week, for about 90 minutes per session. The intervention was delivered by a cardiovascular nurse with a master's degree and a psychosocial nursing specialization. The therapy had three components: (1) physiologic relaxation with computerized biofeedback training focused on altering autonomic tone, specifically to cognitively increase heart rate variability, decrease heart rate and decrease breathing rate; (2) cognitive behavioral therapy aimed at self-management and coping strategies for depression, anxiety, and anger; and (3) health education focused on cardiovascular risk factors.

Based on the theories of Beck's Cognitive Therapy (Beck, 1976) and Lazarus' of stress, appraisal, and coping (Lazarus & Folkman, 1984), the CBT intervention utilized standard practices for self-management of depression (U.S. Department of Health and Human Services, 1993), anxiety, and anger. The physiologic relaxation component of the intervention trained patients to alter cognitively autonomic nervous system responses via deep abdominal breathing, progressive muscle relaxation, autogenic training, and a quieting response. To help participants see the response of these changes, each was done with computerized biofeedback training recording continuous breathing rate, heart rate, blood pressure, and trapezius electromyography (Cowan, 1997). The control group also received the educational component mainly for retention purposes. Both treatment and control groups received health education, which consisted of a 90-minute class on cardiovascular risk factor modification. At treatment end, all subjects passed, at a 70% level, a written exam about basic facts of ventricular fibrillation, the autonomic nervous system, and sudden cardiac arrest. The control group did not receive the psychosocial interventions outlined above. The intervention significantly reduced risk for cardiovascular death by 86%. In the intervention group there were three deaths, compared to eight in the control group. Controlling for other factors, including functional ability, health perception and baseline levels of psychosocial distress, the intervention also reduced depression significantly, as compared to controls.

Lincoln and Flannaghan (2003) tested the effects of CBT on depression in a sample of MI patients with depression as indicated by a score greater than 10 on the Beck Depression Inventory (BDI) or a score greater than 18 on the Wakefield Self-Assessment of Depression Inventory (WDI). The sample included 63 male and 60 female patients (mean age for all groups was 66.1 years) in a hospital setting ($n = 105$), residential care ($n = 11$) and home settings ($n = 7$). Random assignment to the following conditions occurred: CBT therapy ($n = 39$), attention placebo (AP) consisting of a visit from a community psychiatric nurse without therapy ($n = 43$), and standard care ($n = 41$). Participant assessments occurred at baseline, and 3- and 6-month follow-ups. Those in the CBT group were offered 10 weekly one-hour sessions of CBT delivered by the research CPN. Intervention included education, graded task assignment, activity scheduling, and identification and modification of unhelpful thoughts and beliefs. Interventions were tailored to meet the individual's needs. Those in the AP group were offered 10, 1-hour research CPN visits, with no therapeutic intervention. Finally, the standard care, no intervention had contact after baseline measurements with the research CPN. There were no significant differences between the groups in patients' mood, independence in instrumental activities of daily living (IADLs), disability, or satisfaction with care. The researchers do note that because of the small sample size, method of recruitment, and selection criteria, further randomized trials are required.

Rich and colleagues (1995) performed a PNI with an experienced cardiovascular research nurse-led HE component that purposively included patient's family members. Using a sample of patients diagnosed with CHF (age 79 yrs, $SD = 6$), random assignment was made to treatment ($n = 140$) and control ($n = 142$) groups. Assessment occurred at baseline and 90 days post-assessment. The treatment group received a multidisciplinary intervention. Treatment group participants had consultation with social service personnel to facilitate discharge planning and care after discharge. The research nurse provided extensive CHF education to both the patient and the patient's family. A registered dietician did an individualized dietary assessment and a prescribed diet and instruction were given. A geriatric cardiologist examined the patient's medication regimen to reduce unneeded medications and also simplified the overall care regimen. Intensive follow-up treatment occurred via hospital home care services, home visits, and telephone contact. Patients in the control group received usual care from their primary care physicians with no intensive multidisciplinary HE component; however, no standard therapies were withheld. Restricting analysis to first hospitalization survivors, there were more 90-day survivors in treatment group (67%) than that in the control group (54%, p = .04). There was a tendency for the treatment group to experience a 90-day survival without readmission (p = .09). In the treatment group, readmissions for CHF were reduced by 56.2%, and in the control group by 24%. The intervention increased quality of life, as assessed by the Chronic Heart Failure Questionnaire (CHFQ) (p = .001). There were 41 hospital re-admissions in the treatment group compared to 59 patients in the control group. Further, the hospital readmission costs were lower in the treatment group ($3,236 per patient) than those in the control group ($2,178 per patient, p = .03).

TREATMENT SUMMARY

More than 40 years of investigation and mixed findings provide no easy answers to questions concerning psychosocial treatments for older adults with heart diseases. In the 1990s, three meta-analyses all suggested the positive effect of psychosocial treatment on some primary health outcomes. However, because survivor trials tend to need a large sample, the most valid evidence is found in the more recent trials, particularly the ENRICHD trial. In the regarded and well-implemented ENRICHD trial, findings about health outcomes were contrary to expectations. These findings brought considerable attention from both cardiologic and psychosocial communities because of the ENRICHD investigators' immense effort in improving the scientific rigor of clinical trials on psychosocial treatment, including attention to issues of diversity. Several factors seem to account for the lack of significant CBT impacts on medical endpoints, including the use of antidepressants in both treatment and control groups, the unmet difficulties and low motivation in subjects from lower SEM strata, difficulties in altering long-standing low levels of social support, the need for a longer period of intervention (>6 months), and unaddressed pathophysiological and behavioral mechanisms underlying the link between depression and CHD mortality (Frasure-Smith & Lesperance, 2003; The ENRICHD Investigators, 2003). However, a moderate improvement in depression and social support was found for the treatment group.

Findings from the multi-site trial performed in Scotland (Campbell et al., 1998a, 1998b) suggest that PNI and HE interventions may improve health. Mortality rates are not reported, but the treatment group had fewer hospital admissions. This finding must be interpreted with caution because rates of consultation with general practitioners are similar in treatment and control groups, and there is a lack of data about morbidity, the specific treatments that occurred during practitioner consultations, and the costs of care. Further, those in the treatment group showed no improvement in anxiety or depression.

In the GMCB trial, the group intervention suggests an improvement in health-related QOL (Focht et al., 2004; Rejeski et al., 2003). Like the ENRICHD trial, in the GMCB trial QOL improvements also were found in the control group–specifically for men. The Campbell trial and the GMCB trial both suggest that psychosocial interventions can influence improvements in secondary health outcomes, such as adherence to exercise and diet. This leads to the question of whether better secondary health management can lead to improvement in QOL and fewer depressive symptoms.

Smaller trials suggest that PNI and CBT interventions may help patients to return to normal levels of physical activity. They found that control group members avoided activities–suggesting the possibility of increased isolation. Overall, the recent smaller PNI and CBT trials fail to suggest explanations for the mixed findings in the ENRICHD trial. In general, findings in the smaller PNI and CBT trials are mixed and comparisons between trials are difficult to make because of significant differences in intervention protocols.

The SM trials by Blumenthal and colleagues (2002) and by Luskin and colleagues (2002) suggest that SM may help in both physical recovery and long-term health maintenance. A key aspect of the Blumenthal study is the cognitive component to the SM intervention, which implies that the cognitive component of psychosocial interventions is crucial. However, these findings must be interpreted with caution due to the sample size

Perhaps the secondary outcomes, especially mental health and QOL-related measures, are more interesting for mental health professionals, especially social workers. To date, most studies determined a positive role for psychosocial treatment. The support of the CBT findings, including those from the ENRICHD trial, and evidence from two of the meta-analyses support the efficacy of HE and SM, and a combination of these two approaches. However, two large-sample studies in the third meta-analysis (Dusseldorp et al., 1999) yielded negative results for SM and HE interventions with regard to reducing depression and anxiety. A well-designed PNI study, referred to as M-HART (Frasure-Smith et al., 1999), suggests that SM and HE are less effective. The M-HART trial lacked a mental health focus, failed to use skilled mental health service providers, and found a potential intervention-related harm in the mortality of women with MI. Therefore, this negative finding does not eliminate the positive effects of psychosocial inventions. Rather, future research must focus on (a) addressing cardiac mental health with evident techniques, (b) utilizing mental health professionals as intervention providers, and (c) considering demographic risk factors that may interact with psychosocial therapies.

CONCLUSION

With regard to psychosocial interventions, social work practitioners have an important role in enhancing the functioning, QOL, and mental health of older adults. Given the convincing evidence of psychosocial intervention on secondary outcomes, it is promising that social workers may play a highly significant role in this dimension of health care in a rapidly aging yet prosperous society. Considerable evidence suggests that more specified interventions are superior to less specified interventions. Given the immense and increasing impact of CVDs on the lives of Americans, SM, HE, and CBT should be included in social work education. However, current curricula tend to separate health, gerontology, and mental health components to very different foci–such as health disparities, service provision, and individual practice methods. This conventional design fails to prepare future practitioners for the multidisciplinary team approaches that are supported highly by the literature. Social work practitioners may need more specialized health-related mental health training to provide intervention for older adults with CVD.

In conclusion, there are many CHD-related psychosocial factors unaddressed in current research, despite millions of dollars in government and foundation research grants. These factors include anger, hostility, some unidentified components of social support, and pathophysiological and behavioral mechanisms underlying the heart-mind link. Most important, the subgroup analysis in the ENRICHD trial clearly suggested cardiac health disparity in relation to gender, race, and socioeconomic status. These psychosocial components, traditionally not examined in medical trials, but within the expertise of social workers, may affect CHD outcomes. Discrimination (e.g., ageism, racism, and sexism), for example, could trigger anger and hostility; adversity in social strata could exacerbate inequality in accessing the aggressive cardiac treatment; and spirituality- and religion-related factors could contribute to the mental health of older persons who face CHD-related life-or-death challenges. In these areas, the social work profession may have a great opportunity to research the efficacy and cost-effectiveness of CVD-related psychosocial treatments, which in turn will enhance the professional role in cardiac care and education.

TREATMENT RESOURCE APPENDIX

33rd Bethesda Conference: Preventive Cardiology: How Can We Do Better?

http://www.acc.org/clinical/bethesda/beth33/index.htm

Maintained by the American College of Cardiology Foundation, this website provides extensive resources about policy and interventions related to cardiac disease.

American Heart Association

http://www.americanheart.org

This national organization maintains a vast website of information about heart health. Be sure to visit the "Publications & Resources" link. In particular, there is practice information for clinicians and service providers including:

> *Heart at Work: Health Promotion Coordinators Guide.*
> *http://216.185.102.50/haw/.* Unsure about how to conduct an employee wellness program? Here you'll find detailed information and worksheets to help you plan, implement and maintain an effective health promotion program for employees. It's everything a worksite coordinator needs to know!

Content includes:
- Physical activity
- Managing stress
- Nutrition and weight management
- Blood pressure
- Smoking
- Self-assessment for cardiac and stroke risk

> *Heart of Caregiving.* Site for care providers of persons with cardiac disease. *http://www.americanheart.org/presenter.jhtml?identifier=3039829.* The site provides information about caring for oneself as a care provider. The web site is informative, comprehensive, and easy to navigate.

> *American Heart Association; Fitting in Fitness: Hundreds of Simple Ways to Put More Physical Activity into Your Life. http://*

www.americanheart.org/presenter.jhtml?identifier=3040240. Published by: Clarkson Potter/Publishers, a division of Random House, Inc. This fun and inspiring pocket guide throws all those excuses for not exercising out the window. It tells you how to fit exercise into your daily schedule by giving you helpful hints like taking the stairs instead of the elevator at work and doing stretching exercises while you watch TV.

American Heart Association; 365 Ways to Get Out the Fat: A Tip a Day to Trim the Fat Away. Published by: Clarkson Potter/Publishers, a division of Random House, Inc.
This fun pocket guide is filled with tips on shopping, cooking, snacking, and preparing and customizing favorite foods. You'll also find nutrition guidelines to help keep fat and cholesterol under control. It's a must-read for healthier hearts and trimmer waistlines.
http://www.americanheart.org/presenter.jhtml?identifier=3040241

Enhancing Recovery in Coronary Heart Disease (ENRICHD)

http://www.bios.unc.edu/units/cscc/ENRI/

Maintained by the Collaborative Studies Coordinating Center, this website directs you through resources and information about the ENRICHD study, personnel, manuscripts and more.

Heart Info

www.heartinfo.org.

HeartInfo.org provides timely and trustworthy patient guides about heart attack, blood pressure, cholesterol, stroke, diet and more.

National Heart, Lung, and Blood Institute

http://www.nhlbi.nih.gov/health/public/heart/index.htm

The National Institutes of Health page. Contains Fact Sheets about cardiac issues, blood pressure, and diet.

National Institute on Aging

http://www.niapublications.org/pubs/hearts/aginghearts.asp

A 64-page booklet offers an inside look at the latest cardiac research funded by the National Institutes of Health (NIH). Using easy-to-understand diagrams and illustrations of the heart, Aging Hearts and Arteries discusses the link between aging and cardiovascular diseases, such as coronary heart disease and high blood pressure.

SeniorNet

http://www.seniornet.org/php/default.php

SeniorNet's mission is to provide older adults education for and access to computer technologies to enhance their lives and enable them to share their knowledge and wisdom. Provides web-based information on a variety of conditions, including heart and cardiac issues.

Third Age Heart Information

http://www.thirdage.com/healthgate/files/40485.html

Describes how the aging process effects cardiac functioning. Provides guidelines about "heart healthy" issues about diet, exercise, and habits.

REFERENCES

American Heart Association (AHA, 2006a). International cardiovascular death statistics. Retrieved February 1, 2006 from http://americanheart.org/presenter.jhtml?identifier=2011

American Heart Association (AHA, 2006b). Men and cardiovascular diseases. Retrieved February 1, 2006 from http://americanheart.org/presenter.jhtml?identifier=2011

American Heart Association (AHA, 2006c). Statistical fact sheet populations: Baby boomers and cardiovascular diseases–statistics. Retrieved February 1, 2006 from http://americanheart.org/presenter.jhtml?identifier=2011

American Heart Association (AHA, 2006d). Women and cardiovascular diseases. Retrieved February 1, 2006 from http://americanheart.org/presenter.jhtml?identifier=2011

American Heart Association (AHA, 2005). Heart disease and stroke statistics 2005 update. Retrieved June 10, 2005 from http://www.americanheart.org/downloadable/heart/1105390918119HDSStats2005Update.pdf

American Heart Association (2003). Heart disease and stroke statistics 2003 update. Retrieved December 20, 2003 from http://www. americanheart.org/ downloadable/ heart/4 838_HSSTATS2001_1. 0. pdf

Barth, J., Schumacher, M., & Herrmann-Lingen, C. (2004). Depression as a risk factor for mortality in patients with coronary heart disease: A meta-analysis. *Psychosomatic Medicine, 66*(6), 802-813.

Beck, A.T. (1976). *Cognitive therapy and the emotional disorders.* New York: International Universities Press.

Black, J.L., Allison,T.G., Williams, D.E., Rummans, T.A., & Gau, G.T. (1998). Effect of intervention for psychological distress on rehospitalization rates in cardiac rehabilitation patients. *Psychosomatics: Journal of Consultation Liaison Psychiatry, 39*(2), 134-143.

Blumenthal J.A., Babyak, M., Jang, W., O'Connor, C., Waugh, R., Eisenstein, E., Mark, D., Sherwood, A., Woodley, P.S., Irwin, R.J., & Reed, G. (2002). Usefulness of psychosocial treatment of mental stress-induced myocardial ischemia in men. *American Journal of Cardiology.* Jan 15;89(2):164-8.

Blumenthal, J.A., Jang, W., Babyak, M.A., Krantz, D.S., Frid, D.J., Coleman, R.E. et al. (1997). Stress management and exercise training in cardiac patients with myocardial ischemia: Effects on prognosis and evaluation of mechanisms. *Archives of Internal Medicine, 157,* 2213-2223.

Campbell, N.C., Ritchie, L.D., Thain, J., Deans, H.G., Rawles, J.M., & Squair, J.L. (1998a). Secondary prevention in coronary heart disease: A randomized trial of nurse led clinics in primary care. *Heart, 80,* 447-452.

Campbell, N.C., Thain, J., Deans, H.G., Ritchie, L.D., Rawles, J.M., & Squair, J.L. (1998b). Secondary prevention clinics for coronary heart disease: Randomised trial of effect on health. *British Medical Journal, 316*(7142), 1434-7.

Carney, R.M., Freedland, K.E., Veith, R.C., & Jaffe, A.S. (1999). Can treating depression reduce mortality after an acute myocardial infarction? *Psychosomatic-Medicine, 61,* 666-675.

Cowan, M.J., Pike, K.C., Budzynski, H.K.. (2001). Psychosocial nursing therapy following sudden cardiac arrest: Impact on two-year survival. *Nursing Research.* Mar-Apr;50(2):68-76.

Cowan, M.J. (1997). Innovative approaches: A psychosocial therapy for sudden cardiac arrest survivors. In Dunbar, S.B., Ellenbogen, K.A., & Epstein, A.E. (Eds.) *Sudden cardiac death: Past, present, and future.* Armonk, NY: Futura Publishing

Dusseldorp, E., van Elderen, T., Maes, S., Meulman, J., & Kraaij, V. (1999). A meta-analysis of psychoeducational programs for coronary heart disease patients. *Health Psychology, 18*(5), 506-519.

ENRICHD Investigators (2004a). Depression and late mortality after myocardial infarction in the Enhancing Recovery in Coronary Heart Disease (ENRICHD) study. *Psychosom Medicine.* 2004, Jul-Aug;66(4):466-74.

ENRICHD Investigators (2004b). Psychosocial treatment within sex by ethnicity subgroups in the Enhancing Recovery in Coronary Heart Disease clinical trial. *Psychosomatic Medicine.* Jul-Aug;66(4):475-83.

ENRICHD Investigators (2003). Effects of treating depression and low perceived social support on clinical events after myocardial infarction: The Enhancing Recovery in Coronary Heart Disease Patients (ENRICHD) Randomized Trial. *JAMA, 289*(23), 3106-16.

ENRICHD Investigators (2001). Enhancing recovery in coronary heart disease (ENRICHD) study intervention: Rationale and design. *Psychosomatic Medicine, 63*(5), 747-55.

Focht, B.C., Brawley, L.R., Rejeski, W.J., & Ambrosius, W.T. (2004). Group-mediated activity counseling and traditional exercise therapy programs: Effects on health-related quality of life among older adults in cardiac rehabilitation. *Annals of Behavioral Medicine, 28*(1):52-61.

Frasure-Smith, N., & Lesperance, F. (2003). Depression and other psychological risks following myocardial infarction. *Archives of General Psychiatry, 60*, 627-36.

Frasure-Smith, N., Lesperance, F., Juneau, M., Talajic, M., & Bourassa, M.G. (1999). Gender, depression, and one-year prognosis after myocardial infarction. *Psychosomatic Medicine, 61*(1), 26-37.

Hemingway, H., Malik, M., & Marmot, M. (2001). Social and psychosocial influences on sudden cardiac death, ventricular arrhythmia and cardiac autonomic function. *European Heart Journal, 22*, 1082-1101.

Kohn, C.S., Petrucci, R.J., Baessler, C., Soto, D.M., & Movsowitz, C. (2000). The effect of psychological intervention on patients' long-term adjustment to the ICD [implanted cardioverter defibrillator]: A prospective study. *Pacing Clinical Electrophysiology.* Apr. 23(4 Pt 1):450-6.

Krantz, D.S., Sheps, D.S., Carney, R.M., & Natelson, B.H. (2000). Effects of mental stress patients with coronary artery disease: Evidence and clinical implications. *JAMA, 283*, 1800-1802.

Lazarus, R.S., & Folkman, S. (1984). *Stress, appraisal and coping.* New York: Springer.

Lincoln, N.B., & Flannaghan, T. (2003). Cognitive behavioral psychotherapy for depression following stroke: A randomized controlled trial. *Stroke.* Jan;34(1):111-5.

Linden, W., Stossel, C., & Maurice, J. (1996). Psychosocial interventions for patients with coronary artery disease: A meta-analysis. *Archives of Internal Medicine,* April 8. *156* (7), 745-752.

Luskin, F., Reitz, M., Newell, K., Quinn, T.G., & Haskell, W. (2002). A controlled pilot study of stress management training of elderly patients with congestive heart failure. *Preventative Cardiology.* Fall; 5(4):168-72.

Miller, G. E., & Cohen, S. (2001). Psychological interventions and the immune system: A meta analytic review and critique. *Health Psychol, 20*(1), 47-63.

Mullen, P.D., Mains, D.A., & Velez, R. (1992). A meta-analysis of controlled trials of cardiac patient education. *Patient Education and Counseling, 19*(2), 143-62.

Musselman, D.L., Evans, D.L., & Nemeroff, C.B. (1998). The relationship of depression to cardiovascular disease. *Archives of General Psychiatry, 55*, 580-592.

Nemeroff, C.B., Musselman, D.L., & Evans, D.L. (1998:8 Suppl 1). Depression and cardiac disease. *Depression and Anxiety*, 71-9.

Pignay-Demaria, V., Lesperance, F., Demaria, R.G., Frasure-Smith, N., & Perrault, L. P. (2003). Depression and anxiety and outcomes of coronary artery bypass surgery. *Annals of Thoracic Surgery, 75*, 314-321.

Rejeski, W.J., Brawley, L.R., Ambrosius, W.T., Brubaker, P.H., Focht, B.C., Capri, C.G., & Fox, L.D. (2003). Older adults with chronic disease: Benefits of group-mediated counseling in the promotion of physically active lifestyles. *Health Psychology, 22*(4), 414-423.

Rich, M.W., Beckham, V., Wittenburg, C., Leven, C.L., Freedland, K.E., & Carney, R.M. (1995). A multidisciplinary intervention to prevent the readmission of elderly patients with congestive heart failure. *New England Journal of Medicine, 333*(18), 1190-5.

Rozanski A., Blumenthal, J.A., & Kaplan, J. (1999). Impact of psychological factors on the pathogenesis of cardiovascular disease and implications for therapy. *Circulation, 99,* 2192-2217.

U.S. Census Bureau. http://www.census.gov/prod/2004pubs/04statab/pop.pdf

U.S. Department of Health and Human Services (1993). Depression in primary care: Treatment of major depression (AHCPR Publication Number 93-0551). Washington.

van Melle, J. P., de Jonge, P., Spijkerman, T.A., Tijssen, J G., Ormel, J., van Veldhuisen, D.J., van den Brink R.H.S., & van den Bero, M.P. (2004). Prognostic association of depression following myocardial infarction with mortality and cardiovascular events: A meta-analysis. *Psychosomatic Medicine, 66,* 814-822.

Chapter 3

Cancer Treatments

Peter Maramaldi, PhD
Sheryn Dungan, LICSW
Nancy Levitan Poorvu, LICSW

Cancer is of particular importance to gerontology due to the changing nature of the disease. Survival rates are at all time highs as a result of technological advances in early detection and treatment of cancer. Some less aggressive or invasive forms of cancer are now seen as chronic illnesses rather than acute, terminal diseases. As a result, demand is increasing for evidence-based psychosocial interventions designed to improve the health and well-being of people living with cancer. Such interventions consider the biopsychosocial, and spiritual aspects of patients' adjustment to illness, and address the impact of illness on couples and the family system. Several studies reviewed will address the impact of widespread use of technology that now enables psychosocial interventions to be delivered beyond the confines of the treatment center. Others address complementary and alternative therapies designed to augment traditional interventions.

DEMOGRAPHICS AND PREVALENCE

Cancer is the second leading cause of death in the United States following heart disease. Annual projections published by the American Cancer Society (2006) indicate that 570,280 people will die of cancer in 2005–meaning that approximately 1,500 people in the United States are expected to die from some form of cancer every day. During the same year, more than 1.4 million additional people are projected to be newly diagnosed with some form of invasive cancer. Rates and types of cancer differ by gender. Cancers of the breast, lung/bronchus, and colon/rectum will account for 55% of newly diagnosed cancer in women. Prostate, lung/bronchus, and colon/rectum account for 56% of cancers in men. The two most prevalent types of cancer expected to be diagnosed this year are breast cancer for women and cancer of the prostate for men, accounting for 32 and 33% of incident cases respectively (Jemal et al., 2005).

Breast cancer is a major cause of both morbidity and mortality in women. Between 1992 and 2001, Surveillance, Epidemiology, and End Results data (The SEER Program of the National Cancer Institute) indicate that 242,549 cases of invasive female breast cancer were diagnosed. Older women are particularly affected. Of these cases, 23.5% were < 50 years, and 76.5% were >50 years of age. For this same period, the incidence of breast cancer peaked between the ages of 70 and 79 (NCI Surveillance, Epidemiology and End Results, cited in Anderson, Jatoi & Devesa, 2005). Older women may receive different treatment than their younger counterparts. Increasing age has been independently associated with a decreased use of treatment guidelines for definitive surgery, adjuvant chemotherapy, and adjuvant hormonal therapy (Giordano, Hortobagyi, Kau, Theriault & Bondy, 2005).

According to the American Cancer Society, prostate cancer accounts for one third (33%) of the estimated 1,372,910 new cancer cases in the United States in 2005 (Jemal et al., 2005). It remains the most common cancer in American men, with one in six men diagnosed during their lifetime. Through early detection and treatment, only one in 34 will die of the disease and 77% will survive at least 15 years. Prostate cancer is predominantly a disease impacting men ages 65 and older (American Cancer Society, 2006).

In general, older people bear a disproportionate cancer burden in the United States as evidenced by cancer being classified as a disease of older adults (Cohen, 2003; Deimling, Kahana, Bowman & Schaefer, 2002; Ershler, 2003; Goodwin & Coleman, 2003; Kurtz, Kurtz, Stommel, Given & Given, 1999; Nussbaum, Baringer & Kundart, 2003; Overcash, 2004; Sacks & Abrahm, 2003; Wallace, 2001). Despite having the highest incidence rates of almost all cancers, older people have the lowest rates of cancer screening procedures. The data indicates that between 1994-1998, 60% of all newly diagnosed malignant tumors and 70% of cancer deaths occurred in people age 65 and older. Compared with younger segments of the population, cancer incidence rates are 10 times higher for people age 65 and above (Perlich, 2002). Considering that 75 million "baby boomers" born in the United States between 1946 and 1964 will soon age into higher risk groups for various forms of cancer, incidence rates are likely to reach all-time highs.

Cancer impacts the physiological, psychological, emotional, and social aspects of a person's existence. Cancer and cancer treatments are often complicated by existing comorbidities related to age, physical and cognitive impairment, ongoing symptom management and complications of treatments, pain management, related side effects to treatments, possible physical impairments, limited social relationships, psychological and emotional distress, nutritional issues, and financial burdens (Ahmed, 2004; Badura & Grohmann, 2002; Balducci, 2003; Frongillo, Valois & Wolfe, 2003; Haley, 2003; Hayman et al., 2001; Ingram, Seo, Martell, Clipp, Doyle, Montana & Cohen, 2002; Jepson et al., 1999; McCarthy, Phillips, Zhong, Drews & Lynn, 2000; Sharp, Blum & Aviv, 2003). The psychosocial aspects of cancer detection, treatment, and survivorship result in increasing need for support if older adults afflicted with the disease are to achieve positive health outcomes and an acceptable quality of life (Cancer Care, 2003; Coleman, Hutchins & Goodwin, 2004; Deimling, Kahana, Bowman & Schaefer, 2001; Ershler, 2003; Goodwin & Coleman, 2003; Overcash, 2004; Query & Wright, 2003; Vig, Davenport & Pearlman, 2002). The psychosocial impact of the disease and its treatment, demographic shifts toward an aging population, and biomedical advances in screening and treatment technologies which increase rates of survival have highlighted the importance of empirically-based psychosocial interventions to supplement and enhance medical interventions for cancer patients and their caretakers.

THEMES AND NATURE OF THE PROBLEM

Cancer is a category of diseases characterized by uncontrolled and abnormal cell growth that often invades nearby tissue. Cancer cells can spread through the lymphatic system and the bloodstream. There are four main types of cancer: *Carcinoma* begins in the skin or tissues that line the cover of the internal organs; *Sarcoma* begins in the bone, cartilage, fat, muscle, blood vessels, or other connective tissue; *Leukemia* starts in blood-forming tissue such as bone marrow and then flows into the blood; and *Lymphoma* begins in the cells of the immune system (NCI Web page, b). Cancer is not a single disease but more than a hundred diseases that can occur in almost all of the organs and anatomic sites of the human body. Certain types of cancer are more lethal than others and each one has its own unique profile (Cohen, 2003; Hess, 1991; Roy & Russell, 1992; Wallace, 2001).

As a serious illness linked with aging, cancer and the side effects of its treatment may present the added burden of loss of acuity of the senses (e.g., hearing and sight) and impaired cognitive functioning. Exhausting, anxiety-provoking symptoms and aggressive medical treatments often leave people vulnerable to losing their sense of humor, flexibility, and playful spirit (Goodheart & Lansing, 1997). Frustration, anger and blame can be difficult to contain, spilling over and impairing judgment as these feelings frequently are projected outward (Goodheart & Lansing, 1997). The potential for withdrawal, isolation, depression, self-pity, and spiritual crisis in an otherwise mentally healthy, well-functioning person is huge.

Yet, the experience of serious illness can result in renewed strength and value clarification (Frank, 1991). For seriously ill people, connecting to others in a caretaking role can refocus them on their core values. Caring for others can give people the fortitude to continue caring for themselves. Reasons for living can become clearer when the seriously ill person faces the potential for death. With reevaluation of life principles and an increased desire to accomplish cherished goals, people often use periods of remission and wellness for a sense of reinvigorated enthusiasm and wisdom.

Advances in detection and screening have improved dramatically in recent decades. National efforts to monitor cancer in the United States started in the 1930s. Since then, death rates rose steadily for approximately 60 years until a decline occurred in the 1990s when interdisciplinary cancer control efforts appear to have reduced mortality. Despite these lower death rates, the aging of the U.S. population will result in greater numbers of people being diagnosed with cancer. If cancer rates follow current patterns, cancer incidence will double over the next half century with 2.6 million newly diagnosed cases in the year 2050 (Edwards et al., 2002). Although recent years have seen dramatic increases in survival rates, one in four deaths in the United States are attributable to some form of cancer (Jemal et al., 2005).

Since detection provides earlier diagnosis and treatment, a greater number of people are living with a history of cancer. Once diagnosed, an individual is considered to be a "survivor" for the remainder of her/his life. In 2001 (the most recent year for which data is available), it was estimated that 9.8 million people, or 3.5% of the U.S. population, were survivors of cancer. Of the almost 10 million survivors, 14% have lived 20 years or longer after diagnosis (NCI, n.d.a.). As a result of early detection and advances in treatment, many forms of cancer have taken on dimensions of a chronic disease.

The effect of a cancer diagnosis or death goes far beyond the patient, however. In addition to the economic impact on the nation's spiraling health care costs, the impact of cancer includes lost wages, and decreased productivity by patients and caregivers. The psychosocial consequence of cancer radiates far into the constellation of people and systems around the patient her/himself to include caretakers, family members, and the community. This situation presents clinicians and behavioral scientists with new challenges that are difficult to identify, conceptualize and measure. As more people survive the disease and live longer than at any time in the history of cancer surveillance, the psychosocial impact of cancer will increase.

CONSEQUENCES

In coping with a serious illness such as cancer, one is beset by threats to body integrity, to life goals, and to one's sense of immortality (Goodheart

& Lansing, 1997). Any fantasy of invulnerability is lost; the future becomes uncertain, and planning is impossible. Frank (1991) states that illness, with all of the restrictions it imposes, destroys one's sense of freedom. In his view, it is not until one works through the many complex responses and comes to a sense of no longer needing perfect health that freedom is regained. Meanwhile, the unpredictability caused by cancer creates incoherence and presents significant challenges to a person's sense of self. The changes in roles, relationships, employment, family life, and finances that a person facing cancer might confront compound the loss of body integrity that shakes the foundation of the self.

Depending on the type of cancer, the experience may be quite different for the patient and family. In the situation of a breast cancer diagnosis, numerous psychosocial consequences include emotional, psychological, and existential distress that can lead to sexual and relationship difficulties (Wimberly, Carver, Laurenceau, Harris & Antoni, 2005). Although the association is not clear, a diagnosis of prior depression has been found to be a risk factor for decreased survival with this type of cancer (Goodwin, Zhang & Ostir, 2004). In patients with prostate cancer, psychosocial adjustment depends on a range of factors, including a preexisting support network, marital status, previous psychiatric history, retirement, as well as significant life stressors such as loss or illness of a loved one. Annual screening, including digital examination and monitoring of PSA levels, can amplify anxiety. The treatment options for prostate cancer include radical prostatechtomy, radiation, and monitoring the disease through watchful waiting. Along with worries about morbidity, these treatment options for prostate cancer result in side effects that can impact one's sense of self. Urinary incontinence, sexual dysfunction and changes in bowel function present challenges that may significantly diminish quality of life, increase depression and anxiety, and create disturbances in social relationships.

Regardless of the type of cancer, many seriously ill people often withdraw socially in an effort to preserve energy for work and the closest loved ones. For many, it is essential to maintain employment, which can reinforce a sense of normalcy, as well as minimize the financial losses caused by time off, diminished workloads, and increased medical expenses. The pain that often accompanies cancer can be difficult to articulate and, therefore, can be experienced as silencing and lonely. The difficulties in making plans and accepting responsibility contribute to loss of a sense of belonging (Frank, 1991). Cancer can also present anticipated or actual stress for patients as related to the ebb and flow of remission.

EVIDENCE-BASED PSYCHOSOCIAL INTERVENTIONS

The following databases were used in searching for evidence based psychosocial interventions for cancer patients: Medline, CINAHL, and Psych Abstracts. Our findings are organized by cancer type (breast, prostate, or undifferentiated diagnoses), with subcategories by focus on individual, couples, or groups. The majority of interventions have been developed with breast cancer patients. We attribute the abundance of research in breast cancer to established funding from organizations like the National Institutes of Health, Centers for Disease Control, American Cancer Society, the Susan G. Koeman Foundation, and many other national and regional organizations.

In order for a study to be included, the average age of the participants had to be at least 45 years old. One reason that we established this age is because other aging and cancer research have used comparable ages for intervention research at this point in the life course. Secondly, several of the studies have a mixed age group as part of the study protocol, and older adults are included within the interventions. Wherever possible, age ranges are reported to provide as much information about the distribution of ages for the study sample.

Breast Cancer

During the past five years, there have been a number of empirical studies published that describe psychosocial interventions for women with breast cancer. The studies involve a variety of interventions, target populations, and stages of illness. The majority of recent studies of evidence-based interventions utilized some form of group treatment.

Three studies involved supportive-expressive group therapy (SET) as the primary intervention. Study results were somewhat mixed. Bordeleau et al. (2003) randomized women with metastatic breast cancer (N = 215) to a SET group (mean age = 49.4, sd = 8.4 years) plus additional educational materials, or to a control (mean age = 50, sd = 10 years) that provided educational materials only. The groups were held weekly for 90 minutes and co-led by psychiatrists, psychologists, social workers, and nurses. Participants were asked to attend for at least 1 year, if possible. For the SET groups, no change in quality of life was found. In addition, results also revealed that there was deterioration over time in several functional scales such as the profile of mood states (POMS), and a measure of health related quality of life (HrQOL). Declines in these functional areas are normative for a population with advanced metastatic breast cancer, and the researchers posit a few possibilities for this finding. One was a true lack of change that was produced by the SEM intervention in the study population. A rival hypothesis, however, was that the instruments used to evaluate outcome (especially the HrQOL) are typically used in drug trials and may have lacked validity in measuring change through psychosocial treatment.

In a similar study, Classen et al. (2001) randomized 125 women with metastatic or recurrent breast cancer to a weekly 90-minute SET group (mean age = 54 years, sd = 10.7) plus educational materials, or to a comparison (mean age = 58, sd = 10.7) with educational materials only. The weekly therapist-led SET groups continued for 1 year. In this study, women who attended the SET groups had a significantly greater decline in traumatic stress symptoms than did those in the comparison group.

Giese-Davis et al. (2001) also studied the SET intervention on women with metastatic or recurrent disease. In this study, 123 women were randomly assigned to either a control group (mean age = 53.8, sd = 10.49) or a weekly 90-minute SET group (mean age = 52.7, sd = 10.53) co-led by psychiatrists, psychologists, and social workers. The women were encouraged to remain in a group for 1 year. For the SET groups, suppression of negative affect decreased, and restraint of aggressive impulses and behavior increased as compared to baseline. Repression or self-efficacy did not change for either the intervention or control groups.

Education was an important component of several intervention studies. Group interventions utilizing a psychoeducational approach were cited in two studies. Taylor et al. (2003) studied 73 African Americans who had undergone surgery for various stages of breast cancer within the previous 10 months. The intervention group (mean age = 55.78, sd = 11.3) received an individual assessment interview, followed by eight weekly 2-hour psychoeducational group sessions. The control group (mean age = 52.24, sd = 10.9) received the assessment interview only. Results indicated that the intervention benefited women with greater baseline distress and lower income and helped to maintain their baseline functioning. The intervention did not benefit women with low baseline distress and high income.

Helgeson et al. (2000) randomized women (N = 230, mean age = 48, sd = 9.64) with Stage I or II breast cancer, who had received surgery and adjuvant chemotherapy, to three possible interventions, a group emphasizing peer discussion, a group focused on education, a group with a combination of both approaches, or to a control. The educational group showed the greatest benefit in physical functioning for the women who had fewer social supports at the baseline measure. The peer discussion group benefited women with low emotional supports, but was ineffective with those having high levels of emotional support.

Two additional studies illustrate psychoeducational interventions. Angell et al. (2003) described the use of a theoretically-based interactive workbook, the Westbook-Journal (WBJ). The WBJ was developed by the authors and rural breast cancer survivors and contained illustrative stories and a list of resources focused on the rural experience, the disease and treatment education. Opportunities for journal writing were included throughout the workbook to encourage interactivity and emotional release related to the intense emotional experience of breast cancer. One hundred women (mean age = 58.6) with Stage 0 to Stage III breast cancer were randomly assigned to receive the WBJ plus educational materials, or to the comparison that provided educational materials only. The workbook and materials were distributed to the homes of women in a rural area. Assessment was done three months after distribution. There were no main effects for the intervention (WBJ). However, three significant effects were found for the women who did not receive the WBJ: an increase in symptoms of PSTD, an increase in emotional venting, and a decrease in fighting spirit.

In a study of the partners of breast cancer patients, Bulz et al. (2000) randomly assigned partners (N = 34, mean = 51, range = 32-67) to psychoeducational group sessions or to a control. The group intervention consisted of six weekly 1.5-2 hour sessions, focusing on education, and the later four sessions focused on expression of feelings. Outcomes showed that the partners who participated in the intervention had less mood disturbance, greater confidence, and greater marital satisfaction than the control group participants.

Studies have also focused on complementary and alternative medicine (CAM) approaches. Tacon, Caldera and Ronaghan (2004) utilized a non-randomized pretest/posttest design to study the effects of a CAM group on women diagnosed with breast cancer (N = 27, mean age = 53.28, range = 30-78). Eight weekly 1.5-hour group sessions focused on three types of mindfulness practice: bodyscan, sitting meditation, and Hatha Yoga. The intervention produced a significant reduction in levels of stress and in mean state anxiety scores. There was also a significant decrease in helpless/hopelessness and anxious preoccupation, and an increase in what the authors called "fighting spirit."

Simpson et al. (2002) combined a group psychotherapy and a CAM approach in a longitudinal study with women (N = 89) with Stage 0 to

State II breast cancer who had completed treatment. Subjects were randomly assigned to the intervention (n = 46, mean age = 50, sd = 8.4) or to a control (n = 43, mean age = 48.9, sd = 6.8). The intervention consisted of six weekly 1.5-hour group psychotherapy sessions that focused on muscle relaxation, inner relaxation, stress management, mental imagery, goal setting, planning, and achieving change. The comparison group received a standard educational approach. Assessed at one year and two years post-intervention, the intervention showed a positive relationship between social support and psychiatric morbidity at both times. The psychoeducational group did not improve social support, nor did it have an effect on psychiatric morbidity.

Three studies focused on cognitive behavioral approaches to psychosocial interventions. Antoni et al. (2001) studied 100 women with Stage 0 to Stage II breast cancer, who were randomly assigned to a cognitive-behavioral stress management group (CBSM) (mean age = 48.17, sd = 8.97), or to a control (mean age = 52.09, sd = 8.97) that consisted of a one-day seminar. The CBSM groups were held for 2 hours over a 10 week period. Pre- and post-intervention measures at 3 and 9 months were taken. The CBSM group significantly reduced moderate depression and increased optimism about the future. However, the group did not have significant changes in other measures of emotional distress such as anxiety and anger.

Shields and Rousseau (2004) conducted a non-randomized comparison group study on patients (mean age = 52) and their spouses (mean age = 61). The study design compared a two-session workshop, a one-session group, and no intervention. The group intervention was based on the principles of cognitive therapy and marital therapy, targeted at the avoidance of thinking or talking about cancer. Communication exercises, timelines, and mini-lectures were utilized in the workshops. Although the results are preliminary and warrant further study, the two-session workshops showed more positive changes in their quality of life than the one-session group.

Traditional psychotherapy as an intervention was examined in four studies, one with an individual approach, one with a group approach, and two in which therapy was provided over the telephone. Scholten et al. (2001) studied women with a new diagnosis of early breast cancer (N = 41, mean age = 52, sd = 9.0) and women with advanced breast cancer (N = 43, mean age = 62, sd = 8.4). The intervention was psychosocial counseling, the duration and type was determined by individual preferences and needs. Measures of counseling acceptance and quality-of-life were taken at 6 months post-intervention. Women with newly diagnosed early disease showed a high acceptance of counseling and a significant improvement in quality-of-life. However, women with advanced disease showed a low acceptance of counseling and no improvement in quality-of-life. (See Table 1.)

In a large study on telephone therapy, Sandgren and McCaul (2003) provided five weekly 30-minute calls to women with Stage I-III breast cancer (N = 222, mean age = 54.4, sd = 11.8). The women were randomly assigned to calls using a cancer education approach, an emotional expression approach, or to the control (standard care). Pretest and 5-month posttest measures were taken. The group who received cancer education, not the emotional expression approach, showed greater knowledge of lymphedema and greater perceived self-control than the standard care control group. There were no effects for mood or quality-of-life.

In a related study, Stanton et al. (2002) randomly assigned women (N = 60, mean age = 49.53, sd = 12.16) with Stage I or II breast cancer to an intervention of emotional disclosure and benefit finding through written expression. Participants were randomized to one of three groups. One group expressed their deepest thoughts and feelings, a second wrote about the positive benefits of the cancer experience, and a third group wrote facts about the cancer experience. Assessed at 1 and 3 months post-intervention, both the emotional expression and benefits of breast cancer diagnosis treatment groups had reduced the number of medical visits for morbidities. Psychological outcomes such as distress, vigor and perceived quality of life varied as a function of cancer-related avoidance.

Pinto et al. (2003) utilized exercise as an intervention in the study of 24 women (mean age = 52.5, sd = 6.8) diagnosed with breast cancer in the previous 3 years who had completed surgery, chemotherapy, or radiation. The intervention consisted of a 12-week supervised aerobic exercise program. Women were randomized to the exercise group (N = 12), or to a support group (N = 12). The aerobic exercise group showed significant improvement in body image. A decrease in distress was not significant, and the exercise group showed modest improvements in overall fitness.

Prostate Cancer

Reports of evidence-based psychosocial interventions specific to prostate cancer patients are few. However, evidence shows that trained peer support is a viable alternative for men with prostate cancer. The studies that are included in this section focus on both the patients and the interactions with their partners.

Weber et al. (2004) reported a randomized, controlled pilot study testing the effects of a dyadic intervention on social support, self-efficacy, and depression. This study demonstrated the feasibility of providing support by trained lay supportive partners to men who have undergone recent radical prostatectomy. Ten long-term survivors whose procedures had resulted in urinary and sexual dysfunction were recruited to act as support partners. Thirty participants, ages 48-67 (mean age = 58 years) who had recently undergone radical prostatectomy were recruited at their 6-week post-operative visit. Paired with individual support partners, the men met in support dyads for eight weekly sessions. The emphasis was to create a supportive environment where the men could discuss their concerns following radical prostatectomy and regarding survival. The supportive partner kept a log of the meetings, recording the length of the meeting and the focus of the conversation. The logs were also used to monitor the quality of the supportive intervention. There were no adverse effects of participating in the dyadic support partnership. A low attrition rate of 6% indicated the participants' receptivity to this type of intervention. Self-efficacy and social support were measured at baseline and at 8 weeks. Although there was no significant difference in social support or depression over time, the self-efficacy of those receiving the supportive dyadic intervention significantly improved. Although there were no statistical differences between the intervention and the control group at the onset, after 8 weeks of intervention the dyadic support group was significantly less bothered by sexual function in comparison to the men in the control group who received usual care.

Educational groups for men with prostate cancer are generally well-accepted and increase knowledge about the disease, health behaviors and physical functioning. In a randomized controlled study of 250 men who were treated for localized prostate cancer in the Greater Pittsburgh area urology and radiology clinics, participants were assigned to one of three conditions (Lepore et al., 2003). In the control group (mean age = 65.6, sd = 6.6), patients received nothing beyond their standard medical care. In the two intervention groups, one group (mean age = 64.8, sd = 7.7) received education only, and a second group (mean age = 64.8, sd = 8.0) received a lecture plus a 45-minute discussion led by a psychologist for six weekly sessions plus a peer facilitated discussion group. Only the facili-

TABLE 1. Breast Cancer

Author	Intervention	Population	Duration/Frequency	Outcomes
Angell et al., 2003	Interactive Journal, Westbook-Journal	Stage 0–III women (N = 100)	Assessment 3 mos. Post distribution of workbook	Group w/o workbook had increased PTSD, decreased "fighting spirit," and increased emotional venting.
Antoni et al., 2001	Cog-Beh Stress Management groups, RCT	Newly diagnosed, had surgery within 8 weeks (N = 100)	2 hours for 10 weeks	CBSM group had decreased depression, increased optimism about future.
Bordeleau et al., 2003	Supportive Expressive groups	Metastitic Cancer (N = 215)	Weekly, 90 min. for one year	SE group did not have any changes in QOL. Functional declines were experienced over time.
Bulz et al., 2000	RCT Psychoed Grps	Survivors & Partners (N = 34)	6 sessions, 1.5. hours	Partners had less mood disturbance, greater confidence and marital satisfaction
Classen et al., 2001	Supportive Expression groups RCT	Women with metastatic or recurrent breast cancer	3 sessions, 90 min.	Support + education group had decreased stress symptoms over education only group.
Giese-Davis et al., 2002	Support Expressive Group	Metastatic breast cancer (N = 125)	Weekly, 90 min., 1 year	Participants had decreased negative affect, restraint of aggression.
Helgeson et al., 2000	RCT Support Groups	Survivors who received surgery and chemo (N = 230)	8 weekly sessions	Education had greatest benefit for women with low emotion support. Peer discussion beneficial for women with few supports, but not those with high supports
Pinto et al., 2003	Supervised aerobic exercise program	Survivors through year 3 with surgery, radiation or chemo (N = 24)	12 weeks	Exercise group had improved body image and fitness over control or regular activity groups.
Sandgren & McCaul, 2003	Telephone therapy–3 groups: education, emotional support, control	Stage I-III, 1-3 mos post diagnosis	5 sessions, 30 min.	Education group had greater knowledge and control over control.

TABLE 1 (continued)

Author	Intervention	Population	Duration/Frequency	Outcomes
Scholten et al., 2001	Psychosocial counseling RCT	New diagnosed and advanced cancer patients (N = 84)	Determined by needs and desire of each participant	Newly diagnosed = high acceptance of counseling, improved QOL; Advanced = low acceptance and no improvement in QOL.
Simpson et al., 2002	Psychotherapy by psychiatrist and peer survivor	Survivors who completed treatment (N = 89)	6 sessions, 90 min.	Positive relationship between social support and morbidity at 1 and 2 years.
Shields & Rousseau, 2004	Cognitive behavior and Marital two session workshop, one session workshop or control	Patients and spouses (N = 33)	2, 1 or 0 sessions	Two sessions workshop had significant gains over one session.
Stanton et al., 2002	Written expression of emotional and benefits	Stage I or II survivors completing treatment (N = 60)	4 sessions	Emotion and benefit groups had reduced medical benefits.
Tacon, Caldera & Ronaghan, 2004	CAM group of mindfulness practices	Survivors (N = 27)	8 sessions, 1.5 hrs	Decreased anxiety, stress, hopelessness, increase in "fighting spirit."
Taylor et al., 2003	Psychoeducational	African American women, undergoing surgery in past 10 mos (N = 73)	2 hr assessment, 8 sessions, 2 hrs	Greatest emotional distress at baseline had greatest improvement; intervention did not benefit women with low baseline distress and high income.

57

tated education plus peer discussion group resulted in more stable employment and diminished stress relating to sexual dysfunction.

Threats to one's sense of masculinity and sexuality also create challenges for partners, who are in the position of both offering and requiring support. Manne et al. (2004) examined the effects of a 6-week psychoeducational group intervention on the distress, coping, personal growth and marital communication of the partners of men diagnosed with prostate cancer in a randomized, controlled study. Sixty female partners (mean age = 59.6, sd = 9.26) of prostate cancer patients diagnosed with any stage of prostate cancer, who were married or living with that partner were included. The intervention was a closed, structured group intervention. The groups met for one hour per week for six weeks and focused on medical information, nutrition, stress management and coping skills training, maintaining good communication, maintaining intimacy, and survivorship issues. Didactic presentations were combined with group contributions and home practice assignments. No significant differences with regard to the wives' general distress or cancer-specific distress were noted. However, in comparison with the control group, participants receiving the intervention perceived that having a spouse with prostate cancer had made positive contributions to their lives, and reported gains in the use of positive reappraisal coping and reductions in denial coping. (See Table 2.)

Mixed Diagnoses

The psychosocial interventions that have been applied to treatment of patients with different cancer diagnoses are predominantly group treatments. Used to promote hope, self-efficacy, relaxation, and tolerance of medical treatments, these more generic interventions can be used to treat an increasing number of patients in a cost-effective manner. A number of alternative treatments for individuals have been examined, many of which augment traditional individual or group psychotherapies. Innovations in the delivery of interventions reported here include both print and audio materials.

Bennenbroek et al. (2003) assessed the impact of providing patients with increased information in a randomized, controlled study evaluating the use of audiotapes as a delivery method. The participants were 226 newly diagnosed patients (mean age = 60, age range = 29-91) with breast, cervical, head and neck, or prostate cancer, who had been treated over the past 4 to 7 weeks with curative intent. Recruited from the radia-

TABLE 2. Prostate Cancer

Author	Intervention	Population	Duration/Frequency	Outcomes
Lepore et al., 2003	Educational Groups	Patients with localized prostate cancer (n = 250)	Six sessions, 1 hour	Both education and education+peer discussion groups had more knowledge about disease and functioning. Education+peer had more stable employment and diminished stress about sexual dysfunction.
Manne et al., 2004	Psychoeducational Groups	Wives of patients (N = 60)	Six weekly sessions, 1 hour	No difference between intervention and control on distress. Intervention increased coping.
Weber et al., 2004	One-one support with cancer survivor	Patients who had radical prostatectomy	8 weekly sessions, 60 minutes	Depression lower for intervention group at 4 weeks over control, no difference at 8 weeks.

tion therapy departments of three hospitals in The Netherlands, the patients were randomly assigned to a procedural group (n = 59), emotional group (n = 55), coping group (n = 56), or to a control (n = 56) with no structured group experience. Audiotapes of 25 minutes duration were designed to increase subjective understanding for the procedural group; to validate emotions for the emotional group; and to increase self-efficacy in the coping group members. Self-efficacy increased for all groups. In addition, all participants reported validation of their emotions, and increased learning about radiation therapy.

In a randomized, controlled study evaluating the impact of increasing patients' access to information, Stiegelis et al. (2004) utilized a coping booklet given to patients. Two-hundred-nine newly diagnosed cancer patients who received external radiotherapy with a curative intent were recruited from three cancer facilities in The Netherlands. Patients in the experimental arm were given a booklet containing general and specific information about cancer and treatment, information about possible coping strategies and social comparison information, which consisted of short stories of other patients. The booklet was designed to address the negative relationship between loss of control and psychological distress. All patients completed a questionnaire at home 1 week prior to beginning radiation and again 3 months after radiation. The aspects of psychological distress assessed included tension, anger, depression, fatigue, and vigor. Two weeks after completing radiotherapy, patients were randomized to a group (mean age = 60.3, sd = 12.5) who received a booklet and a second group (mean age = 60.6, sd = 11.7) who did not. Significant main effects were evident for tension, anger and depression. Patients evaluated as low in control reported less tension, anger, and depression when they received information than when they did not receive information. Patients who did not receive a booklet showed more psychological distress when they were high in illness uncertainty, which supports the need for increased information.

Stress, mood disturbance, anxiety, depression, anger, and confusion have been targeted by alternative CAM interventions, including meditation, progressive muscle relaxation, guided imagery and exercise. Speca et al. (2000) reported on a randomized controlled trial of a meditation group that met weekly for 1.5 hours for 7 weeks, which was supplemented with additional home meditation practice. A convenience sample of 90 cancer patients (any type) at any point in their illness was gathered from a clinic in a Calgary, Alberta, Canada hospital. Patients were assigned to the treatment group (mean age = 54.9, sd = 10.5) that started immediately, or to the control group (mean age = 48.9, sd =

13.2) that placed patients on a 2-week waiting list. Mood disturbance and symptoms of stress were measured before and after completion of the treatment group. The patients in the meditation group had lower scores on total mood disturbance and symptoms of stress, including depression, anxiety, anger and confusion, at the end of the treatment as compared to controls.

In a related investigation, Carlson et al. (2001) used a longitudinal design to determine effectiveness of the same mindfulness meditation-based stress reduction program on mood disturbance, anxiety, depression, anger, and confusion. In this study, 50 of the original 90 patients in the Speca et al. (2000) research were included (mean age = 52, sd = 12.5). Utilizing a pre- and post-intervention design, measures included the Profile of Mood States (POMS) and the Symptoms of Stress Inventory (SOSI). The results showed that less mood disturbance and fewer symptoms of stress were maintained at 6 months post intervention.

Sloman (2002) evaluated the effects of relaxation and guided imagery on the anxiety, depression, and quality of life of 50 men and women in Sydney, Australia who had advanced cancer and who were receiving palliative care at home (mean age = 54.5, range = 27-79). In this randomized pre- and posttest design controlled study, patients were offered relaxation, guided imagery, or a combination of both during a 30 minute session for 3 weeks. A trained community nurse explained how the tape-recorded intervention would be presented, and then played the tape. At the end of each session, the patients were instructed to repeat the procedure twice weekly at home. During the 3 weeks of the intervention, the nurse visited each patient to encourage and monitor the twice-weekly sessions. A control group received regular nursing care with the nurse timing her visits, which consisted of discussion of medical treatment, to coincide in frequency and duration for the same amount of time as she spent with the treatment group. None of the interventions resulted in decreased anxiety. Positive effects were found for depression and quality of life in all intervention groups.

Progressive muscle relaxation has been reported to positively impact issues of psychological distress, anxiety and quality of life. In a randomized, controlled study of 116 female and male patients with any type of cancer who had been diagnosed within the previous month, Baider et al. (2001) assessed the effect of progressive muscle relaxation and guided imagery. The intervention was offered in six weekly group sessions lasting one hour each, with eight to 10 participants. Assessments were done at the completion of the group and at 3 and 6 months. Comparisons were made among the treatment group (n = 63, mean age = 53.3, sd =

15.51), the control group (n = 27, mean age = 54.5, sd = 14.23), and the refusal to participate group (n = 26, mean age = 52.1, sd = 16.99). Patients who refused to participate were somewhat less distressed at the pretest than those who participated in the study. A small positive effect of the intervention on psychological distress remained present at 6 months for the treatment group.

By comparison, a significant reduction in anxiety and increase in general quality of life was reported when using progressive muscle relaxation training (PMRT) with colorectal patients after stoma surgery. Cheung, Molassoitis, and Chang (2003) recruited 59 patients of Chinese origin from the Departments of Surgery of two regional Hong Kong hospitals, covering patients in two different geographic areas in Hong Kong. In a randomized controlled study of PMRT, patients were assigned to an experimental group (mean age = 60.1, sd = 10.91) that received routine care and PMRT, or to a control group (mean age = 56.4, sd = 13.53) that received only routine care. All of the patients had undergone either temporary or permanent stoma surgery for cancer treatment. Both males and females were included in this study as well. In the experimental group, PMRT was carried out for a 20-minute period, and patients were required to tense and relax different muscle groups in combination with deep breathing. Ten major muscle groups were included. Subjects were taught to use the controlled breathing pattern and ways to decrease the tensing time using face-to-face verbal instructions. A tape containing instructions was given to the patients for practice sessions along with a written and pictorial manual of PMRT to supplement the instructor's training. The frequency of the home practice sessions was recorded in a log. Subjects were contacted every 2 weeks to monitor the progress of their practice sessions after discharge. A significant difference in state-anxiety over 10 weeks was found between the two groups, with the experimental group reporting significantly lower levels of anxiety compared than the control group. A significant time effect was noticed, with anxiety decreasing over time. The use of PMRT significantly increased the generic quality of life in the experimental group, especially in the domains of physical health, psychological health, social concerns and environment. These results make a strong recommendation for PMRT to be integrated into long-term care of colorectal cancer patients as a cost-effective intervention that requires minimal training.

Foot reflexology, consisting of a 30-minute foot massage, was evaluated by Stephenson, Weinrich and Tavakoli (2000). The participants in this study were 23 patients (mean age = 68.7, sd = 2.69), who were diagnosed with breast or lung cancer, spoke English, and were able to give consent. The setting was an inpatient medical/oncology unit of a hospital in the Southeastern U.S. Patients were excluded if they reported no anxiety prior to the intervention. Using a quasi-experimental, pre/post, cross-over trial, patients were randomized into a treatment group, those receiving a foot massage by a nurse, and a control group, those receiving only the usual nurse interaction. While not effective for treating pain, the patients in the experimental group experienced significantly decreased anxiety following reflexology, with the greatest decrease in the lung cancer patients.

Courneya et al. (2003) studied the effects of adding an exercise program to traditional group psychotherapy. The participants were 108 cancer survivors (mean age = 51.55, sd = 10.15) at the Cross Cancer Institute in Canada, who were enrolled in one of 22 group psychotherapy classes. The inclusion criteria were a confirmed diagnosis of cancer, ability to speak English, and passing a Physical Activity Readiness Questionnaire. Group psychotherapy classes were held weekly, for 90-minute sessions for 10 weeks. In a randomized, controlled trial, patients were assigned to a psychotherapy group plus a home-based, moderate exercise program (n = 60), or to a psychotherapy group without exercise (n = 48). The exercise program involved moderate aerobic exercise 3 to 5 times a week. The combined program of psychotherapy and exercise improved quality of life in cancer survivors beyond group psychotherapy alone. There was a significant benefit for physical and functional well-being, but no change in the indicators of emotional or social well-being.

Psychotherapy groups using cognitive and psychoeducation models have been evaluated for their impact on couples and family caregivers. Kuijer et al. (2004) evaluated group interventions led by a psychologist, which consisted of five 90-minute sessions. Fifty-nine couples, married or cohabitating, with a diagnosis of cancer in one partner, and a life expectancy of at least 6 months, participated in the study. The patients were recruited from several hospitals and two cancer information centers in the region of Rotterdam, The Netherlands. Couples were randomly assigned to an experimental group (n = 32, mean age of patient = 50, sd = 12; mean age of partner = 49, sd = 10) and a wait-list control group (n = 27, mean age of patient = 49, sd = 10; mean age of partner = 50, sd = 11). The experimental group intervention included perspective taking, cognitive restructuring, and behavioral exercises with additional homework assignments. Measures were taken prior to the intervention and again at 3 months and 6 months. The experimental group reported lower levels of perceived inequalities in their relationship (e.g., either underinvestment or overinvestment from the cancer-free partner), higher levels of relationship quality, and lower levels of psychological distress.

Scott, Halford and Ward (2004) conducted a study in three hospital oncology clinics in Brisbane, Australia, that utilized a randomized, mixed method design. Ninety-four couples in which the female partner had either localized breast cancer (n = 57) or gynecological cancer (n = 37) participated. The average age for the patients was 51 years (sd = 9.8) and 53 years (sd = 10.0) for their partners. Couples were assigned to one of three treatment conditions: the couple-coping training (CanCOPE), an individual patient-coping training, or medical information education. The couple-coping training consisted of a five-session, 2 hour couples-based intervention with two 30-minute phone calls, utilizing couple-coping training. The couples in the CanCOPE group reported significant improvements in supportive communication, reduced psychological distress, enhanced coping efforts, and improved sexual adjustment.

Family caregivers who provided home care for patients with any type of advanced cancer were included in a study reported by Cameron et al. (2004), which utilized a non-randomized, one-sample pretest/posttest design. People with severe visual, hearing or cognitive impairments were excluded from the study. People who were able to speak and read English, and give informed consent were included. The setting was a large tertiary care hospital in Canada. The brief problem-solving intervention consisted of an hour session with the caregiver alone. It included a slide presentation and education regarding a five-step problem-solving approach. Pretest measures and posttest measures at 4 weeks after completion of the intervention were taken. One significant difference between participants (N = 34, mean age = 53.6, sd = 16.7) and non-participants (N = 27, mean age = 50.4, sd = 16.1) was that participants had been caregivers for a shorter time. Follow-up at 4 weeks showed a decrease in emotional tension and an increase in confidence and positive problem-solving for the treatment group (See Table 3.).

One additional study investigated the impact of sharing patients' psychosocial information (collected on a computer touch screen) with their health care provider teams (McLachlan et al., 2001). The purpose was to determine whether making patient-reported cancer needs, quality of life and psychosocial information available to health care provider teams would provide more coordinated and targeted psychosocial inter-

TABLE 3. Mixed Diagnosis

Author	Intervention	Population	Duration/Frequency	Outcomes
Baider et al. (2001)	Progressive muscle relaxation	Cancer patients diagnosed within the previous month (N = 116)	6 weekly group sessions, 1 hour	A small positive effect of the intervention on psychological distress remained present at six months.
Bennenbroek et al. (2003)	Audio tapes	Newly diagnosed patients with breast, cervical, head and neck, or prostate cancer, who had been treated over the past four to seven weeks with curative intent (N = 226)	Audiotapes of twenty-five minutes duration	Self-efficacy increased for all of the groups. All reported learning more about radiation therapy.
Carlson et al. (2001)	mindfulness meditation-based stress reduction program	Longitudinal analysis of Speca study (N = 50)	6 months	Less mood disturbance and that fewer symptoms of stress were maintained at six months post intervention.
Cheung, Molassoitis & Chang, 2003	Progressive muscle relaxation training (PMRT)	Colorectal patients who underwent surgery (N = 59)	20 min. sessions	PMRT increased QOL, PMRT group had reduced anxiety compared to controls.
Scott, Halford & Ward, 2004	CanCOPE couple's intervention	Women with breast or gynecological concern about to start treatment and partners (N = 94)	5 sessions, 2 hours, 2 30 min. phone calls	CanCOPE resulted in improved communication, reduced stress, improved coping and sexual adjustment.

Author	Intervention	Population	Duration/Frequency	Outcomes
Sloman (2002)	relaxation and guided imagery	Patients receiving palliative care (N = 50)	30 min.	No difference between treatment and control on anxiety, all had decreased depression and increased QOL.
Speca et al. (2000)	Meditation group	Any diagnosed cancer patient (N = 90)	7 weeks, 1.5	Meditation group had lower scores on total mood disturbance and symptoms of stress, including depression, anxiety, anger, and confusion at the end of the treatment.
Stiegelis et al. (2004)	A coping booklet	Newly diagnosed cancer patients receiving radiotherapy (N = 229)	3 months	Significant main effects were evident for tension, anger and depression.
Stephenson, Weinrich & Tavakoli, 2000	Foot reflexology	Breast or lung inpatients (N = 23)	30 min. massages	Decreased anxiety, greatest decreased in lung cancer patients. No significant difference between intervention and controls however.

ventions. The hypothesis was that this coordinated approach would result in reduced cancer needs, improved quality of life (QOL) and increased satisfaction with care for patients. Four hundred fifty people (median age = 61, range = 18 to 92) with cancer of any types, who were not attending their first consultation and with adequate proficiency in the English language were considered for participation. In a randomized trial, 66% had the experimental treatment and 33% did not. The intervention consisted of having information regarding cancer needs, QOL, and psychosocial information relayed to the treatment teams by coordination nurses, who then formulated individual management plans. Patients were assessed 2 and 6 months after randomization for changes in their cancer needs, QOL, and psychosocial functioning. There were no significant differences on any of these variables, or satisfaction with care, between the groups. The conclusion was that making patient reported cancer needs, QOL and psychosocial data available to the health care team does not reduce these variables.

TREATMENT SUMMARY

Looking collectively at the literature on psychosocial intervention for cancer care, the majority of empirically-tested approaches were conducted with breast cancer patients. Most of the interventions included some form of group treatment, which promotes mutual aid among breast cancer survivors and is also cost effective. A frequent approach involved the use of complementary and alternative medicine (CAM) approaches. CAM approaches varied and included realization techniques, meditation, imagery, and yoga. Designed to supplement regular medical treatment and education, these interventions showed some level of success with patients afflicted with this form of cancer. Outcome indicators used in most of the studies were well-established measures of health-related quality of life (HrQOL) and perceptions of mood states (POMS). Although the interventions had mixed outcomes, improvements in some elements of HrQOL and mood states were evidenced in all of the studies using these measures.

Regardless of the type of diagnosis, several studies used psychoeducational interventions to increase patients' awareness of their disease. In some cases, patients reported changes in perceptions about their cancer, and even seeing some benefits of the cancer experience in their lives. These interventions took various forms including group treatments, journal-writing, audiotapes or an employing standardized curriculum. Clearly, outcome evidence indicates that providing information about the disease and treatment process produces positive outcomes for people who are managing a cancer diagnosis.

Psychoeducational interventions also had positive effects with caregivers. For those in care provision roles, these interventions yielded improvements in communication and perceptions of the quality of the patient/caregiver dyad. These findings were reported across different types of cancer diagnoses. Therefore, psychoeducational interventions can have positive impacts within family systems and caregiving relationships as well as with the identified patient.

CONCLUSION

A common thread in the literature concerning the experience of illness is that serious, life-threatening, and chronic illnesses alter a person's sense of self (Frank, 1991; Goodheart & Lansing, 1997). Each person's journey through serious illness is unique and creates the possibility of both positive and negative experiences and changes. As can be seen through this review, evidence-based psychosocial interventions for older adults living with cancer and their caregivers, can diminish the deleterious effects of the disease and, in some cases, result in some form of gain from the experience.

Although cancer is widely studied by a broad range of disciplines from cell biology to behavioral medicine, the literature on evidence-based psychosocial interventions aimed at improving the health and well-being of cancer patients is relatively sparse. As a result of the aging of the U.S. population and the technological advances in early detection and treatment of cancer, there are an increasing number of people impacted by the disease, and the behavioral interventions designed to improve the health and well-being of cancer survivors will take on increasing importance. The void of empirically tested interventions will be filled with a new wave of studies similar to, and based upon, those reported in this article.

The studies reported in this article illustrate that empirically tested psychosocial interventions with cancer patients and their caretakers are feasible, measurable, and capable of producing favorable outcomes. To this end, readers interested in developing, adapting, or replicating interventions with cancer patients are encouraged to use the work reported here as a foundation, to look to emerging discoveries, and to adapt interventions to the populations and clinical context where interventions are needed.

TREATMENT RESOURCE APPENDIX

American Cancer Society: *http://www.cancer.org/docroot/home/index.asp*

Provides information about diagnosis, support, treatment, and resources for cancer. Also includes data about cancer statistics and latest types of treatment.

American Cancer Society (2004) Powerpoint Presentation: *http://www.cancer.org/downloads/PRO/Cancer%20Statistics%202004.ppt*

A powerpoint presentation that presents cancer statistics by different sociodemographic characteristics including race/ethnicity, gender, and age.

BreastCancer.Org: *http://www.breastcancer.org/*

Provides information about risks, symptoms, diagnosis, recovery and support that is specific to a breast cancer diagnosis.

Cancer and Aging Program: *http://www.cancerandaging.uiowa.edu/*

The mission of the Cancer and Aging Program (CAP) is to foster basic and clinical research and address issues uniquely associated with cancer in the elderly. This site is part of the University of Iowa's Center on Aging Program and provides opportunities for funding, as well as research initiatives in cancer in older adults.

Cancer Facts for People over 50: *http://www.mamashealth.com/cancer/oldcancer.asp*

Provides information about particular risks with the aging population. Describes various screening mechanisms for different types of cancers.

Cancer Research: *http://cancerres.aacrjournals.org/*

Journal of the American Association for Cancer Research. Cancer Research publishes significant, original studies in all areas of basic, clinical, translational, epidemiological, and prevention research devoted to the study of cancer and cancer-related biomedical sciences.

Center for Disease Control: *http://www.cdc.gov/cancer/*

CDC's section on cancer prevention and control initiatives. Includes statistics, fact sheets, community-based initiatives, funding opportunities, and screening information.

Sandy D. Hutchison, Suzanne K. Steginga, Jeff Dunn (2005)
The tiered model of psychosocial intervention in cancer:
A community based approach. John Wiley and Sons.

Clinical practice guidelines for the management of psychosocial distress in people with cancer have been produced in Australia and North America and these provide direction for the provision of psychosocial care for patients with cancer and their families. This report describes a tiered intervention model to operationalise psychosocial care in oncology in the community and outlines a framework for integrating services across sectors.

National Cancer Institute, Institute of Health:
http://www.cancer.gov/

Provides summary information about all types of cancer. Includes reports about the latest clinical trials by type of cancer and type of treatment. Also has summaries about various funding opportunities in cancer research. The site also contains an extensive list of resources for practitioners, patients, and family members and several are in Spanish as well as English. Included are booklets, posters, and videos–such as:

- *Coping with Advanced Cancer.* This is a booklet for patients with end stage cancer. It discusses treatment options such as palliative care, clinical trials, hospice care and home care, as well as symptom control. It also addresses emotional concerns including feelings, communicating with friends and family, and living the rest of life to its fullest and with meaning.

- *Facing Forward Series: Life After Cancer Treatment.* Covers posttreatment issues such as follow-up medical care, physical and emotional changes, changes in social relationships, and workplace issues. To educate and empower cancer survivors as they face the challenges associated with life after cancer treatment.
- *Moving Beyond Breast Cancer (Video or DVD).* For women as they finish breast cancer treatment. Features stories of breast cancer survivors in various stages of life who share their concerns and perspectives to help other women know what to expect
- *When Someone You Love Is Being Treated for Cancer.* The focus of the booklet is to provide care givers with coping strategies to help them deal with the stress and anxiety associated with caring for cancer patients. Discusses communication skills, ways to get support, feelings, helping with medical care, and the need for self-care.

All can be found at:

https://cissecure.nci.nih.gov/ncipubs/searchResults.asp?subject2=Coping +with+Cancer

ONCO Link *http://www.oncolink.upenn.edu/library/library.cfm?c=5*

This site contains a wealth of information about cancer, treatment, and cancer related research. An invaluable aspect is the opportunity to access peer reviewed journals, including full text articles. The journal offerings include *Breast Cancer Research and Treatment, Cancer* (journal of the American Cancer Society), *Evidence-Based Oncology, Journal of the American Medical Association* (JAMA), *Lancet Oncology, Nature, Pain Research & Management* among many others.

REFERENCES

Ahmed, S. M. (2004). Is Ageism a factor in cancer screening?, *Annals of Family Medicine,* retrieved on December 21, 2004 from World Wide Web, http://annfammed.org/cgi/eletters/2/5/481

American Cancer Society (2006). *Prostate Cancer Detailed Guide.* Found on the World Wide Web: http://documents.cancer.org/117.00/117.00.pdf

Anderson, W.F., Jatoi, I, & Devesa, S. S. (2005). Distinct breast cancer incidence and prognostic patterns in the NCI's SEER program: Suggesting a possible link between etiology and outcome. *Breast Cancer Research and Treatment,* 90(2), 127-137.

Angell, K., Kreshka, M., McCoy, R., Donnelly, P., Turner-Cobb, J., Graddy, K., Kraemeer, H. & Koopman, C. (2003). Psychosocial intervention for rural women with breast cancer. *Journal of General Internal Medicine,* 18(7), 499-507.

Antoni, M., Lehman, J., Kilbourn, K., Boyers, A., Culver, J., Alferi, S., Yount, S., Mcgregor, B., Arena, P., Harris, S., Price, A. & Carver, C. (2001). Cognitive-behavioral stress management intervention decreases the prevalence of depression and enhances benefit finding among women under treatment for early-stage breast cancer. *Health Psychology,* 20(1), 20-32.

Badura, A. S. & Grohmann, J. M. (2002). Psychological issues in pain perception and treatment in the elderly, *Annals of Long-Term Care,* 10(7), 29-34.

Baider, L., Peretz, T., Hadani, P. & Koch, U. (2001). Psychological intervention in cancer patients: A randomized study. *General Hospital Psychiatry,* 23, 272-277.

Balducci. L. (2003). New Paradigms for Treating Elderly Patients with Cancer: The comprehensive geriatric assessment and guidelines for supportive care. *The Journal of Supportive Oncology,* 1(Supp.2), 30-37.

Bennenbroek, F., Brunk, B., Stiegelis, H., Hagedoorn, M., Sanderman, R., Van Den Bergh, A. & Botke, G. (2003). Audiotaped social comparison information for cancer patients undergoing radiotherapy: Differential effects of procedural, emotional and coping information. *Psycho-Oncology.* 12, 567-579.

Bordeleau, L., Szalai, J., Ennis, M., Leszcz, M., Speca, M., Sela, R., Doll, R., Chochinov, H., Navarro, M., Arnold, A., Pritchard, A., Bezjak, A., Llewellyn-Thomas, H., Sawka, C. & Goodwin, P. (2003). Quality of life in a randomized trial of group psychosocial support in metastatic breast cancer: Overall effects of the intervention and an exploration of missing data. *Journal of Clinical Oncology,* 21(10), 1944-1951.

Bultz, B., Speca, M., Brasher, P., Greggie, P. & Page, S. (2000). A randomized controlled trial of a brief psychoeducational support group for partners of early stage breast cancer patients. *Psycho-Oncology,* 9, 303-313.

Cameron, J., Shin, J., Williams, D. & Stewart, D. (2004). A brief problem-solving intervention for family caregivers to individuals with advanced cancer. *Journal of Psychosomatic Research,* 57,137-143.

Cancer Care (2003). *Working with an Older Person Who Has Cancer,* Retrieved on December 21, 2004 from World Wide Web, http://www.cancercare.org/news/NewsPrint.cfm?ID = 3553&c = 394.

Carlson, L., Ursuriak, Z., Goodey, E., Angen, M. & Speca, M. (2001). The effects of a mindfulness meditation-based stress reduction program on mood and symptoms of stress in cancer outpatients: 6-month follow-up. *Supportive Care in Cancer,* 9, 112-123.

Cheung, U., Molassiotis, A. & Chang, A. (2003). The effect of progressive muscle relaxation training on anxiety and quality of life after stoma surgery in colorectal cancer patients. *Psycho-Oncology,*12, 254-266.

Classen, C., Butler, L., Koopman, C., Miller, E., DiMicelli, S., Giese-Davis, J., Fobair, P., Carlson, R., Kraemar, H. & Spiegel, D. (2001). Supportive-expressive group therapy and distress in patients with metastatic breast cancer. *Archives of General Psychiatry,* 58, 494-501.

Cohen, H. J. (2003). Cancer in the elderly: An overview. In C. K. Cassel, R. M. Leipzig, H. J. Cohen, E. B. Larson, & D. E. Meier (Eds.), *Geriatric Medicine: An Evidence Based Approach* (4th ed., pp. 361-373), New York: Springer.

Coleman, E. A., Hutchins, L. & Goodwin, J. (2004). An overview of cancer in the older adult. *MEDSURG Nursing*, 13(2), 75-109.

Courneya, K., Friedenreich, C., Sela, R., Quinney, A., Rhodes, R. & Handman, M. (2003). The group psychotherapy and home-based physical exercise (group-hope) trial in cancer survivors: Physical fitness and quality of life outcomes. *Psycho-Oncology*, 12, 357-374.

Deimling, G. T., Kahana, B., Bowmon, K. F. & Schaefer, M. L. (2002). Cancer survivalship and psychological distress in later life. *Psycho-Oncology*, 11, 479-494.

Edgar, L., Rosberger, Z. & Collet, J. (2001). Lessons learned: Outcomes and methodology of a coping skills intervention trial comparing individual and group formats for patients with cancer. *International Journal of Psychiatry in Medicine*, 31(3), 289-304.

Edwards, B. K., Howe, H. L., Ries, L. A. G., Thun, M. J., Rosenberg, H. M., Yanick, R., Wingo, P. A. Jemal, A. & Feigal, E. G. (2002). Annual report to the nation on the status of cancer, 1973-1999. *Cancer*, 94(10), 2766-2792.

Ershler, W. B. (2003). Cancer: A disease of the elderly. *The Journal of Supportive Oncology*, 1(2), 5-10.

Frank, A. W. (1991). *The wounded storyteller: Body, illness and ethics*. Chicago & London: The University of Chicago Press.

Frongillo, E. A., Valois, P. & Wolfe, W. S. (2003). Using a concurrent events approach to understand social support and food insecurity among elders. *Family Economics and Nutrition Review*, 15(1), 25-32.

Giese-Davis, J., Koopman, C., Fobair, P., Benson, J., Kraemer, H. & Spiegel, D. (2002). Change in emotion-regulation strategy for women with metastatic breast cancer following supportive-expressive group therapy. *Journal of Consulting and Clinical Psychology*, 70(4), 916-925.

Giordano, S. H., Hortobagyi, G. N., Shu-Wan, C. K., Theriault, R. L., & Bondy, M. L. (2005). Breast cancer treatment guidelines in older women, *Journal of Clinical Oncology*, 24(4), 783-791.

Goodheart, C. D. & Lansing, M. H. (1997). *Treating people with chronic disease: A psychological guide*. Washington, DC: American Psychological Association.

Goodwin, J. S., Zhang, D. D., & Ostir, G. V. (2004). Effect of depression on diagnosis, treatment, and survival of older women with breast cancer. *Journal of the American Geriatrics Society*, 52, 106-111.

Goodwin, J. A. & Coleman, E. A. (2003). Exploring measures of functional dependence in the older adult with cancer. *MEDSURG Nursing*, 12(6), 359-366.

Haley, W. E. (2003). Family Caregivers of elderly patients with cancer: Understanding and minimizing the burden of care. *The Journal of Supportive Oncology*, 1(Supp.2), 25-29.

Hayman, J. A., Langa, K. M., Kabeto, M. U., Katz, S. J., DeMonner, S. M., Chernew, M. C., Slavin, M. B. & Fendrick, A. M. (2001).Estimating the cost of informal caregiving for elderly patients with cancer. *Journal of Clinical Oncology*, 19(13), 3219-3225.

Helgeson, V., Cohen, S., Schultz, R. & Yasko, J. (2000). Group support interventions for women with breast cancer: Who benefits from what? *Health Psychology*, 19(2), 107-114.

Hess, J. W. (1991). Health promotion and risk reduction for later life. In R. F. Young & E. A. Olson (Eds.), *Health, Illness, and Disability in Later Life: Practice Issues and Interventions* (pp. 25-43). Newbury Park, CA: SAGE Publications, Inc.

Ingram, S. S., Seo, P. H., Martell, R. E., Clipp, E. C., Doyle, M. E., Montana, G. S. & Cohen, H. J. (2002). Comprehensive assessment of the elderly cancer patient: The feasibility of self-report methodology. *Journal of Clinical Oncology*, 20(3), 770-775.

Jemal, A., Murray, T., Ward, E., Samuels, A., Tiwari, R. C., Ghafoor, A., Feuer, E. J., & Thun, M. J. (2005). Cancer statistics, *CA Cancer Journal for Clinicians*, 55, 10-30. Found on the World Wide Web: http://caonline.amcancersoc.org/cgi/reprint/55/1/10

Jepson, C., McCorkle, R., Adler, D., Nuamah, I. & Lusk, E. (1999). Effects of home care on caregivers' psychosocial status, *Journal of Nursing Scholarship*, 31(2), 115-120.

Kuijer, R., Buunk, B., Jong, G., Ybema, J. & Sanderman, R. (2004). Effects of a brief intervention program for patients with cancer and their partners on feelings of inequity, relationship quality and psychological distress. *Psycho-Oncology*, 13, 321-334.

Kurtz, M. E., Kurtz, J. C., Stommel, M., Given, C. W. & Given, B. (1999). The influence of symptoms, age, comorbidity and cancer site on physical functioning and mental health of geriatric women patients. *Women & Health*, 29(3), 1-12.

Lepore, S., Helgeson, V., Eton, D. & Schulz, R. (2003). Improving quality of life in men with prostate cancer: A randomized controlled trial of group education interventions. *Health Psychology*, 22(5), 441-452.

Manne, S., Babb, J., Pinover, W., Horwitz, E. & Ebbert, J. (2004). Psychoeducational group intervention for wives of men with prostate cancer. *Psycho-Oncology*, 13, 37-46.

McCarthy, E. P., Phillips, R. S., Zhong, Z., Drews, R. E. & Lynn, J. (2000). Dying with cancer: Patients' function, symptoms, and care preferences as death approaches. *Journal of the American Geriatric Society*, 48(5).

McLachlan, S., Allenby, J., Wirth, A., Kissane, E., Bishop, M., Beresford, J. & Zolcberg, J. (2001). Randomized trial of coordinated psychosocial interventions based on patient self-awareness versus standard care to improve the psychosocial functioning of patients with cancer. *Journal of Clinical Oncology*, 19(21), 4117-4125.

National Cancer Institute (n.d.a.). Office of Cancer Survivorship [OCS]. Retrieved February 10, 2005 from http://dccps.nci.nih.gov/ocs/ocs_factsheet.pdf

Nussbaum, J. F., Baringer & Kundart, A. (2003). Health, communication, and aging: Cancer and older adults. *Health Communication*, 15(2), 185-192.

Overcash, J. A. (2004). Using narrative research to understand the quality of life of older women with breast cancer, *Oncology Nursing Forum*, 31(6), 1153-1159.

Perlich, P. (October 2002). *Utah Minorities: The Story Told by 150 Years of Census Data*. Retrieved July 2, 2003 from Bureau of Economic and Business Research, David S. Eccles School of Business, University of Utah Web site, http://www.business.utah.edu/bebr/onlinepublications/Utah_Minorities.pdf

Pinto, B., Clark, M., Maruyama, N. & Feder, S. (2003). Psychological and fitness changes associated with exercise participation among women with breast cancer. *Psycho-Oncology*, 12, 118-126.

Query, Jr., J. L. & Wright, K. (2003). Assessing communication competence in an on-line study: Toward informing subsequent interventions among older adults with cancer, their lay caregivers, and peers. *Health Communication,* 15(2), 203-218.

Roy, F. H. & Russell, C. R. (1992). *The encyclopedia of aging and the elderly care.* New York: Facts on File.

Sacks, N. R. & Abrahm, J. L. (2003). Cancer. In R. S. Morrison & D. E. Meier (Eds.), *Geriatric Palliative Care* (pp. 123-133). New York: Oxford University Press.

Sandgran, A. & McCaul, K. (2003). Short-term effects of telephone therapy for breast cancer patients. *Health Psychology*, 22(3), 310-315.

Scholten, C., Weinlander, G., Krainer, M., Frischenschlager, O. & Zielinski, C. (2001). Difference in patient acceptance of early versus late initiation of psychosocial support in breast cancer. *Supportive Care in Cancer,* 9(6), 459-464.

Scott, J., Halford, W. & Ward, B. (2004). United we stand? The effects of a couple coping intervention on adjustment to early stage breast or gynecological cancer. *Journal of Consulting and Clinical Psychology,* 72 (6), 1122-1135.

Sharp, J. W., Blum, D. & Aviv, L. (2003). Elderly men with cancer: Social work interventions with prostate cancer, *Cancer Care*, Retrieved on December 21, 2004 from World Wide Web, http://cancercare.org/news/NewsPrint.cfm?ID = 3251&c = 395

Shields, C. & Rousseau, S. (2004). A pilot study of an intervention for breast cancer survivors and their spouses. *Family Process*, 43 (1), 95-107.

Simpson, J., Carlson, L., Beck, C. & Patten, S. (2002). Effects of brief intervention on social support and psychiatric morbidity in breast cancer patients. *Psycho-Oncology*. 11, 282-294.

Sloman, R. (2002). Relaxation and imagery for anxiety and depression control in community patients with advanced cancer. *Cancer Nursing*, 25(6), 432-435.

Speca, M., Carlson, L., Goodey, E. & Angen, M. (2000). A randomized, wait list controlled clinical trial: The effect of a mindfulness meditation-based stress reduction program on mood and symptoms of stress in cancer outpatients. *Psychosomatic Medicine,* 62, 613-622.

Stanton, A., Danoff-Burg, S., Sworowsji, L., Collins, C., Branstetter, A., Rodrigues-Hanley, A., Kirk, S. & Austenfeld, J. (2002). Randomized controlled trial of written emotional expression and benefit finding in breast cancer patients. *Journal of Clinical Oncology,* 20(20), 4160-4168.

Stephenson, N., Weinrich, S. & Tavakoli, A. (2000). The effects of foot reflexology on anxiety and pain in patients with breast and lung cancer. *Oncology Nursing Forum*, 27 (1), 67-72.

Stiegelis, H., Hagadoorn, M., Sanderman, R., Bennenbroek, F., Buunk, B., Van Den Bergh, A., Botke, G. & Ranchor, A. (2004). The impact of an informational self-management intervention on the association between control and illness uncertainty before and psychological distress after radiotherapy. *Psycho-Oncology*, 13, 248-259.

Tacon, A., Caldera, Y. & Ronaghan, C. (2004). Mindfulness-based stress reduction in women with breast cancer. *Families, Systems & Health*, 22 (2), 193-203.

Taylor, K., Lamdan, R., Siegal, J., Shelby, R., Moran-Klimi, K. & Hrywna, M. (2003). Psychological adjustment among African American breast cancer patients: One-year follow-up results of a randomized psychoeducational group intervention. *Health Psychology*, 22 (3), 316-323.

Vig, E. K., Davenport, N. A. & Pearlman, R. A. (2002) Good Deaths, Bad Deaths, and Preferences for the End of Life: A qualitative study of geriatric outpatients. *Journal of the American Geriatric Society*, 50(9), 1541-1548.

Wallace, R. B. (2001). Prevention of cancer in elderly. In E. A. Swanson, T. Tripp-Reimer & K. Buckwalter. *Health Promotion and Disease Prevention in the Older Adults: Interventions and Recommendations* (pp. 146-155). New York: Spring Publishing Company.

Weber, B., Roberts, B., Resnick, M., Deimling, G., Zausznieski, J., Musil, C. & Yarandi, H. (2004).The effect of dyadic intervention on self-efficacy, social support, and depression for men with prostate cancer. *Psycho-Oncology*, 13(1), 47-60.

Wimberly, S. R., Carver, C. S., Laurenceau, J-P, Harris, S. D. & Antoni, M. H. (2005). Perceived partner reactions to diagnosis and treatment of breast cancer: Impact on psychosocial and psychosexual adjustment. *Journal of Consulting and Clinical Psychology*, 73(2), 300-311.

Chapter 4

Arthritis Pain

Eunkyung Yoon, PhD
John B. Doherty, PhD

Arthritic pain is a common and disabling problem for many older adults. There is widespread evidence that despite its prevalence and debilitating effects on the physical, emotional and cognitive status of older adults, arthritic pain remains under treated in those age 65 and older (Affleck, Tennen, Keefe, Lefebvre, & Kashikar-Zuck, 1999; American

Geriatrics Society [AGS], 1998). This condition significantly and negatively impacts older adults' quality of life and is a critical problem that requires the attention of gerontological social work. This chapter provides a brief summary of arthritic pain in older adults. It also discusses the treatment efficacy of cognitive-behavioral therapy and psycho-educational programs for older adults with this type of pain.

DEMOGRAPHICS AND PREVALENCE OF ARTHRITIC PAIN IN OLDER ADULTS

Arthritis is one of the most prevalent chronic health problems and the nation's leading cause of disability among older Americans (Arthritis Foundation, 2005). Arthritis and other rheumatic conditions affected 70 million U.S. adults in 2001 (Centers for Disease Control and Prevention [CDC], 2003). The CDC (2003) also predicted that if arthritis prevalence rates remain stable, the number of affected persons aged over 65 years will nearly double by 2030, from 21.4 million in 2005 to 41.1 million in 2030. Arthritis collectively refers to more than 100 different diseases that affect the body in or around joints. Although rheumatoid arthritis affects 3 million Americans annually and is the most disabling form of the disease, osteoarthritis impacts an estimated 21 million adults and is the most common form of arthritis (CDC, 2005). This chapter focuses on chronic pain caused by these two common forms of arthritis.

The population prevalence and characteristics of pain complaints are difficult to ascertain and to compare across studies for several reasons. The selection of the population for study, information gathering methods, response rates, age distributions and the nature of the questions asked contribute to this difficulty (Crombie, Croft, & Linton, 1999). In addition, "throbbing," "burning," "aching," and "stinging," which are common descriptors of pain, can mean different things to different individuals. Taken together, pain is a personal and subjective experience that is influenced by age, gender, race, ethnicity, and psychosocial factors (National Institute of Arthritis and Musculoskeletal and Skin Disease [NIAMSD], 2002).

Epidemiological studies have recorded a peak in pain's prevalence by the age of 65 (Brattberg, Parker, & Thorslund, 1997; Helme & Gibson, 2001). Although persons over 65 have more than double the prevalence of joint pain when compared to samples of younger adults, recent research has indicated a decline after the mid-70s (Mobily, Herr, & Clark, 1994). In a study by Andersson, Ejlertsson, and Leden (1993), joint pain's prevalence decreased from 20% in males ages 75-79 to less than 8% in males more than 90 years old. Women's joint pain prevalence also dropped from 35% to 29% in both of the same age categories, respectively.

Pain prevalence is related to gender. Since women are disproportionately represented in older population cohorts, this fact could affect age-specific estimates of pain prevalence. Several epidemiological studies have shown that women have a significantly higher prevalence of pain than men of comparable age (e.g., Andersson et al., 1993; Helme & Gibson, 2001). The magnitude of gender differences in pain prevalence may depend on the nature of the condition under examination. Rheumatoid arthritis, osteoarthritis, headaches, and fibromyalgia are more common in women, whereas gout, alkalosis, spondylitis and coronary heart disease are more common in men (Arthritis Foundation, 2005). Psychosocial support, education, and life-style factors may potentially influence pain prevalence reports based on gender (NIAMSD, 2002).

While arthritis affects people of all races, some racial and ethnic differences in the experience of arthritic pain have been demonstrated in recent research (Baker, 2005; Kramer, Wray, & Ferrell, 1996; Tan, 2005). While African-Americans and Caucasians have similar prevalences of arthritic pain, African-Americans also reported significantly higher instances of work and general activity limitations and greater severity of joint pain than Caucasians (Baker, 2005; Tan, 2005). A randomized telephone survey found that the psychosocial dimensions of arthritic pain also differed between African-Americans and Caucasians (Ruehlman, 2005). This nationwide study found that African-Americans reported greater pain-related interference and more coping difficulties than Caucasians. Research conducted in selected reservation communities across the U.S. found that certain autoimmune rheumatic diseases are more prevalent among American Indians than among either non-Indians or Alaskan Natives, and that this difference is most likely genetic in origin (Peschken & Esdaile, 1999). In a national study, American Indians reported significantly more frequent pain experiences than other ethnic Americans and arthritis was the greatest predictor of that pain (Kramer et al., 1996).

Research that compared older nursing home residents with community-dwelling elders revealed that institutionalized older adults reported higher levels of pain prevalence (Ferrell, 1995; Fox, Raina, & Jadad,

1999). In these studies, arthritic pain was reported mostly in the back and joints. The overall prevalence of pain in institutionalized older adults has been reported to be as high as 45%-80% (Ferrell, 1995). It is noteworthy that depression, a common condition in institutionalized older adults, is likely to influence their pain reports (Davis, 1997; Davis, Cortez, & Rubin, 1990; Lin, Katon, Korff et al., 2003). Helme and Gibson (2001) found that 96% of depressed patients and 80% of all others reported pain in a geriatric hospital setting. Finally, substantial barriers such as dementia, pain due to non-arthritic causes, and increased sensitivity to medication side effects often make pain assessment and management more difficult in nursing homes (Ferrell, 1995).

THE NATURE OF ARTHRITIC PAIN IN OLDER ADULTS

Pain is defined as an unpleasant experience associated with actual or potential tissue damage to a person's body (AGS, 2002). From a neurological perspective, pain is a complex phenomenon derived from sensory stimuli or injury and modified by individual memory, expectations, and emotions (AGS, 2002). Although there are no objective biological markers of pain, an individual's description and self-report usually provide accurate, reliable, and sufficient evidence for the presence and intensity of pain (Weiner, Herr, & Rudy, 2002).

There are two basic forms of physical pain: acute and chronic (National Institute of Arthritis and Musculoskeletal and Skin Disease [NIAMSD], 2002). Acute pain resulting from disease, inflammation, or injury to tissue is of short duration, and its causes can usually be diagnosed and treated. Chronic pain is continuous and persists for more than three months. The cause of chronic pain is not always evident but can be the result of conditions such as arthritis and fibromyalgia. Chronic pain is one of the most debilitating effects of arthritis (NIAMSD, 2002).

Among a variety of arthritic conditions, osteoarthritis (OA) is a progressive disease that affects at least 80% of adults over the age of 50 (National Institute of Health, 2001). This condition results from the weakening of joint cartilage, usually in weight-bearing joints such as the knee, hips, and spine. The risks for OA include factors that contribute to excessive joint loading or stress (e.g., obesity) or traumatic injuries that damage cartilage or bone. There is no current cure for OA.

A second major condition is rheumatoid arthritis (RA). More than 3 million people in the United States have RA. Generally, it affects about twice as many women as men. Although RA can develop in childhood, in most cases it develops between the ages of 25 and 50 years. Patients with RA often experience painful and disabling joint conditions. This condition can adversely affect multiple organ systems and is associated with premature mortality (Simon, Lipman, Allaire, Caudill-Slosberg, & Gill, 2002). In addition, RA produces 42% more daily pain than OA (Affleck et al., 1999).

A number of psychological factors that influence pain in arthritis have been identified including coping variables and pain control/appraisal variables. There is strong evidence that pain-coping strategies can be assessed in a reliable fashion in both osteoarthritis (OA) and rheumatoid arthritis (RA) patients (Keefe, Abernethy, & Campbell, 2005; Keefe, Caldwell, & Queen, 1987; Keefe, Dunsmore, & Burnett, 1992). This line of study suggests that more active coping strategies are related to improved adjustment to arthritis, while more passive strategies result in poorer adjustment. There is evidence that pain-coping variables are important in explaining individuals' adjustments even after controlling for pain levels (Rhee, Parker, Smarr, Petroski, & Johnson et al., 2000; Turk & Monarch, 2002).

CONSEQUENCES OF ARTHRITIC PAIN IN OLDER ADULTS

Chronic arthritic pain is a frequent cause of distress and disability among older adults (AGS, 2002). For the individual suffering from arthritis, poorly managed chronic pain frequently generates feelings of hopelessness and despair. Ultimately, the consequences of disease may result in significant disruptions in individual and family functioning (Grossberg, Sherman, & Fine, 2000; LeFort et al., 1998).

There are numerous consequences of arthritic pain among older adults. Depression, anxiety, decreased socialization, sleep disturbance, impaired ambulation and increased health-care utilization and costs have been found to be associated with the presence of arthritic pain in older people (AGS, 2002). There is general agreement that depressive symptoms are both common in arthritis patients and associated with reduced health status (Lin et al., 2003). Higher depression rates have been shown to be related to more intense pain, greater fatigue, and reduced quality of life for persons with arthritis (Parker, Smarr, Slaughter, Johnston, Priesmeyer et al., 2003). In a multidimensional health assessment study of 688 consecutive patients with pain, the majority of patients reported difficulty in performing activities of daily living. Fifty-eight percent experienced problems running errands, 68% had difficulty climbing stairs and 79% had difficulty in walking two miles. Sleep difficulties were reported by 75% of the patients, 61% reported elevated anxiety and 57% reported depression (Pincus, Swearingen, & Wolfe, 1999).

The economic impact of chronic pain on the American health-care system and American society as a whole is considerable. An estimated $79 billion is spent annually in the United States on treating and managing chronic pain (Rowat, Jeans, & LeFort, 1994). According to Gatchel and Turk (1999), pain accounts for over 80% of all physician visits and affects more than 50 million Americans. Each year, an estimated 177,000 patients seek treatment in pain centers in the United States alone. More than $100 billion is lost in annual productivity, including lost earnings, increased health care utilization and payment of disability benefits (LeFort, Gray-Donald, Rowat, & Jeans, 1998). Clearly, the cost of managing and treating persistent pain is high, both personally and from a social resource perspective.

REVIEW OF EMPIRICAL LITERATURE

Persistent disease-related pain is amenable to psychosocial interventions (Keefe et al., 2005). Although medical or surgical approaches can be helpful in managing arthritic pain, these have several limitations. Surgery or radiation may produce tissue damage that results in persistent pain. Medications also may have significant side effects such as constipation or fatigue that limit their use over sustained periods. These side effects may be particularly problematic in many older adults who suffer from a multiplicity of chronically painful diseases. Given this multiplicity and chronicity, it is critical to note that psychosocial factors affect and are affected by arthritic pain in older patients.

Psychological approaches can build upon and enhance individual self-reliance. Recent clinical guidelines for chronic disease management emphasize the important role that self-help plays in the overall management of these conditions (American Geriatrics Society, 2002; American Pain Society Quality of Care Committee, 1995). Many studies have confirmed the possibility that psychosocial interventions designed to enhance pain control and appraisal may benefit OA and RA patients (Branch, Lipsky, Nieman, & Lipsky, 1999; Keefe et al., 1992;

Mullen, Laville, Biddle, & Lorig, 1987). Cognitive-behavioral treatment and biofeedback have been found to be especially beneficial in arthritic pain management.

While most outcome studies have examined the effectiveness of pharmacological treatment, surgery, and physical exercises, psychosocial outcome studies have focused primarily on two types of interventions—cognitive behavioral therapy and psychoeducation programs. Since these two interventions have been among the most frequently examined, the following two sections present summary evidence of their effectiveness for managing chronic arthritic pain in older adults. A systematic computerized literature search (at EBSCOHOST and PRO-QUEST) was conducted with the use of PUBMED, PSYCINFO, PSYCARTICLE, MEDLINE, AGELINE, and ERIC. Major search terms were chronic pain, arthritis, rheumatology, chronic joint symptoms, older adults, evidence-based practice, intervention, meta-analysis, clinical trials, randomized controlled trials, patient education, and cognitive behavioral therapy. Further studies were subsequently identified by cross-referencing and manually checking abstracts. Studies published before May 2005 are included in this chapter.

Cognitive-Behavioral Treatments

In the mid 1980s, cognitive-behavioral models of pain were proposed that could be easily applied to persons having disease-related pain (Turk & Monarch, 2002). According to the cognitive-behavioral model, cognitive responses such as thoughts, beliefs, and expectations play a key role in perceptions of and adjustments to pain. While a traditional biomedical model has long dominated the understanding of disease-related pain, some health-care professionals such as psychologists and social workers have recently started to explore the utility of cognitive-behavioral approaches to persistent pain conditions related to ongoing disease such as arthritis, cancer, and sickle cell disease (Keefe et al., 2005). The cognitive-behavioral model is presented along with the outcome studies that have evaluated its effectiveness for arthritis pain relief.

There have been several studies that examined the effectiveness of cognitive-behavioral interventions. A combined pharmacologic and cognitive-behavioral study was conducted with 54 patients whose average age was 54.6 years (SD = 11.4 years). They had been diagnosed with both major depression and RA and were randomly assigned to one of three groups: (1) a cognitive-behavioral group, in which the patients received their ongoing rheumatological care, anti-depressant medication and instruction in depression management; (2) an attention-control group, in which the patients received their ongoing rheumatological care, anti-depressant medication and participated in a general patient education program; or (3) a pharmacological control group, in which the patients received only their ongoing rheumatological care and anti-depressant medication (Parker et al., 2003). These interventions were provided individually to each patient over a 10-week period. The intervention sessions were one and one-half hours long and included a 15-month follow-up program. The findings showed that the patients who received only the anti-depressant medication improved just as much in the acute phase of treatment for depression as did the members of the other groups (Parker et al., 2003). In another study in which all participants were age 18 and older, 47 patients with rheumatoid arthritis received their regular rheumatological care and also completed 10 weekly two-hour stress management training sessions. These sessions taught various cognitive-behavioral strategies such as relaxation, coping skills and problem-solving techniques. A 49-member control group received their regular rheumatological care and also participated in a general patient education program. A 45-member standard care control group received only their regular rheumatoligical care (Rhee et al., 2000). This study reported significant decreases in pain and depression for those patients who received the cognitive-behavioral training.

Coping skills training (CST) is another type of intervention in pain management and is based on the cognitive-behavioral model (Keefe et al., 2005; Kerns, Otis, & Marcus, 2001). The effectiveness of coping skills training interventions has been confirmed in several empirical studies with older adults. In a randomized trial of this 10-session protocol (Keefe & Williams, 1990), 99 older adults with persistent OA knee pain were randomly assigned to a 10-sesssion coping skills training protocol that included diversion strategies, goal-setting strategies, and cognitive approaches to minimizing pain experiences. A second group participated in a 10-session arthritis information/educational protocol, and a third group received standard care. Older patients who received pain coping skills training showed greater improvement in pain and psychological status compared to the two other groups. Patients who reported increases in perceived pain control throughout the course were significantly more likely to show improvements in pain levels and physical functioning at a six-month follow-up.

An additional study also investigated CST for chronic knee pain relief (Fry & Wong, 1991). In this research, the long-term effect of pain management training in community-dwelling older adults ages 63 to 82 was examined. This one-group study with repeated measures supported the effectiveness of coping skills training for reducing pain and anxiety, as well as increased life satisfaction and adjustment at 16- and 24-week follow-ups. These findings suggest that coping skill training can benefit patients with OA and that changes in pain control are related to long-term treatment outcomes (Fry & Wong, 1991; Keefe & Williams, 1990).

Several studies have confirmed that family members may also benefit from Coping Skills Training (CST) that helps them manage their loved one's chronic pain conditions. Methods of CST-based adjustment can be provided to caregivers including spouses and family members. A long-term follow-up study was conducted with 88 OA patients age 40-64 years who had been randomly assigned to one of three treatment conditions: (1) spouse-assisted CST; (2) a conventional CST intervention with no spousal involvement; and (3) an arthritis education spouse support control condition (Keefe et al., 1999). At a 12-month follow-up, patients in the spouse-assisted CST condition had significantly higher overall self-efficacy and showed greater improvement than those in the two comparison groups. Patients who reported improved marital relationships as a result of the training had lower levels of psychological and physical disability, and improved pain levels at a 12-month follow-up.

A comparative pre- and post-test study was conducted with 59 RA patients on comparing behavioral therapy with and without family support (Radojevic, Nicassio, & Weisman, 1992). Comparisons between the two groups indicated that a behavioral coping skills protocol involving family support was more effective in reducing pain intensity and psychological strain than an educational protocol that did not include family involvement. Taken together, studies on coping skill training support the proposition that arthritis patients may benefit from coping skills training protocols that involve their family caregivers.

Psycho-Educational Interventions

The Arthritis Self-Management Program (ASMP) is a comprehensive, accessible, community-based approach to pain management. It is a standardized 12-session psycho-educational group program that uses a detailed, widely disseminated protocol from the United States National Arthritis Foundation (Lorig, 1992). The ASMP has been implemented by both generalist health-care providers and by trained lay leaders at a cost ranging from zero to $600 per course as compared to $3,000 for a short-term outpatient group program at a pain clinic (Turk & Monarch, 2002). A more recent and shorter format, the Chronic Pain Self-Management Program (CPSMP) (Lorig & Holman, 2003), is delivered in six two-hour sessions in community settings such as local churches and schools, or through outpatient groups in geriatric hospital settings. The CPSMP emphasizes group problem-solving, mutual support, and experimentation in various pain management techniques. Each participant receives a workbook, relaxation tapes and pamphlets about chronic pain, nutrition and walking.

The ASMP has demonstrated efficacy in decreasing pain, depression and disability and in reducing post-intervention health-care costs for as many as four years (Lorig, Mazonson, & Holman, 1993). A longitudinal study of 211 adults ages 51-74 on the effectiveness of ASMP found that pain declined an average of 20% and visits to physicians declined a mean of 40%, while patients reported a 9% improvement in coping with their physical disabilities over the four years of the study. The estimated health-care savings were $648 per RA patient and $189 per OA patient over the four-year time period. As this study suggests, health education about chronic arthritis may add significant and sustained benefits to conventional therapies while simultaneously reducing costs (Lorig et al., 1993; Mazzuca, Brandt, Katz, Hanna, & Melfi, 1999).

The ASMP has been effectively implemented in other countries. For example, a quasi-experimental study reported the positive effect of an ASMP on residents in a home for 42 elderly people in Hong Kong (Yip, Sit, & Wong, 2004). Twenty-one residents were part of the intervention group that received the ASMP curriculum, as well as Tai Chi movements during the final three sessions. Sixteen residents were placed on a wait list for the intervention and comprised the control group. Data were collected at baseline and at 16 weeks after completing the intervention. At posttest, the residents in the self-management program had significant improvement in self-efficacy for arthritis management, muscle strength and reduced arthritic pain as compared to the control group.

In a study with Spanish-speaking participants in California, the effectiveness of the Spanish ASMP was evaluated with 141 Hispanic participants age 18 and older. The mean age of the participants was 50.7 years (SD = 14.4) (Wong, Harker, Lau, Shatzel, & Port, 2004). Most of the participants (84%) were born in Mexico, and only spoke Spanish

(60%). Data were collected at baseline, six weeks after intervention, and six months post-intervention. Compared to baseline scores, significant improvement was found at the six-month period in pain relief, self-efficacy, self-care behavior, arthritis knowledge and overall general health. This study indicates that the ASMP is effective with Spanish-speaking participants.

The effectiveness of the shorter format, the Chronic Pain Self Management Program (CPSMP), has also been supported empirically. Lorig, Ritter, Stewart, Sobel, Brown, and Bandura (2001) conducted a longitudinal analysis of health and self-efficacy outcomes for the CPSMP program. At one- and two-year intervals, participants from the CPSMP provided data on health status and utilization. From an original sample of 831, 82% at the one-year interval and 76% at the two-year interval provided data. Compared with baseline, health utilization (emergency room visits, physician visits) was reduced. Health distress scores were also reduced. In addition, self-efficacy scores increased significantly during this two-year time period.

Other brief psychoeducational programs have also been effective in reducing pain. For example, a program of self-care education for inner-city patients with OA was evaluated, comparing an education group (n = 105) to a control group (n = 106) (Mazzuca, Brandt, Katz, Chambers, Byrd, & Hanna, 1997). Within the study sample, 69% were African American, 85% were women, most (74%) lived alone, and the participants had a mean age of 62 years. Those in the education group received individualized instruction that emphasized non-pharmacological pain management interventions. Those in the control group viewed a 20-minute slide presentation that is a regular part of an arthritis public awareness program. Data were collected at baseline and at 12 months post-intervention. At the 12-month mark, the education group had significantly lower scores for disability and resting knee pain. In addition, the education group had fewer primary care visits (528 compared to 616), and fewer median visits per participant (5 versus 6). Overall, the average cost per patient to deliver the intervention was calculated to be $58.70.

Another low-cost protocol involved a telephone-based educational intervention designed for OA patients (Rene, Weinberger, Mazzuca, Brandt, & Katz, 1992). On a bi-weekly basis, telephone counselors reviewed patients' medications and their side effects, pain levels, early warning signs of other chronic diseases, outpatient visits and ways to make sure they made their scheduled visits. The counselor also provided education about pain management and suggestions about medical treatment. The evaluation revealed that these 409 patients who received telephone counseling reported significant improvements in pain and physical disability when compared to symptom-monitoring control and usual-care control groups over the course of one year.

The effects of symptom-monitoring telephone intervention on the health outcomes of patients with RA or OA were compared with usual care over a nine-month period (Maisiak, Austin, & Heck, 1996). Four hundred and five patients were randomized into a treatment group that received telephone counseling, or a group that only included monitoring of arthritis symptoms. A third (control) group received only standard care protocols for RA or OA. At post-intervention, the treatment group, but not the monitoring group, had significantly better health status scores. In addition, the average number of medical visits by OA (but not RA) patients in the treatment group also decreased.

As self-management courses in arthritis have been shown to improve outcomes and to decrease medical resource utilization, the effectiveness of a mail-delivered arthritis self-management program was examined (Fries, Carey, & McShane, 1997). This intervention consists of a health assessment questionnaire at three-month intervals, with computer-generated recommendation letters and reports individualized to age, diagnosis, educational level, disability, pain, medication and other patient-specific variables. This randomized controlled trial of 375 program participants and 434 controls (mean age = 64 years) reported that at six months, outcomes of function (4.7%), decreased pain (9%), global vitality (7%), and joint count (28%) were improved in the program group compared with the controls. Annual physician visits decreased by 16% in the program group compared with the control group, and days confined to home decreased by 52% in the mail program group. Accordingly, a mail-delivered arthritis self-management program can positively affect patient outcomes and can decrease medical resource utilization.

An Internet-based support group provided another way to reach pain patients who otherwise might not benefit from such programs. A randomized study was conducted to test the efficacy of an e-mail discussion group in the management of chronic pain (Lorig, Laurent, Deyo, Marnell, & Minor, 2002). Five hundred and eighty people with OA were randomly assigned to a closed, moderated e-mail discussion group or to a no-treatment control condition. All patients in the e-mail discussion group were on a listserv through which they received e-mail messages from all the other members of their group. The discussion was guided by two moderators and a physician, physical therapist and psychologist. All participants in the e-mail discussion condition also received a book and videotape based on self-help pain management principles. This study revealed that at the end of the one-year online treatment period, participants in the e-mail discussion group showed significant improvements in pain, disability, role function, health distress, self-efficacy, and self-care when compared to the control participants. The participants in the e-mail discussion group also reduced their physician office visits by 46% in the last six months of the study, a pattern that supports the cost effectiveness of the intervention. These findings suggest that an e-mail discussion intervention may have benefits for persons suffering from persistent pain.

A recent meta-analysis was undertaken to assess the effect of arthritis self-management education programs (Warsi, LaValley, Wang, Avorn, & Solomon, 2003). Studies were included if the intervention contained a self-management education component, a concurrent control group was included, and pain and/or disability were assessed as end points. The MEDLINE and HealthStar databases were used in this meta-analysis, examining the period from 1964 to 1998 that produced 17 studies. The majority of intervention approaches were either social cognitive in focus (e.g., Bandura) (n = 8) or cognitive behavioral (n = 4). Seven studies had mixed populations (OA, RA or other chronic conditions such as fibromyalgia), while seven included only participants with RA and three included only participants with OA. The results of the 17 outcome studies indicate fairly small effect sizes both for pain reduction (0.12) and for disability status (0.7). These results suggest that arthritis self-management education programs may produce fairly small gains in the areas of pain and disability.

TREATMENT SUMMARY

Based upon clinical evidence, cognitive-behavioral treatment models (CBT) can have a major positive impact on pain treatment. Several reasons appear to account for successes with CBT protocols (Rowat et al., 1994; Skinner, Erskine, Pearce, Rubenstein, Taylor, & Foster, 1990; Turk & Monarch, 2002). First, this model is flexible and can easily be used with persons who have both disease-related pain and nonmalignant chronic pain conditions. Second, CBT integrates information about biological, psychological and social influences on pain. Third, the CBT model has produced standardized treatment protocols that teach patients specific cognitive and behavioral pain coping skills. Cognitive-behavioral treatments are commonly administered in individual or group outpatient treatment sessions. Models for couples and family treatment have also been described (Keefe et al., 1987; Keefe, Caldwell, Baucom, Salley, & Robinson, 1999). Treatment is usually limited to no more than ten 60- to 90-minute sessions (Kerns et al., 2001).

The other intervention method outlined in this chapter, psychoeducation, has also gained support via the outcome literature. The efficacy of psychoeducational approaches that are used as an adjunct to traditional medical and physical therapies for the management of chronic pain is well-established (LeFort et al., 1998; Lorig, 1992). As an example of a low-cost, accessible and effective intervention that will help people find ways to better manage arthritic pain, the community-based self-management educational programs have been shown to have a demonstrable positive effect on a variety of pain-related and quality of life variables over long periods of time. Many clinical trials and meta-analyses also suggested that the Arthritis Self-Management Program (ASMP) may be a practical, cost-effective program on which to base educational programs for those with other types of chronic non-malignant pain (Lorig et al., 2002; Superio-Cabuslay, Ward, & Lorig, 1996). Because it has a standard protocol, psychoeducation has the potential to be reliably delivered at low cost in varied urban and rural community settings and be more widely accessible to a greater number of older people suffering from chronic pain. The positive effect of multiple program delivery methods via mail, telephone and the Internet has been demonstrated (Fries et al., 1997; Rene et al.,1992).

Overall, cognitive-behavioral treatment has relatively strong empirical support as an effective treatment for persistent pain conditions, either as a single intervention or in the context of multidisciplinary and multi-modality treatment programs. Specifically, coping skills training is an effective individual, group, and family-oriented intervention in managing chronic arthritic pain. Empirical evidence has also demonstrated that educational approaches can make important contributions to our understanding and treatment of arthritis-related pain. Lorig's (1992) self-help program is an excellent example of how a self-management intervention can be implemented in a cost-effective fashion and can reach a wide range of older persons who have pain. Additionally, telephone or Internet-based support groups are economically promising interventions for people experiencing chronic arthritic pain. Tables 1 and 2 summarize several exemplary studies highlighting the effectiveness of both cognitive-behavioral treatments (on individual, couple, or group

TABLE 1. Cognitive-Behavioral Intervention and Outcome Summary

Author/year	Population	N	Intervention	Outcome
Astin (2002)	Meta-analysis (RA)	25	CBT, biofeedback	Effective post-intervention for decreasing pain and functional disability, and increasing psychological status, coping and self-efficacy.
Ersek (2003)	Chronic pain	45	CBT, Educational booklet group	CBT yielded greater improvement in physical role functioning and pain intensity than educational group.
Fry (1991)	OA	69	CBT (MF, PF, EF)	Overall, CBT Reduced pain and anxiety, increased satisfaction and adjustment. PF and EF intervention more effective than MF.
Keefe (1990)	OA Knee pain	99	CBT, PE, RCT	CBT showed more significant improvements in pain and psychological disability compared to those receiving the PE or standard care.
Keefe (1999)	OA Knee pain	88	Spouse-assisted CBT, RCT	Spouse-assisted CBT had significantly higher overall self-efficacy than other control condition.
Parker (2003)	RA	54	CBT, RCT, Medications	Medication better than CBT in managing depression.
Radojevic (1992)	RA	59	CBT, Educational Protocol, Family therapy	CBT involving family support was more effective in reducing pain and strain than educational protocol in persons without family involvement.
Rhee (2000)	RA	92	CBT, CG	CBT decreased in pain and depression.

TABLE 2. Psycho-Educational Intervention and Outcome Summary

Author/year	Population	N	Intervention	Outcome
Fries (1997)	Arthritis	375	Mail delivered ASMP	Positive effect in reduced overall pain and decreased doctor visits.
Lorig (1993)	OA and RA	341	ASMP–4 year follow up	20% reduced pain and 40% reductions in visits to physicians, but 9% increased physical disability.
Lorig (2002)	Mixed pain	580	E-mail discussion group, RCT	More adaptive coping, reduced emotional distress.
Lorig (2004)	Mixed pain	831	CDSMP	ER/outpatient visits and health care distress were reduced and self-efficacy improved.
Maisiak (1996)	RA & OA	405	Telephone monitoring	Improved overall health and reduced doctor visit by OA patients.
Mazzuca (1999)	OA	211	CCT, Self-care education	Education reduced frequency and cost of primary care visits (88%).
Mullen (1987)	Meta-analysis	15	Psycho-education	Relatively small pooled effect size (.20 for pain, .27 for depression, &.09 for disability).
Peters (1992)	OA	52	CG, RCT of pain management program	Analgesic use, activity levels and pain ratings are the criteria for 'success'– 68% of inpatients, 61% of outpatients, and 21% of control subject met all 3 criteria.
Rene (1992)	OA	409	Telephone counseling, CG	Telephone counseling yielded significant improvements in pain and physical disability over usual care group.
Superio-Cabuslay (1996)	Meta-analysis	19	Patient education, NSAID	Patient education provides additional benefits that are 20-30% as great as the effects of NSAID treatment for pain relief in OA and RA.
Warsi (2003)	Meta-analysis	17	ASMP	The summary effect size was .12 for pain and .07 for disability.
Wong (2004)	Arthritis	141	Spanish ASMP	Improved pain, self-efficacy, self-care behavior, arthritis knowledge, and general health.
Yip (2004)	LTC residents in HK	42	ASMP, CG	Increased self-efficacy and reduced pain.

ASMP = Arthritis self-management program, CPSMP = Chronic pain self-management program, CBT = Cognitive-behavioral therapy, PF = Problem-focused (coping), EF = Emotion-focused (coping), MF = Mixed focused (intervention), CCT = Controlled clinical trial, CG = Control group, PST = Problem-solving treatment, PE = Psycho-education, RCT = Randomized controlled trial, WL = Waiting list.

levels) and community-based psychoeducational programs (on group levels in local churches, or via telephone and Internet support groups).

CONCLUSION

Over the past 20 years, researchers have started to explore innovative pain management interventions for older adults. The importance of psychological and social factors in chronic pain management has encouraged the development and application of psychosocial treatment approaches to this complex clinical problem. A range of alternative psychological treatments exists, and many of these specific approaches have empirical support for their effectiveness. In particular, cognitive-behavioral therapy and psychoeducational self-help programs appear to be promising for pain management among older adults (e.g., Bradley, 1996; Fry & Wong, 1991; Kerns et al., 2001; Lorig & Holman, 2003). These approaches incorporate cognitive and behavioral coping skills training and encourage the adoption of a self-management attitude towards pain.

When ambulatory older adults are diagnosed with symptomatic arthritis, education about the natural progression, treatment, and self-management of the disease should be offered at least once within six months of diagnosis. This is because such education has been shown to produce improvements in physical functioning and pain (Lorig & Holman, 2003; MacLean, 2001). The educational component of treatment should address the unspoken fears that many older patients have about their condition (e.g., fear that health-care providers do not believe their pain is real). This educational effort must be interdisciplinary in nature and should include a biopsychosocial and behavioral review of the results by the treatment providers.

However, there are several limitations in the effectiveness of these psychosocial treatments. First, it remains unclear which of these interventions are more or less effective than others. Since many of these treatments were multi-modal and integrated a variety of psychosocial approaches, it is difficult to determine which particular components or combinations of components may have been responsible for the observed treatment effects. Accordingly, it would be useful to design trials that directly compared such psychological treatments to pharmacological approaches. Second, an additional question is the extent to which the effects of these psychological interventions produce long-term effects. For some outcomes, such as pain and disability, the treatment effects appeared to diminish over time when compared to treatments for depression and arthritic pain, which appeared to increase in effectiveness over time. Future trials should explore the potential value of building booster/relapse prevention strategies into the trial designs.

There are obvious barriers to psychological pain management in intervention research with older adults. First, researchers often have difficulty in recruiting and retaining older patients for clinical trials. Second, patients may be reluctant to admit that factors such as stress and/or mood influence their pain since they fear that their pain will be prematurely dismissed and not regarded as a real condition. Spouses and other significant others may also discount the value of psychologically-based pain management interventions. Accordingly, it is important to recognize the influence of the patient's significant others as well as the positive contribution that family education can play in the treatment process. Finally, some health-care professionals who are treating the patient may be unsupportive or actively critical of the person's involvement in psychological pain management interventions. Educational efforts directed at health-care professionals, such as the 1999 Joint Commission on Accreditation of Healthcare Organizations Pain Standards, are playing an important role in helping these professionals appreciate the impact that psychological factors and psychosocial interventions can have on disease-related pain (AGS, 2002).

There are several potential directions for future research. First, more intervention research is needed in which the treatment setting more closely resembles actual clinical situations. Before starting the psychological interventions, it is critical for practitioners and researchers to gather pertinent information necessary for assessing the relationship between the dimensions of pain, distress, disability, and the social context in which they occur. In recognizing that aging-related developmental changes may affect responses to various assessment instruments, the chosen assessment tools should reflect a cognitive-behavioral conceptualization of pain and should assess those areas considered important to understanding a patient's experience of pain (Weiner & Hanlon, 2001). Second, given the increasing evidence supporting cognitive-behavioral pain management interventions in rheumatoid arthritis, effectiveness studies with this particular patient population would be beneficial. In collecting data on the potential health-care cost savings of these treatments, such trials could have public health-care policy implications. Third, research should address the roles that psychological and social factors play in health disparities in disease-related pain. There is growing evidence that members of minority groups are more prone to adverse health outcomes from arthritic pain. However, it is also true that less is known about the psychological and social mechanisms that may underlie these health disparities. Fourth, more psychosocial treatments should be made accessible to persons of lower socioeconomic status. Future studies should explore other potential psychological barriers (e.g., low self-efficacy, depression) and social mediators (e.g., lower social support) that may contribute to disparities in pain-related treatment outcomes among older adults living alone and in poverty. Fifth, further chronic pain studies are needed within defined racial and ethnic groups. A culturally heterogeneous population will require different cultural interpretations affecting treatment decisions and the self-management of chronic disease.

TREATMENT RESOURCE APPENDIX

Keefe, F.J., Abernethy, A.P., & Campbell, L.C. (2005). Psychological approaches to understanding and treating disease-related pain. *Annual Reviews of Psychology, 56,* 601-630.

A summary of a coping skills training protocol is presented. This article provides a session-by-session summary of various activities for techniques to assist arthritic patients with pain management.

Kerns, R.D., Otis, J.D., & Marcus, K.S. (2001). Cognitive-behavioral therapy for chronic pain in the elderly. *Clinics in Geriatric Medicine, 17*(3), 503-523.

A summary of common components of cognitive-behavioral therapy for chronic pain. These typically involve education, communication skills, problem-solving, distraction, relaxation, goal-setting, and cognitive reconstruction.

Loring, A.K. (1992). *Arthritis self-help course: Leader's manual and reference materials.* Atlanta, GA: Arthritis Foundation.

This manual assists practitioners with leading a course on arthritis pain management. The manual includes information on nutrition, depression, exercise, fatigue management, and medications. www.arthritis.org/condition/paincenter/

Web Sites

Arthritis Foundation
www.arthritisinsight.com/medication/alternative

The web site of the Arthritis Foundation provides arthritis education and introduces the concept of an individualized pain management plan. The site includes a place to order books on arthritis, and other resources such as information about arthritis and depression. There are several resources about the management of arthritic pain, including the emotional issues involved such as feelings of grief and loss. In addition, strategies to live with chronic pain can be found such as guided imagery and breathing exercises.

National Institute of Arthritis and Musculoskeletal and Skin Diseases
www.niams.nih.gov

One of the Institutes of Health, NIAMS provides information about clinical trials, research in this area, and training that is taking place. This web site is provided by the National Institute of Arthritis and Musculoskeletal and Skin Diseases. It presents information about arthritis, treatments and current research.

Centers for Disease Control
www.cdc.gov/arthritis/data_statistics/arthritis_related_statistics.htm

This web site of the Centers for Disease Control and Prevention summarizes arthritis-related statistics based on two broad categories, self-reported data and health-care data. The site presents prevalence and types by age, ethnicity, and gender along with related references.

National Center for Complementary and Alternative Medicine
http://www.nccam.nih.gov

This site provides scientific evidence for alternative treatments of many health conditions, including arthritis. Information can be obtained about the types of alternative treatment that are available for arthritis, such as magnetic therapy and botanicals, and the evidence about the helpfulness (or lack thereof) of each.

Johns Hopkins Medicine Treatment Center
http://www.hopkins-arthritis.org/mngmnt/mngmnt.html

This site is hosted by Johns Hopkins University Division of Rheumatology. Various information and interventions for arthritis pain and discomfort are provided. Topics include yoga, dealing with sleep disturbances, and managing weight. An interesting aspect of the site is information that is specific about various forms of the disease such as rheumatoid arthritis, osteoarthritis or conditions which are a consequence of Lyme Disease.

The Arthritis Society of Canada
http://www.arthritis.ca

ASC has a well-developed web site that provides resources and information for health promotion in the areas of arthritis management and chronic pain. The site contains a section on Tips for Living Well that can assist in making decisions about the various approaches to living with the condition. There are also links to a self-management program that is taught throughout the provinces and includes topics such as:

- exercising with arthritis
- managing pain
- eating healthy
- preventing fatigue
- protecting joints
- taking arthritis medications
- dealing with stress and depression
- working with your doctor and health-care team
- evaluating alternative treatments
- outsmarting arthritis: problem solving

REFERENCES

Affleck, G., Tennen, H., Keefe, F.J., Lefebvre, J.C., & Kashikar-Zuck, S. (1999). Everyday life with osteoarthritis or rheumatoid arthritis: Independent effects of disease and gender on daily pain, mood, and coping. *Pain, 83*(3), 601-9.

American Geriatrics Society (1998). Clinical practice guidelines: The management of chronic pain in older persons. *Journal of American Geriatrics Society, 46,* 635-651.

American Geriatrics Society (2002). The management of persistent pain in older persons: AGS panel on persistent pain in older persons. *Journal of American Geriatrics Society, 50,* S205-224.

American Pain Society Quality of Care Committee (1995). Quality improvement guidelines for the treatment of acute pain and cancer pain. *Journal of the American Medical Association, 274*(23), 1874-90.

Andersson, H.I., Ejlertsson, G., & Leden, I. (1993). Chronic pain in a geographically defined population: Studies of differences in age, gender, social class, and pain localization. *Clinical Journal of Pain, 9,* 174-188.

Arthritis Foundation (2005). The facts about arthritis. Retrieved on May 16, 2005 from http:www.arthritis.org.

Baker, T.A. (2005). Intra-race differences among black and white Americans presenting for chronic pain management: The influence of age, physical health, and psychosocial factors. *Pain Medicine, 6*(1), 29-39.

Bradley, L.A. (1996). Cognitive-behavioral therapy for chronic pain. In R.J. Gatchel & D.C. Turk (Eds.), *Psychological approaches to pain management: A practitioner's approach* (pp. 131-145). New York: Guilford Press.

Branch, V.K., Lipsky, K., Nieman, T., & Lipsky, P.E. (1999). Positive impact of an intervention by arthritis patient educators on knowledge and satisfaction of patients in a rheumatology practice. *Arthritis Care and Research, 12*(8), 370-375.

Brattberg, G., Parker, M.G., & Thorslund, M. (1997). A longitudinal study of pain: Reported pain from middle age to old age. *Clinical Journal of Pain, 13,* 144-51.

Centers for Disease Control and Prevention (2003). Public health and aging: Projected prevalence of self-reported arthritis or chronic joint symptoms among persons aged over 65 years in United States of 2005-2030. *Morbidity and Mortality Weekly Report, 52*(21), 489-491.

Centers for Disease Control and Prevention (2005). Arthritis related statistics. Retrieved on October 29, 2005, from http://www.cdc.gov/arthritis/data_statistics/arthritis_related_statistics.htm

Crombie, I.K., Croft, P.R., & Linton, S.J. (1999). *Epidemiology of pain.* Seattle, WA: IASP Press.

Davis, G.C. (1997). Chronic pain management of older adults in residential settings. *Journal of Gerontological Nursing, 23*(6), 16-22.

Davis, G.C., Cortez, C., & Rubin, B.R. (1990). Pain management in older adults with rheumatoid arthritis and osteoarthritis. *Arthritis Care and Research, 3,* 127-131.

Ferrell, B.A. (1995). Pain evaluation and management in the nursing home. *Annals of Internal Medicine, 123,* 681-687.

Ferrell, B.A., & Ferrell, B.R. (1991). Pain management in the home. *Clinics in Geriatric Medicine, 7,* 765-776.

Fox, P.L., Raina, P., & Jadad, A.R. (1999). Prevalence and treatment of pain in older adults in nursing homes and other long term care institutions: A systematic review. *Canadian Medical Association Journal, 160*(3), 329-44.

Fries, J.F., Carey, C., & McShane, D.J. (1997). Patient education in arthritis: Randomized controlled trial of a mail-delivered program. *Journal of Rheumatology, 24*(7), 1378-83.

Fry, P.S., & Wong, P.T. (1991). Pain management training in the elderly: Matching interventions with subjects coping style. *Stress Medicine, 7,* 93-98.

Gatchel, R.J., & Turk, D.C. (Eds.) (1999). *Psychosocial factors in pain: Critical perspectives.* New York: Guilford Press.

Gowans, S.E., deHueck, A., Voss, A.D., & Richardson, M. (1999). A randomized, controlled trial of exercise and education for individuals with fibromyalgia. *Arthritis Care and Research, 12*(2), 120-128.

Grossberg, G.T., Sherman, L.K., & Fine, P.G. (2000). Pain and behavioral disturbances in cognitively impaired older adults: Assessment and treatment issues. *Annals of Long Term Care, 8,* 22-24.

Helme, R.D., & Gibson, S.J. (2001). The epidemiology of pain in elderly people. *Clinics in Geriatric Medicine, 17*(3), 417-430.

Keefe, F.J., Abernethy, A.P., & Campbell, L.C. (2005). Psychological approaches to understanding and treating disease-related pain. *Annual Reviews of Psychology, 56,* 601-630.

Keefe, F.J., Dunsmore, J., & Burnett, R. (1992). Behavioral and cognitive-behavioral approaches to chronic pain: Recent advances and future directions. *Journal of Consulting Clinical Psychology, 60,* 528-43.

Keefe, F.J., Caldwell, D.S., Baucom, D., Salley, A., & Robinson, E. (1999). Spouse-assisted coping skills training in the management of knee pain in osteoarthritis: Long-term follow-up results. *Arthritis Care and Research, 12*(2), 101-111.

Keefe, F.J., Caldwell, D.S., & Queen, K.T. (1987). Pain coping strategies in osteoarthritis patients. *Journal of Consulting Clinical Psychology, 55,* 208-212.

Keefe, F.J., & Williams, D. (1990). A comparison of coping strategies in chronic pain patients in different age groups. *Journal of Gerontology, 45,* 161-165.

Kerns, R.D., Otis, J.D., & Marcus, K.S. (2001). Cognitive-behavioral therapy for chronic pain in the elderly. *Clinics in Geriatric Medicine, 17*(3), 503-523.

Kramer, B.J., Wray, L.A., & Ferrell, B.A. (1996). Gender, ethnicity and pain. *Gerontologist, 36*(1), 308-314.

LeFort, S.M., Gray-Donald, K., Rowat, K.M., & Jeans, M.E. (1998). Randomized controlled trial of a community-based psychoeducation program for the self-management of chronic pain. *Pain, 74,* 297-306.

Lin, E., Katon, W., Korff, M.V., Tang, L., Williams, J. et al. (2003). Effect of improving depression care on pain and functional outcomes among older adults with arthritis: A randomized controlled trial. *Journal of the American Medical Association, 290*(18), 2428-2803.

Lorig, K.R. (1992). *Arthritis self-health course: Leader's manual and reference materials.* Atlanta, GA: Arthritis Foundation.

Lorig, K.R., Mazonson, P.D., & Holman, H.R. (1993). Evidence suggesting that health education for self-management in patients with chronic arthritis has sustained health benefits while reducing health care costs. *Arthritis & Rheumatism, 36*(4), 439-446.

Lorig, K.R., & Holman, H. (2003). Self-management education history, definition, outcomes and mechanisms. *Annals of Behavioral Medicine, 26*(1), 1-7.

Lorig, R.K., Ritter, P., Stewart, A.L., Sobel, D.S., Brown, B.W., & Bandura, A. (2001). Chronic disease self-management program: 2-year health status and health care utilization outcomes. *Medical Care, 39*(11), 1217-23.

Lorig, R.K., Laurent, D.D., Deyo, R.A., Marnell, M.E., & Minor, M.A. (2002). Can a back pain e-mail discussion group improve health status and lower health care costs? *Archives of Internal Medicine, 162*(7), 792-96.

MacLean, C.H. (2001). Quality indictors for the management of osteoarthritis in vulnerable elders. *Annals of Internal Medicine, 135*(8), 711-721.

Maisiak, R., Austin, J., & Heck, L. (1996). Health outcomes of two telephone interventions for patients with rheumatoid arthritis or osteoarthritis. *Arthritis Rheumatology, 39*(8), 1391-1399.

Mazzuca, S.A., Brandt, K.D., Katz, B.P., Chambers, M., Byrd, D., & Hanna, M.P. (1997). Effects of self-care education on the health status of inner-city patients with osteoarthritis of the knee. *Arthritis Rheumatology, 40*(8), 1466-74.

Mazzuca, S.A., Brandt, K.D., Katz, B.P., Hanna, M.P., & Melfi, C.A. (1999). Reduced utilization and cost of primary care clinic visits resulting from self-care education for patients with osteoarthritis of the knee. *Arthritis & Rheumatism, 42*(6), 1267-1273.

Mobily, P.R., Herr, K.A., & Clark, M.K. (1994). An epidemiologic analysis of pain in the elderly: The Iowa 65 + Rural Health Study. *Journal of Aging and Health, 6,* 139-150.

Mullen, P.D., Laville, E.A., Biddle, A.K., & Lorig, K. (1987). Efficacy of psycho-educational intervention on pain, depression, and disability in people with arthritis: A meta-analysis. *Journal of Rheumatology, 14* (Suppl. 15), 33-39.

National Institute of Arthritis and Musculoskeletal and Skin Disease [NIAMSD] (2002). Arthritis pain. Retrieved on March 20, 2005 from www.niams.nih.gov/hi/topics/arthritis/arthpain.html

National Institute of Health. (2001). National Institute of Arthritis and Musculoskeletal and Skin Disease. Handout on health: Osteoarthritis. Retrieved on March 20, 2005 from http:www.niams.nih.gov/hi/topics/arthritis/oahandout.htm.

Parker, J.C., Smarr, K.L., Slaughter, J.R., Johnston, S.K., Priesmeyer, M.L. et al. (2003). Management of depression in rheumatoid arthritis: A combined pharmacologic and cognitive-behavioral approach. *Arthritis & Rheumatism, 15,* 766-777.

Peschken, C.A., & Esdaile, J.M. (1999). Rheumatic disease in North America's indigenous peoples. *Seminar in Arthritis Rheumatology, 28,* 368-91.

Pincus, T., Swearingen, C., & Wolfe, F. (1999). Toward a multidimensional health assessment questionnaire (MDHAQ). *Arthritis & Rheumatism, 42*(10), 2220-2230.

Radojevic, V., Nicassio, P.M., & Weisman, M.H. (1992). Behavioral intervention with and without family support for rheumatoid arthritis. *Behavioral Therapy, 23*(1), 13-30.

Rene, J., Weinberger, M., Mazzuca, S.A., Brandt, K.D., & Katz, B.P. (1992). Reduction of joint pain in patients with knee osteoarthritis who have received monthly telephone calls. *Arthritis & Rheumatism, 35*(15), 511-15.

Rhee, S.H., Parker, J.G., Smarr, K.L., Petroski, G.F., Johnson, J.C., Hewett, J.E. et al. (2000). Stress management in rheumatoid arthritis: What is the underlying mechanism? *Arthritis Care and Research, 13*(6), 435-442.

Rowat, K., Jeans, M.E., & LeFort, S.M. (1994). A collaborative model of care: Patient, family and health professionals. In: P.D. Wall & R. Melzack (Eds.), *Textbook of pain* (pp. 1381-1386). Edinburgh: Churchill Livingstone.

Ruehlman, L.S. (2005). Comparing the experiential and psychosocial dimensions of chronic pain in African Americans and Caucasians: Findings from a National Community Sample. *Pain Medicine, 6*(1), 49-61.

Simon, L., Lipman, A.G., Allaire, S.G., Caudill-Slosberg, M., & Gill, L.H. (2002). *Guideline for the management of acute and chronic pain in osteo and rheumatoid arthritis.* Glenview, IL: American Pain Society.

Skinner, J.B., Erskine, A., Pearce, S., Rubenstein, I., Taylor, M., & Foster, C. (1990). The evaluation of a cognitive treatment program in outpatients with chronic pain. *Journal of Psychosomatic Research, 34,* 13-19.

Superio-Cabuslay, E., Ward, M.M., & Lorig, K.R. (1996). Patient education interventions in osteoarthritis and rheumatoid arthritis: A meta-analytic comparison with non-steroidal anti-inflammatory drug treatment. *Arthritis Care and Research, 9,* 292-301.

Tan, G. (2005). Ethnicity, control appraisal, coping, and adjustment to chronic pain among black and white Americans. *Pain Medicine, 6*(1), 18-29.

Turk, D.C., & Monarch, E.S. (2002). Biopsychosocial perspective on chronic pain. In D.C. Turk & R.J. Gatchel (Eds.), *Psychological approaches to pain management: A practitioner's handbook* (2nd ed., pp. 3-29). New York: Guilford Press.

Warsi, A., LaValley, M.P., Wang, P.S., Avorn, J., & Solomon, D.H. (2003). Arthritis self-management education programs: A meta-analysis of the effect on pain and disability. *Arthritis Rheumatology, 48,* 2207-13.

Weiner, D.K., Herr, K., & Rudy, T.E. (2002). *Persistent pain in older adults.* New York: Springer Publishing Company.

Weiner, D.K., & Hanlon, J.T. (2001). Pain in nursing home residents: Management strategies. *Drugs & Aging, 18*(1), 13-29.

Wong, A.L., Harker, J.O., Lau, V.P., Shatzel, S., & Port, L.H. (2004). Spanish arthritis empowerment program: A dissemination and effectiveness study. *Arthritis & Rheumatism, 51*(3), 332-336.

Yip, Y.B., Sit, J.W., & Wong, Y. (2004). A quasi-experimental study on improving arthritis self-management for residents of an aged people's home in Hong Kong. *Psychology, Health, & Medicine, 9*(2), 235-246.

Chapter 5

Diabetes Treatments

Vaughn A. DeCoster, MSW, PhD, LCSW

With the aging of many countries, physical inactivity, and growing rates of obesity, there has been a dramatic rise in the incidence of diabetes. Diabetes and its treatment is a holistic and dynamic experience, shaping many aspects of a person's life and well-being. From lacerated fingers, blood sugar irritability, and regimented meal times to incapacitating glucose lows, vision impairment, and erectile problems, diabetes becomes a daily factor of life. These and other consequences influence the performance of social roles, requiring accommodation by employers and changes in family routines. For instance, operating vehicles or aircraft, habits of skipping meals, pickup games of basketball with grandkids, or spontaneous fishing trips alone–all require some form of change or limitation. Managing this condition demands considerable lifestyle adjustments, some by choice (diet, exercise, stress management) and others by necessity (insulin injections, renal dialysis treatment, rehab after an amputation). Emotionally, people must cope with a chronic, progressive, debilitating disease that typically reduces life expectancy by 15 years. In essence, diabetes adds additional complications and barriers to living. With holistic treatment and adequate resources, however, it can be a source of strength and a motivating factor for health improvement. Despite the biopsychosocial nature of this chronic disease, medications tend to be the principal intervention among medical professionals. Pharmacological treatment, though, does not assist with the psychosocial consequences of this disease nor the required lifestyle changes to achieve adequate blood sugar control.

Epidemiologically, diabetes morbidity is highest among lower socioeconomic, minority, and elder populations, which are groups already at-risk for other biopsychosocial challenges (Centers for Disease Control & Prevention [CDC], 2005). Hence, it is likely that many of the clients who frequent social work practice have diabetes themselves or care for someone who does. Unfortunately, social work practice and research involvement with this disease is limited. Social work clinicians make up less than 1% of registered diabetes professionals. Considering the psychological, social, and familial effects, social workers have remarkable potential to make a difference in the lives of people living with diabetes (DeCoster, 2001). Over the past 15 years, diabetes researchers and clinicians have begun to develop interventions addressing the psychosocial aspects of diabetes. The majority of these interventions fall within the knowledge base and clinical abilities of social work practitioners. This paper systematically reviewed psychosocial intervention studies with older adults, identifying and summarizing treatment protocols.

DEMOGRAPHICS/PREVALENCE

The increase in life expectancy throughout the world is changing the age demographics of populations. Currently in the United States, adults

65 and older comprise 13% (36 million) of its citizens, and it is expected that the number of older adults will nearly double by 2030 to 20% (71.5 million) of the population (He, Sengupta, Velkoff, & DeBarros, 2004). Although this aging trend will stabilize thereafter, adults 85 and older will increase from 4.2 million in 2000 to nearly 21 million by 2050 (Horiuchi, 2000; Oeppen & Vaupel, 2002).

One consequence of aging is an increase in the incidence of chronic diseases. The likelihood of being diagnosed with diabetes increases as people age. Among adults 20-39 years of age the incidence of diabetes is 2.2%, 9.9% among 40-59 year-olds, rising to 18.3% among those 60 years of age and older. Including pre-diabetes raises the count to 40%, or nearly 17 million elders who are diagnosed or at greater potential for a diagnosis of diabetes (American Diabetes Association [ADA], 2005). When considering gender and racial differences, the rates tend to increase for minority women. Between the ages of 65 and 74, 32% of African American and 29.8% of American Indian and Alaskan Native women are diagnosed with diabetes (National Institute of Diabetes and Digestive and Kidney Diseases [NIDDKD], 1998; National Center for Health Statistics [NCHS] & CDC, 2005). An exception, 34% of Hispanic males in this same age range have diabetes, in comparison to 28% Hispanic women (NCHS & CDC, 2005).

Nonetheless, the epidemic of diabetes among seniors is multifactorial in etiology (Goldberg & Coon, 1987). Nearly 30% of adults in the United States are clinically obese, with a body mass index of 30 or more (NCHS, 2005). Obesity, especially abdominal obesity, increases the risk for diabetes, which is an effect that is even more pronounced among older adults (Bray, 1992). As Catalano, Bergman, and Ader state (2005) ". . . youth affords significant protection against obesity-induced insulin resistance" (p. 11). Coinciding with obesity, 40% of adults are physically inactive, a trend that increases with age, climbing to over 60% of adults 75 and older (Lethbridge-Çejku & Vickerie, 2005). According to LaMonte, Blair, and Church (2005) ". . . the most proximal behavioral cause of insulin resistance is physical inactivity . . ." (p. 1205). Together, obesity and inactivity are significantly associated with diabetes and other comorbid conditions (Sullivan, Morrato, Ghushchyan, & Wyatt, 2005). Hence, an aging body compounds the effects of obesity and physical inactivity in the onset of diabetes among older adults.

NATURE OF THE PROBLEM

Diabetes mellitus is a series of endocrine disorders affecting tens of millions of Americans. There are essentially four classifications: gestational, pre-diabetes, Type 1, and Type II. *Gestational diabetes* occurs during pregnancy and involves abnormal glucose tolerance, i.e., blood sugars rise higher than normal and decrease to normal levels slower than usual. Insulin is either not produced, or body cells do not respond to the insulin that is produced. Normal glucose tolerance typically returns after childbirth. Recently, experts acknowledged a condition called *pre-diabetes*, which is elevated blood glucose levels that are above normal levels (fasting plasma glucose between 100-125 mg/dl; higher would justify a diabetes diagnosis). Depending on the test used to diagnosis it, this condition is also referred to as impaired glucose tolerance or impaired fasting glucose (IGT, IFG). IGT/IFG affects an estimated 41 million adults in the United States and places them at greater risk for diabetes and cardiovascular disease (ADA, 2005). Eventually, many with gestational or pre-diabetes will convert to Type 1 or Type II diabetes. *Type 1 diabetes* is the most frequent childhood chronic disease, although the majority with this disease are adults. The pancreas ceases insulin production, requiring insulin injections to live. Once referred to as juvenile diabetes, advances in treatment have extended the once limited life expectancies to well-beyond 60-70 years of age. *Type II diabetes* accounts for 95% of all diagnoses. Either the pancreas produces insufficient amounts of insulin, or the body's cells become insulin resistant. Elevated blood sugars harden and scar blood vessels allowing cholesterol deposits to collect, and elevate blood pressure, thus destroying micro-vascular systems feeding optic, gastrointestinal, and peripheral nerve endings, as well as overworking the kidneys in their effort to remove the blood sugars.

Risk Factors, Diagnosis, and Treatment

Risk factors for diabetes include obesity, giving birth to an infant weighing greater than nine pounds, family history, being of African-American, Native-American, or Hispanic ancestries, and being 65 years of age or older. The signs and symptoms of diabetes include unexpected and rapid weight loss or gain, light headedness, fatigue, poor concentration, increased thirst and urination, blurred vision, and personality changes such as anxiousness or irritability. Physicians diagnose diabetes after two fasting plasma glucose tests equal to or greater than 126 mg/dl or a single oral glucose tolerance test result of 200 mg/dl or higher (ADA, 2005). The majority of adults learn that they have diabetes during routine physicals or community health screenings.

Diabetes treatment seeks to maintain glucose levels to as close to normal ranges as possible (70-130 mg/dl, glycosolated hemoglobin, and A1C [average blood sugar level for past 3 months]–7% or less), an approach proven to prevent or delay short- and long-term consequences of disease progression (ADA, 1999; Cerveny, Leder, & Weart, 1998; The Diabetes Control and Complications Trial [DCCT], 1993; Herman & Eastman, 1998). Typically, treatment plans involve a combination of pharmacological and lifestyle changes including diet, physical activity, and stress management (ADA, 1999; Davidson, Davidson, & Richard, 1998; DeCoster, 2001). As most people know, achieving these lifestyle changes is quite difficult regardless of age. Diabetes education, normally taught by diabetes nurse educators, is the approach typically used to help patients make these changes. The results have been less than promising, unfortunately, as evidenced by continued poor control and proliferation of diabetes complications (Clement, 1995; Glasgow & Eaking, 1996; Peters et al., 1996; Van den Arend et al., 2000). In response, experts are calling for new approaches to diabetes treatment, especially in regards to behavioral and lifestyle change (for a review see DeCoster, 2001). According to Williams and Zeldman (2002), ". . . if diabetes self-management education is to become more effective, interventions need to be theory-based, to increase patient involvement in their care, and to encompass a broader array of evidence-based outcomes" (p. 151).

CONSEQUENCES OF THE PROBLEM

Diabetes has been found to be a precipitating factor for the onset and progression of other acute and chronic health conditions such as heart attacks, strokes, hypertension, kidney failure, and Alzheimer's disease (National Institute of Diabetes and Digestive and Kidney Diseases, NIDDK, 2004). Traditional diabetes medical treatment efforts are unable to keep pace with these growing numbers and, to some extent, are found to be recurrently ineffective, as evidenced by poor glycemic control among most elders and rising rates of complications (Clement, 1995; Glasgow & Eaking, 1996; Peters et al., 1996; Van den Arend et al., 2000; Williams & Zeldman, 2002). Ultimately, diabetes reduces life expectancy by 15 years and is the sixth cause of death in the United

States (Kochanek, Murphy, Anderson, & Scott, 2004; NIDDK, 2004). Direct health care costs for treating diabetes reached $92 billion dollars in 2002 alone (ADA, 2005). Older adults with diabetes consume more long-term care resources, are placed in nursing homes at an earlier age, and use adult day services more so than those without diabetes (Ahmed, Allman, & DeLong, 2003; Balkrishnan et al., 2003). Health-care systems, policymakers, and practitioners are searching for more useful and cost-effective methods to address this emerging diabetes epidemic among elders.

One promising treatment is islet transplantation which generates new pancreatic cells to produce insulin when it is successful (McCarthy, 2000). Unfortunately, this intervention is in the early stages of development, is available in only a select few communities, and requires remarkable glycemic control prior to transplantation and immunosuppressant treatment afterwards. New medication advances such as Symlin, an injectable medication to help control blood sugar for adults with type 1 and type II diabetes, Glimepiride (Amaryl), Repaglinide (Prandin), Acarbose (Precose) and miglitol (Glycet) also show promise (United States Food and Drug Administration, FDA, 2005). Insulin pumps offer convenience and greater precision in glucose management, delivering precise dosages of insulin via a small catheter, simulating a more natural release without repeated injections. In addition to these medical and pharmacological advances, interventions using or targeting psychosocial elements of this disease are emerging at a greater rate.

Only in the recent past have diabetes experts recognized the importance of psychosocial factors in the control of diabetes among older adults. As Funnell and Merritt note (1993), older adults ". . . experience unique challenges because of the physical and functional changes that may be imposed by the aging process and the prevalence of multiple chronic illnesses and complications" (p. 45). For instance, insufficient family and social support, dementia, depression, low income, access to health care, continuing multiple caregiving roles, low utilization of specialty diabetes care providers–all have been found to be significant psychosocial factors in diabetes management among older adults (Bell et al., 2005; Connell, 1991; Funnell & Merritt, 1993, 1998; Lloyd, Wing, Orchard, & Becker, 1993; Samuel-Hodge, Skelly, Headen, & Carter-Edwards, 2005; Sinclair, Girling, & Bayer, 2000; Wen, Shepherd, & Parchman, 2004). Recent psychosocial treatments show promise as effective approaches for changing health and lifestyle behaviors, blood glucose (glycemic) control, and delaying costly and harmful micro-macro vascular damage. Importantly, these non-medical approaches use less invasive and relatively inexpensive methods capable of reaching more of this affected aged population. Beyond physiologic benefits, many of these treatments improve psychological and social quality of life and well-being as well. As with any treatment innovation, much of the efforts concentrate on exploratory research, basic knowledge construction, theory development, and pilot testing intervention protocols. The quality of work in this area is mixed, requiring a close review to extract those approaches suitable for practice. Although two previous reviews of evidence-based practice in diabetes self-care exist (Norris, Engelgau, & Narayan, 2001; Sarkisian et al., 2003), neither specifically addressed interventions targeting older adults (aged 60 years or more) nor concentrated on psychosocial approaches. The purpose of this study is to systematically review psychosocial intervention studies focused on older adults, and to identify and summarize treatment protocols.

REVIEW OF EMPIRICAL LITERATURE

This study systematically identified, reviewed, and summarized psychosocial interventions for older adults living with diabetes. Adopting methods used in a previous intervention review (DeCoster & Cummings, 2005), four steps were followed: define study inclusion criteria, systematically search literature, identify types of interventions and outcomes, then review significant outcomes.

This project's inclusion criteria were evidence-based psychosocial intervention studies addressing some aspect of diabetes, published in English language peer-reviewed scientific journals sometime over the past 20 years (1985-2005). The target population was older adults, defined as predominately 60 years of age or older. For the systematic literature search, the researcher conducted a boolean search of six electronic databases (CINAHL-nursing and allied health, Medline, ProQuest, PsychInfo, Social Service Abstracts, and Sociological Abstracts). After trial searches using various combinations of terms, the following keywords were used in both singular and plural tenses: diabetes and older adults or elders or seniors. From this first list, article titles were reviewed for duplicates and ineligible titles, e.g., studies clearly focused only on pathophysiology or pharmacology. After this second listing of titles, abstracts were read to further eliminate ineligible studies, those focused on basic or descriptive research only. Papers were then read from this third list and included if they met these criteria: (1) Paper included totally, or in-part, a psychosocial oriented intervention; (2) Intervention was considered within the domain of social work practice knowledge or skill; and (3) Researchers empirically evaluated the intervention, with outcome measures included. The remaining 17 eligible studies were then summarized and analyzed (see Table 1 for a review).

The 17 studies are organized into one of three methods of intervention category: group, individual, or classroom.

Group Interventions

A half-dozen studies employed group-based intervention methods to improve such things as problem-solving skills, support, or commitment to personal change. Alley and Brown (2002) implemented an ongoing, open-ended, problem-solving support group (n = 18) for older members of a Kaiser Permanente health maintenance organization. Constructed and implemented by social workers, this one-year pilot program was based on the task-centered group work model, with participants as experts, and also incorporated social support and education. To evaluate the intervention, they used a single survey administered after 12 months during one of the twice-monthly regular meetings. Fourteen respondents uniformly reported improved problem-solving skills. The study lacked more objective assessment instruments but did show unanimous positive feedback from participants and self-reported improvements in diabetes self-management.

DeCoster and George (2005) pilot-tested a peer-lead, community-based, self-help group, termed the Diabetes Club. Founded on an empowerment theoretical approach and using evidence-based methods, meetings typically focused on problem-solving, resource sharing, mutual support, and assessment of diabetes management progress. Held at a senior activity center in Fayetteville, Arkansas, Club members directed group content and activities, purposively assuming greater control of meetings with a graduated reduction in professional involvement. Using a quasi pre-post test design, social work researchers re-administered baseline measures at six months for the convenience sample of 13 participants. Findings revealed significant improvements in efficacy, self-care behaviors, and glycemic control.

A self-directed support group was added to an existing six-session diabetes program for veterans in North Chicago by Gilden, Hendryx, Clar, Casia, and Singh (1992). Facilitated by a social worker, monthly group sessions focused on coping skills, continuing education, discussions, and organized social activities. Researchers used a non-randomized, pre-post test before and after the education component, then after the support-group. Intervention and control groups were matched by

TABLE 1. Review of Interventions and Significant Positive Outcomes

Author/date	Population	N	Intervention	Significant Outcomes *
Alley, 2002	CDS, family/friends	11	SG & PS	Self-reported problem-solving skills
Chumbler, 2004	CDV	79	CM & TH	Instrumental activities daily living, functional independence, mental status
DeCoster, 2005	Sr. activity center CDS	13	ET, PS & SG	Self-efficacy, diabetes self-care behaviors, A1C
Durso, 2003	CDS	7	TH	Diabetes knowledge
Gilden, 1992	CDV	22	ET & SG	Knowledge, quality of life, depression, A1C
Gilliland, 2002	Native American CDS, family/friends	104	ET & SG	A1C
Glasgow, 1992	CDS	102	ET, EX & PS	Diet, exercise time, weight loss, A1C
Glasgow, 1997	CDS	206	ET, GS & PS	Diet, serum cholesterol
Kochevar, 2001	Native American CDS, family/friends	22	EX	Perceived physical & emotional health, appearance, activity oriented chores, exercise, BP, respirations
Mayer, 2001	Rural CDS	28	Diet, ET & GS	Weight, body mass index, fasting blood glucose levels
Miller, 2001	CDS	92	Diet, ET & GS	FBG, A1C, cholesterol
Pratt, 1987	CDS	79	ET, GS, SG & PS	Weight, feelings of peer support
Ridgeway, 1999	PCCP	38	ET & GS	FBG, A1C, cholesterol, weight
Trozzolino, 2003	Visually impaired CDS	24	TG & ET	Diabetes stressors, knowledge, A1C
Tu, 1993	Post-discharge CDS	27	CM &TH	SBGM, Rx use, diet knowledge
White, 1986	Obese CDV	32	Diet, GS & TG	FBG, A1C
Williams, 2004	Depression, PCCP	417	CM & PS	Depression, overall functioning, exercise

Populations: CDS = Community dwelling seniors; CDV: Community dwelling veterans; PCCP = Primary care clinic out-patients

Interventions: CM = Case management; ET = Education and/or training; EX = Exercise; GS = Goal setting; PS = Problem solving; SG = Support group; TG = Psych-Treatment Group; TH = Telehealth

Outcomes: A1C = Glycosolated hemoglobin (measures average blood sugar level for past 3-months, considered the gold-standard in diabetes research); BP = Blood pressure; FBG = Fasting blood glucose

* Listed outcomes are statistically significant improvements in intervention targets.

age and duration of diabetes. Eleven veterans received both education and the 18-month support group, twelve received only education and delayed entry into the support group condition, and a third group of eight served as a control group, receiving neither treatment. At two years, elders receiving the combined education/support group showed significant improvements in diabetes knowledge, quality of life, depression, and A1C levels.

Pratt, Wilson, Leklem, and Kingsley (1987) conducted a peer support/nutritional education group among Oregon elders (n = 79) with diabetes. A registered dietician taught eight weekly diet education classes with two additional sessions at one and two months after the initial series. Intervention sites, not individual subjects, were randomly assigned to one of three conditions (quasi-experimental design): education and peer support, education only, or control. The peer support condition included a support group following the didactic lessons. The support groups encouraged peer interactions, sharing experiences, normalization, group problem-solving, positive reinforcement, and personal goal setting. Using a pre-post test design, participants in the education-peer support condition showed a significant reduction in weight at the end of the eight-week intervention, then a slight, but insignificant gain, at 16 weeks. Self-reported feeling of emotional support also increased for the support group condition.

A psychoeducational therapy group for older adults with vision loss was evaluated by Trozzolino, Thompson, Tansman, and Azen (2003). The researchers tested this 12-week program by randomly assigning 48 clients in Birmingham, Alabama, to treatment or control conditions. The intervention consisted of one group session on basic diabetes self-care, one on diet, and 10 on cognitive-behavioral factors related to treatment adherence (e.g., attitude, assertiveness, relationships with providers, social support, emotion, and coping styles). From a pre-post design, the intervention produced significant improvements in A1C levels, diabetes knowledge, and reduced diabetes related stressors.

Psychologists White, Carnahan, Nugent, Iwaoka, and Dodson (1986) compared a group management intervention with a traditional advice-education program among 41 veterans with obesity and diabetes in Arizona. Patients randomly assigned to the treatment met for 10 one-hour sessions in the first month, biweekly sessions during the second, then monthly for the remaining period in this six-month study. Based on reference group theory that relies heavily on the group process, a therapeutic group management process was implemented that focused on diet and exercise change. Founded on past research showing success at group decision-making and diet change, subjects assessed progress, shared ideas, advice, and support. After three months, a significant decline in serum glucose and A1C was found for the intervention group. At six months, this decline did not continue, however, neither did these values increase for the intervention group as they did for the comparison group.

Individual Interventions

Five projects employed individual intervention methods in case management efforts, promotion of general treatment adherence, or specifically with setting dietary goals. Chumbler, Mann, Wu, Schmid, and Kobb (2004) tested care coordination using distance monitoring equipment (home-telehealth) with 226 male veterans living in rural areas of North Florida and South Georgia. All subjects had a chronic illness and one-third had diabetes. Participants used one of three analog phone-line devices: (1) hand-held in-home messaging device requiring daily user inputs to a series of disease management questions; (2) audio-video telemonitor with biometric monitoring of blood pressure, heart rate, weight, oxygen saturation, and heart and lung sounds; and (3) videophone without monitoring capability. Care coordinators assessed patients at different intervals, depending on the assigned device. The study used a "case-control design" (p. 132), randomly assigning 111 to one of the three treatment conditions and 115 to the control condition. Comparisons of baseline and 12-month scores revealed significant improvements in instrumental activities of daily living, activities of daily living, and motor and cognitive functional independence for the treatment (telehealth) group. In a telephone survey at one year, 97% of home-telehealth participants wanted to continue, the majority reporting the that technology was easy to use, made them feel more secure, and was helpful in managing their disease.

Durso, Wendel, Letzt, Lefkowitz, Kaseman, and Seifert (2003) promoted medication and self-care adherence among seven older adults with type II diabetes with a web-based telecommunications system. These researchers used a propriety program (Personal Diabetes Management System, PDMS, by Adherence Technologies) to send automated interactive messages concerning key self-care behaviors, and diabetes education, and containing prompts to call care providers at a scheduled time. Researchers programmed the system through a web-based interface and received health data via cellular or home phone. Participants received a cellular phone, and were instructed in its use and PDMS during a dedicated clinic visit with additional help provided as needed. Pre-post test results after the three-month trial revealed improvements in diabetes knowledge, A1C levels, and body-mass indexes for half of the group.

In 1997, Glasgow, La Chance, Toobert, Brown, Hampson, and Riddle tested a brief intervention targeting diet behaviors among 206 older clients, most with type II diabetes, at an internal medicine clinic in Oregon. In a single session, clinic patients randomly assigned to the treatment condition (n = 108) completed a computer assessment on diet barriers, met with a counselor to discuss goal setting and problem-solving, and then received dietary self-help materials. The control group (n = 98) received only usual medical care. At 12 months, treatment group participants showed significant improvements in food habits, calories consumed per day, percent of calories from fat, and serum cholesterol levels.

Tu, McDaniel, and Gay (1993) assessed a post-education telephone follow-up program for older adults after completion of an inpatient diabetes program. Subjects (n = 15) randomly assignment to the treatment condition were telephoned 24-48 hours after discharge from a Birmingham, Alabama, hospital and then weekly for three weeks to assess diabetes self-care knowledge and practices. The control group (n = 12) received a follow-up call six-weeks post-discharge and usual medical care. Using a pre-post design, data obtained at six weeks showed significant improvements in self-blood glucose monitoring, prescription adherence, self-care knowledge and activities for the treatment group but not for those in the control condition.

Targeting depression in older patients across 18 primary care clinics, Williams et al. (2004) randomly assigned 417 diabetes patients to test a depression care management program. The intervention group received a 20-minute educational video, booklet, and met with a "depression care manager" (p. 1017), either a nurse or psychologist. In individual sessions care managers completed a psychosocial history, reviewed treatment options (medications or psychotherapy), and followed up with a treatment team. Following regimen protocols (IMPACT), antidepressants or a series of six to eight structured psychotherapy sessions that focused on problem-solving were administered, but diabetes self-care was not addressed in the program. On average, patients had nine in-person sessions and six telephone contacts with the care manager. The comparison group received usual medical care. Trained interviewers surveyed subjects by telephone at three, six, and 12 months. Depression and overall functional impairment (physical and emotional health) both improved across all time periods for diabetes patients in the treatment group with no significant improvements found for patients in the control condition.

Classes

Six projects used a traditional classroom approach to provide culturally sensitive training, diet problem-solving, or promote physical activity. Gilliland, Azen, Perez, and Carter (2002) conducted a nonrandomized community-based life-style intervention for older Native Americans (n = 104). Conducted at Indian Health Service clinics in New Mexico, sites were assigned to one of three conditions: family and friends intervention, one-on-one intervention, or control, delayed intervention. The researchers presented culturally appropriate diabetes education and skill building activities to both intervention arms, adding a social support component to the family and friends condition. A diabetes mentor led five sessions at six-week intervals, using a narrative, story telling, educational approach. At one year, all groups showed increases in A1C, which is an unwanted rise in three-month blood sugar levels. This change suggests a decline in glycemic control, yet increases for the intervention groups were not statistically significant. No other improvements were found for intervention conditions, either separately or combined.

From prior research with focus groups, Glasgow, Toobert, Hampson, Brown, Lewinsohn, and Donnelly (1992) developed and tested their Sixty Something diabetes self-management program in Eugene, Oregon. One-hundred and two community dwelling older adults were randomly assigned to immediate or delayed intervention conditions. Instructors addressed problem-solving skills related to diet and exercise behaviors in eight weekly classes. Classes then met at two follow-up sessions in two-week intervals, selecting self-care topics to review. Trained exercise leaders conducted two exercise sessions during the eighth week, but only 60% attended. At six months, the immediate intervention group showed a significant decrease in calories consumed per day and percent of calories from fat, and an increase in minutes of physical activities. They also had significant weight loss and improvement in A1C and problem-solving skills. None of these outcomes were seen in patients assigned to the control condition.

Kochevar, Smith, and Bernard (2001) tested a community-based intervention to increase activity levels among urban living American Indian elders (n = 22) in Oklahoma. Sixteen were randomly assigned to a 40-minute mobility and flexibility class which met two days a week for six weeks. The remaining six subjects served as a non-exercise control group, agreeing not to participate in any exercise programs during the course of the project. Ten class participants completed the treatment program, attending eight of 12 classes. Significant post-intervention improvements were found in self-reported feelings about appearance, chore-based and dedicated exercised activities, and in physical and emotional health. The participants also showed significant reductions in blood pressure and respirations. No improvements were found for control subjects.

A weight management program for older adults in rural, underserved communities was pilot tested by Mayer-Davis et al. (2001) in South Carolina. Participants (n = 28) were randomly selected from a primary care organization's registry of diabetes patients to complete the Pounds Off with Empowerment (POWER) program. The POWER program used evidence-based strategies to reduce fat and caloric intake and to increase physical activity and was comprised of an eight-week program with weekly training meetings. Two meetings were one-on-one sessions, with the remainder structured as group sessions. Treatment participants also completed diet/physical activity self-monitoring logs. Participants were randomly assigned to complete this intensive lifestyle intervention or to a control group condition. Formal evaluation, including pre-post session knowledge tests and a satisfaction survey, was conducted after each session. No differences were found between conditions and all patients showed significant reductions in weight, body mass index, and fasting blood glucose levels.

Miller, Edwards, Kissling, and Sanville (2002) investigated the effectiveness of a nutritional intervention specifically designed for older adults. A total of 98 subjects in North Carolina were randomly assigned to control or treatment conditions. The intervention consisted of theory-based diabetes education modules using an adult learning instructional approach that incorporated activities, insight, and personal goal setting. Ten weekly sessions were held, each lasting between one-and-a-half to two hours. Using a pre-post test design, researchers found significant improvement in blood sugar levels (fasting blood sugar, A1C) and cholesterol levels after completion of the intervention for the experiment but not the control group.

Ridgeway, Harvil, Harvil, Falin, Forester, and Gose (1999) developed a practical education/behavior modification program, consisting of classes taught in a primary care clinic in East Tennessee. The one-and-a-half hour monthly behavior/education classes were held for six months, using a standardized diabetes education program, titled Life

Skills. At these classes, patients were updated on their weight, blood pressure, and laboratory results. Diabetes educators held one-on-one sessions, personalizing diet and exercise prescriptions, setting goals, and establishing behavioral contracts. Physicians provided input on patient needs and demonstrated support by brief appearances at some monthly meetings. Fifty-six patients were randomly assigned to either the intervention or control condition. At the end of the classes (6-months) the treatment group showed significant improvements in fasting blood glucose and cholesterol levels, A1C, and diabetes knowledge. However, six-month post-intervention found that these improvements continued only for weight. Researchers noted no improvements for the control group.

TREATMENT SUMMARY

Slightly over fifty percent (58%, 10) of the studies used education or task groups to deploy psychosocial treatment. Over one-third (41%, 7) utilized individual modalities (e.g., care management, follow-up sessions, personal diabetes goal setting) in combination with group methods. Three studies used traditional didactic approaches. Intervention modalities did not appear to influence success. Interventions ranged from computer-assisted diabetes self-care assessment and feedback, food label education and physical activity/exercise programs to varying levels of care management, brief structured psychotherapy, group decision-making and problem-solving. Examining the intervention foci for the 17 reviewed studies, results indicate that a fourth (24%, 10) concentrated on continuity of care issues such as managing patient diabetes self-care, soliciting patient self-monitored outcomes (e.g., self-blood glucose testing, diet, weight), reinforcing contracted diabetes life-style plans/goals, or offering ongoing diabetic technical support and guidance. A fifth (21%, 10) focused on diabetes training such as teaching diabetes self-care knowledge or skills. Psychological support was the third most frequent focus (21%, 9), typically via small self-help or peer support groups. Considering the academic disciplines of the primary authors, a third (29%, 5) of the studies were conducted primarily by medicine, followed by psychology (23%, 4), then geriatrics/gerontology and social work (12%, 2 for each). Nursing, rehabilitation, public health, and exercise physiology each contributed one eligible study. Many interventions were interdisciplinary and relied on additional psychosocial paradigms and knowledge bases beyond those within their professional discipline.

Although only two studies were from social work (Alley & Brown, 2002; DeCoster & George, 2005), many of the interventions were within the scope of social work knowledge and skills for undergraduate and graduate level practitioners. Interventions commonly relied on basic group facilitation skills, case/care management, active listening, age sensitive training techniques, task-centered methods, and some psychoanalytic capabilities. As far as diabetic knowledge, six (Chumbler et al., 2004; Gilden et al., 1992; Glasgow et al., 1992; Glasgow et al., 1997; Miller et al., 2001; and Trozzolino et al., 2003) require basic training in diabetes self-care, which is easily obtained by observing a reputable diabetes patient training program lasting 4-5 days or by studying clinical guidelines. Four (Durso et al., 2003; Gilliland et al., 2002; Pratt et al., 1987; and Tu, McDaniel, & Gay 1993) interventions could be conducted conjointly with a registered dietician or certified diabetes educator, the latter of which could be from any discipline. However, as Alley and Brown (2002) emphasize, the principle challenges working in diabetes as social workers are the political battles and competition for resources among other health disciplines, not the complexity of the disease and patient cases.

CONCLUSION

From the initial 1118 titles on diabetes and older adults, 17 (1.5%) met the criteria as evidence-based psychosocial interventions. Reviewed psychosocial treatments usually targeted one or more of three elements: continuity of care, diabetic self-care training, and/or psychological support. The majority of efforts were lead by medicine and psychology, although many efforts were interdisciplinary. Intervention protocols were within the knowledge and skill range of undergraduate and graduate level social workers, using case management, health education, or group work techniques.

Diabetes is a remarkably complex chronic disease with patients remaining predominately responsible for implementing treatment though self-management of the disease. Considering the power patients have in diabetes treatment regimens, many traditional health-care practitioners and researchers may elect to concentrate on areas over which they have greater control, i.e., psychopharmacology. As Brown and Furstenberg state, "Health professionals, though they have technical expertise . . .

can do little by themselves to create or maintain [lifestyle] change" (1992, p. 90). For this reason, professionals should expand their treatment focus to include educational efforts to help those with diabetes make informed decisions about health behaviors.

A degree of ageism may exist in diabetes care. As Funnell, Arnold, Fogler, Merritt, and Anderson state, diabetes researchers and practitioners may believe ". . . that older adults are unable to participate in educational programs or require excessive amount of education and support to carry out more intensive regimens" (1997, p. 163), which is a concern raised by other scholars as well (Banerjee, Banerjee, & Sarkar, 1998; Glynn et al., 1999). Although diabetes affects nearly 17 million seniors, research on psychosocial interventions remains sparse. This could be the result of reducing the importance for this disease among a patient population with numerous other medical conditions or the predominance of the medical model inhibiting the entry of other disciplines. It could also be associated with the challenge of working with aging subjects. For instance, recruiting and retaining older adults is often more difficult in research studies (Coonrod, Betschart, & Harris, 1994).

Overall, more behavioral research is needed to improve the health and quality of life of older adults with diabetes. The work in this area has yet to fully address the self-management challenges of elders nor has it coalesced into a model explaining how psychosocial aspects relate to self-management and glycemic control. An integrated model explaining life outcomes with diabetes is one desirable product of such research. According to Williams and Zeldman (2002), ". . . if diabetes self-management education is to become more effective, interventions need to be theory-based, to increase patient involvement in their care, and to encompass a broader array of evidence-based outcomes" (p. 151). Second, disciplines other than medicine need to become more involved in diabetes research to expand the conceptual scope and intervention breadth, a position asserted by some experts in diabetes (Vinicor, 2002). Third, since diabetes is a chronic disease, more longitudinal interventions and evaluative research studies are needed. Lastly, community and participant-based projects are required to realize the potential of the patients and families becoming experts in diabetes self-care and management.

Considering the frequency of diabetes, it is likely that social work clients across most areas of practice are affected by this illness, either directly or indirectly through their relationship with someone who has diabetes. As asserted by DeCoster (2001), social workers are abdicating the potential to be change agents for people with diabetes, and are missing opportunities to improve glycemic control and well-being. Although reimbursement for services may be an issue, many health-care organizations and insurers welcome new approaches and disciplines demonstrating successful outcomes, once political obstacles are cleared as suggested by Alley and Brown (2002). As seen in social work's dominance in mental health and substance abuse treatment (NASW, 2005), practitioners often remain under the influence of psychiatry/ medicine, failing to fully implement the social work paradigm (Aviram, 2002). In many ways, these interventions demonstrate the potential of treating the whole person, validating the bio-psycho-social approach, a long-standing principle in the social work paradigm. These interventions provide multiple tools for social work involvement in diabetes and, hopefully, will serve as stimuli for creative application and empirical investigations to support greater inclusion of social work in the treatment of diabetes.

TREATMENT RESOURCE APPENDIX

American Diabetes Association
www.diabetes.org

The American Diabetes Association is the leading diabetes advocacy association and provides overviews on the disease, treatment, research, advocacy and legal resources, and community/local events. In particular, resources on the site include:

- A brief diabetes risk assessment instrument that provides you with your current level of risk for Type II diabetes
- Information if you are a recently diagnosed Type I or Type II diabetic
- Information about weight and diabetes including how to get started, stay motivated and take off the pounds
- Exercise information and tips, including how to integrate exercise into your already packed day!
- Part of the web site resources for members of cultural groups that are high risk for diabetes including people who are African American, Asian/Pacific Islanders, Hispanic, and Native American. Material is printed in both English and languages that are native to those cultures.

National Center for Chronic Disease Prevention and Health Promotion
www.cdc.gov/diabetes

The CDC site also contains excellent information about diabetes including public health resources, fact sheets, geographical (GIS) diabetes maps, short courses, and listings for state-based diabetes prevention and control programs. Several pamphlets and brochures are available off the site including:

- *Taking charge of your diabetes.* Comprehensive information that describes what problems diabetes can cause, how to work with a health-care team to prevent problems, why it is important to get your blood glucose and blood pressure closer to normal, and how to find out about resources in your community to help you prevent problems.
- *Recipes and meal planning.* An English and Spanish guide to making decisions about foods and meal preparation. Introduces the diabetic food pyramid, and includes recipes, portion sizes, among other things.

National Diabetes Education Program
www.ndep.nih.gov

Information is given about this national, multi-agency initiative, with patient education materials on diabetes and pre-diabetes, resources for professionals, awareness programs, and partnerships. There are several free publications that can be downloaded off the site, including:

- *Four Steps to Control Your Diabetes.* Information about the condition, health concerns, health resources, and a diabetes recording system is included.
- *Tips for Helping a Person with Diabetes.* Information and fact sheet about issues if a loved one has diabetes. Includes ways to get information, and the importance of talking about your situation and your feelings.
- *Team Care: Comprehensive Lifetime Management for Diabetes.* Quality diabetes care involves more than just the primary provider. Find out more about implementing multidisciplinary team care for people with diabetes in all clinical settings and how to reduce the human and economic toll of diabetes through a continuous, proactive, planned, patient-centered, and population-based approach to care.

- *The Power to Control Diabetes Is in Your Hands Community Outreach Kit.* This resource kit provides information on diabetes and older adults and suggestions on how to promote the *Power to Control* campaign with ideas for educational activities, media events and promotional campaigns.

National Institute on Diabetes and Digestive and Kidney Diseases
www.niddk.nih.gov

Similar to the other sites listed, this organization has a wide range of publications (several publications in Spanish) and resources on financial help, listing national organizations serving patients and professionals.

U.S. Food & Drug Administration
www.fda.gov/diabetes

Updates on diabetes pharmacological and treatment advances as well as essential information on food and meal planning, insulin, self-blood glucose monitoring devices and lancets, and complications, numerous downloadable publications. The site posts the latest information about diabetes management and consumer-related issues for testing and medications.

WebMD
www.webmd.com

Health and diabetes information on numerous topics, message boards with diabetes professionals.

For research and reviews of diabetes from a social work perspective see Auslander et al., 1990; Auslander et al., 1993; Auslander et al., 1997; DeCoster, 2001; DeCoster, 2003; DeCoster & Cummings, 2004; or DeCoster & Cummings, 2005.

REFERENCES

Ahmed, A., Allman, R., & DeLong, J. R. (2003). Predictors of nursing home admission for older adults hospitalized with heart failure. *Archives of Gerontology and Geriatrics, 36,* 117-126.

Alley, G. & Brown, L. (2002). A diabetes problem solving support group: Issues, process and preliminary outcomes. *Social Work in Health Care, 36,* 1-9.

American Diabetes Association. (1999). Implications of the United Kingdom prospective diabetes study. *Diabetes Care, 22* (Suppl 1), S27-S31.

American Diabetes Association. (2005). *National Diabetes Fact Sheet.* Retrieved December 5, 2005, from http://diabetes.org/main/info/facts/facts_natl.jsp

Auslander, W., Anderson, B., Bubb, J., Jung, K., & Santiago, J. (1990). Risk factors in diabetic children: A prospective study from diagnosis. *Health & Social Work, 15,* 133-42.

Auslander, W., Bubb, J., Rogge, M., & Santiago, J. (1993). Family stress and resources: Potential areas of intervention in children recently diagnosed with diabetes. *Health & Social Work, 18,* 101-113.

Auslander, W., Thompson, S., Dreitzer, D., & Santiago, J. (1997). Mothers' satisfaction with medical care: Perceptions of racism, family stress, and medical outcomes in children with diabetes. *Health & Social Work, 22,* 190-199.

Aviram, U. (2002). The changing role of the social worker in the mental health system. *Social Work in Health Care, 35,* 615-632.

Balkrishnan, R., Rajagopalan, R., Camacho, F., Huston, S., Murray, F., & Anderson, R. (2003). Predictors of medication adherence and associated health care costs in an older population with type 2 diabetes mellitus: A longitudinal cohort study. *Clinical Therapeutics, 25,* 2958-2971.

Banerjee, S., Banerjee, M., & Sarkar, R. (1998). Diabetes mellitus and aging. *Journal of the Indian Medical Association, 96,* 147-164.

Bell, R., Smith, S., Arcury, T., Snively, B., Stafford, J., & Quandt, S. (2005). Prevalence and correlates of depressive symptoms among rural older African Americans, Native Americans, and whites with diabetes. *Diabetes Care, 28,* 823-829.

Bray, G. (1992). Obesity increases risk for diabetes. *International Journal of Obesity and Related Metabolic Disorders, 16, Suppl 4,* S13-17.

Brown, J. & Furstenberg, A. (1992). Restoring control: Empowering older patients and their families during health crisis. *Social Work in Health Care, 17,* 81-101.

Catalano, K., Bergman, R., & Ader, M. (2005). Increased susceptibility to insulin resistance associated with abdominal obesity in aging rats. *Obesity Research, 13,* 11-20.

Centers for Disease Control and Prevention. *National Diabetes Fact Sheet: General Information and National Estimates on Diabetes in the United States, 2005.* Atlanta, GA: U.S. Department of Health and Human Services, Centers for Disease Control and Prevention.

Cerveny, J., Leder, R., & Weart, C. (1998). Issues surrounding tight glycemic control with type 2 diabetes mellitus. *Annals of Pharmacotherapy, 32,* 896-905.

Chumbler, N., Mann, W., Wu, S., Schmid, A., & Kobb, R. (2004). The association of home-telehealth use and care coordination with improvement of functional and cognitive functioning in frail elderly men. *Telemedicine Journal and e-Health, 10,* 129-137.

Clement, S. (1995). Diabetes self-management education. *Diabetes Care, 18,* 1204-1214.

Connell, C. (1991). Psychosocial contexts of diabetes and older adulthood: Reciprocal effects. *The Diabetes Educator, 17,* 364-371.

Coonrod, B., Betschart, J., & Harris, M. (1994). Frequency and determinants of diabetes patient education among adults in the U.S. population. *Diabetes Care, 17,* 852-858.

Davidson, M., Davidson, A., & Richard, Z. (Eds.) (1998). *Diabetes Mellitus: Diagnosis and Treatment* .

DeCoster, V. (2001). The psychosocial challenges of type 2 diabetes and the roles of health care social work: A neglected area of practice. *Health & Social Work, 26*, 26-37.

DeCoster, V. & Cummings, S. (2004). Coping with type 2 diabetes: Do race and gender matter? *Social Work in Health Care, 40*, 37-53.

DeCoster, V. & Cummings, S. (2005). Helping adults with diabetes: A review of evidence based interventions. *Health & Social Work, 30*, 259-264.

DeCoster, V. & George, L. (2005). A community based self-help intervention for elders living with diabetes. *The Journal of Educational Gerontology, 31*, 699-713.

The Diabetes Control and Complications Trial (DCCT) Research Group (1993). The effect of intensive treatment of diabetes on the development and progression of long-term complications in insulin-dependent diabetes mellitus. *New England Journal of Medicine, 329*, 977-986.

Durso, S., Wendel, I., Letzt, A., Lefkowitz, J., Kaseman, D., & Seifert, R. (2003). Older adults using cellular telephones for diabetes management: A pilot study. *MESURG Nursing, 12*, 313-317.

Funnell, M., Arnold, M., Fogler, J., Merritt, J., & Anderson, L. (1997). Participation in a diabetes education and care program: Experience from the diabetes care for older adults project. *The Diabetes Educator, 23*, 163-167.

Funnell, M. & Merritt, J. (1993). The challenges of diabetes and older adults. *The Nursing Clinics of North America, 28*, 45-60.

Funnell, M. & Merritt, J. (1998). The older adult with diabetes. *Nurse Practitioner Forum, 9*, 98-107.

Gilden, J., Hendryx, M., Clar, S., Casia, C., & Singh, S. (1992). Diabetes support groups improve health care of older diabetic patients. *Journal of the American Geriatrics Society, 40*, 147-150.

Gilliland, S., Azen, S., Perez, G., & Carter, J. (2002). Strong in body and spirit: Lifestyle intervention for Native American adults with diabetes in New Mexico. *Diabetes Care, 25*, 78-83.

Glasgow, R. & Eakin, E. (1996). Dealing with complexity: The case of diabetes self-management. In B. Anderson & R. Rubin (Eds.), *Practical Psychology for Diabetes Clinicians.* (pp. 53-62). Alexandria, VA: American Diabetes Association.

Glasgow, R., Toobert, D., Hampson, S., Brown, J., Lewinsohn, P., & Donnelly, J. (1992). Improving self-care among older patients with type II diabetes: The "Sixty Something . . ." study. *Patient Education Counseling, 19*, 61-74.

Glasgow, R., La Chance, P., Toobert, D., Brown, J., Hampson, S., & Riddle, M. (1997). Long term effects and costs of brief behavioral dietary intervention for patients with diabetes delivered from the medical office. *Patient Education and Counseling, 32*, 175-184.

Glynn, R., Monane, M., Gurwitz, J., Choodnoviskiy, I., & Avorn, J. (1999). Aging, comorbidity, and reduced rates of drug treatment for diabetes mellitus. *Journal of Clinical Epidemiology, 52*, 781-790.

Goldberg, A. & Coon, P. (1987). Non-insulin dependent diabetes mellitus in the elderly. Influence of obesity and physical inactivity. *Endocrinology and Metabolism Clinics of North America, 16*, 843-865.

He, W., Sengupta, M., Velkoff, V., & DeBarros, K. (2004). *65 + in the United States: 2004. Current Population Reports, Special Studies.* Washington, DC: U.S. Government Printing Offices.

Herman, W. & Eastman, R. (1998). The effects of treatment on the direct costs of diabetes. *Diabetes Care, 21* (Suppl. 3), C19-24.

Horiuchi, S. (2000). Greater lifetime expectation. *Nature, 405,* 744-750.

Kochanek, K., Murphy, S., Anderson, R., & Scott, C. (2004). Deaths: Final data for 2002. *National Vital Statistics Report, 53.* Washington, DC: National Center for Health Statistics.

Kochevar, A., Smith, K., & Bernard, M. (2001). Effects of a community-based intervention to increase activity in American Indian elders. *Journal–Oklahoma State Medical Association, 94,* 455-460.

LaMonte, M., Blair, S., & Church, T.S. (2005). Physical activity and diabetes prevention. *Journal of Applied Physiology, 99,* 1205-1213.

Lethbridge-Çejku, M., & Vickerie, J. (2005). Summary health statistics for U.S. adults: National Health Interview Survey, 2003. *National Center for Health Statistics. Vital Health Stat 10 (225) 2005.* Washington, DC: U.S. Government Printing Offices.

Lloyd, C., Wing, R., Orchard, T., & Becker, D. (1993). Psychosocial correlates of glycemic control: The Pittsburgh Epidemiology of Diabetes Complications (EDC) Study. *Diabetes Research and Clinical Practice, 21,* 187-195.

Mayer-Davis, E., D'Antonio, A., Martin, M., Wandersman, A., Parra-Medina, D., & Schulz, R. (2001). Pilot study of strategies for effective weight management in type 2 diabetes: Pounds off with empowerment (POWER). *Family & Community Health, 24,* 27-35.

McCarthy, M. (2000). Canadian group reports best results yet with islet-cell transplants. *Lancet, 355,* 2140-2148.

Miller, C., Edwards, L., Kissling, G., & Sanville, L. (2002). Nutrition education improves metabolic outcomes among older adults with diabetes mellitus: Results from a randomized controlled trial. *Preventive Medicine, 34,* 252-259.

National Association of Social Workers (2005). *General Fact Sheets: Social Work Profession.* Retrieved December 5, 2005, from http://www.naswdc.org/pressroom/features/general/profession.asp

National Center for Health Statistics (2005). *Health, United States, 2004 with Chart Book on Trends in the Health of Americans.* Hyattsville, MD: National Center for Health Statistics.

National Center for Health Statistics (NCHS), Centers for Disease Control and Prevention (CDC) (2005). *Data Warehouse on Trends in Health and Aging.* Retrieved December 5, 2005, from www.cdc.gov/nchs/agingact.htm

National Institute of Diabetes and Digestive and Kidney Diseases (1998). *Diabetes in African Americans Fact Sheet.* Bethesda, MD: U.S. Department of Health and Human Services, National Institutes of Health.

National Institute of Diabetes and Digestive and Kidney Diseases (2004). *NIDDK Recent Advances & Emerging Opportunities: Diabetes, Endocrinology and Metabolic Disease.* Bethesda, MD: U.S. Department of Health and Human Services, National Institutes of Health.

Norris, S., Engelgau, M., & Narayan, K. (2001). Effectiveness of self-management training in type 2 diabetes: A systematic review of randomized controlled trials. *Diabetes Care, 24,* 561-587.

Oeppen, J. & Vaupel, J. (2002). Broken limits to life expectancy. *Science, 296,* 1029-1031.

Peters, A., Legorreta, A., Ossorio, R., & Davidson, M. (1996). Quality of outpatient care provided to diabetic patients: A health maintenance organization experience. *Diabetes Care, 19,* 601-606.

Pratt, C., Wilson, W., Leklem, J., & Kingsley, L. (1987). Peer support and nutrition education for older adults with diabetes. *Journal of Nutrition for the Elderly, 6,* 31-43.

Ridgeway, N., Harvil, D., Harvil, L., Falin, T., Forester, G., & Gose, O. (1999). Improved control of type 2 diabetes mellitus: A practical education/behavioral modification program in a primary care clinic. *Southern Medical Journal, 92,* 667-672.

Samuel-Hodge, C., Skelly, A., Headen, S., & Carter-Edwards, L. (2005). Familial roles of older African-American women with type 2 diabetes: Testing of a new multiple caregiving measure. *Ethnicity & Disease, 15,* 436-43.

Sarkisian, C., Brown, A., Norris, K., Wintz, R., & Mangione, C. (2003). A systematic review of diabetes self-care interventions for older, African American, or Latino adults. *The Diabetes Educator, 29,* 467-479.

Sinclair, A., Girling, A., & Bayer, A. (2000). Cognitive dysfunction in older subjects with diabetes mellitus: Impact on diabetes self-management and use of care services. *Diabetes Research and Clinical Practice, 50,* 203-2012.

Sullivan, P., Morrato, E., Ghushchyan, V., & Wyatt, H. (2005). Obesity, inactivity, and the prevalence of diabetes and diabetes-related cardiovascular comorbidities in the U.S., 2000-2002. *Diabetes Care, 28,* 1599-1603.

Trozzolino, L., Thompson, P., Tansman, M., & Azen, S. (2003). Effects of a psychoeducational group on mood and glycemic control in adults with diabetes and visual impairments. *Journal of Visual Impairment & Blindness, 97,* 230-239.

Tu, K., McDaniel, G., & Gay, J. (1993). Diabetes self-care knowledge, behaviors, and metabolic control of older adults–The effect of a posteducational follow-up program. *The Diabetes Educator, 19,* 25-30.

United States Food and Drug Administration (2005). *FDA Talk Paper: FDA Approves New Drug to Treat Type 1 and Type 2 Diabetes.* Retrieved December 5, 2005, from http://www.fda.gov/bbs/topics/ANSWERS/2005/ANS01345.html

Van den Arend, I., Stolk, R., Krans, H., Grobbee, D., & Schrijvers, A. (2000). Management of type 2 diabetes: A challenge for patient and physician. *Patient Education and Counseling, 40,* 187-194.

Vinicor, F. (2002). *Diabetes from a national perspective: The Centers for Disease Control and the World Health Organization.* Paper presented at the Tennessee Governor's Forum on Diabetes, Nashville, TN.

Wen, L., Shepherd, M., & Parchman, M. (2004). Family support, diet, and exercise among older Mexican Americans with type 2 diabetes. *The Diabetes Educator, 30,* 980-993.

White, N., Carnahan, J., Nugent, A., Iwaoka, T., & Dodson, M. (1986). Management of obese patient with diabetes mellitus: Comparison of advice education with group management. *Diabetes Care, 9,* 490-496.

Chapter 6

HIV/AIDS Treatments

Charles A. Emlet, MSW, PhD
R. Andrew Shippy, MA

DEMOGRAPHIC/PREVALENCE TRENDS IN HIV/AIDS

Cumulative estimates indicate that over 60 million individuals have been infected with HIV, the virus that causes AIDS. In 2004 alone, there were an estimated 4.9 million new HIV infections (UNAIDS/WHO, 2005). Although fewer people are being diagnosed with AIDS in the U.S. and deaths continue to decline, the number of adults age 50 and older who are living with HIV/AIDS is larger than ever. Although the overall HIV infection rate slowed from 1996-2000, infection rates increased in the older population. According to the Centers for Disease Control and Prevention, AIDS cases among Americans over 50 have quintupled since 1990, from 16,288 to 90,513 (2003a), with older adults now representing approximately 20% of all persons living with HIV. The "graying" of the HIV epidemic is also evidenced by trends related to median age of AIDS-related issues. In examining data from the Centers for Disease Control and Prevention between 1994 and 2000, we can see slow but consistent increase in age on a number of important indicators. During this period, the median age at diagnosis with AIDS has risen from 37 to 39 years. The median age of individuals with AIDS has risen three years while the median age at death has increased from 39 to 43 years of age (Center for Disease Control and Prevention, 2003b). In New York City, the epicenter of the HIV epidemic in the United States, 25% of the people living with HIV are age 50 or older, and 64% are over age 40. Nearly 20% of new HIV diagnoses were among people over age 50 (NYC Department of Health and Mental Hygiene, 2005).

It is likely that older people will continue to comprise an increasingly larger proportion of individuals diagnosed with HIV/AIDS, reflecting both the ineffective prevention efforts targeting older adults (Ory & Mack, 1998) and the highly effective antiretroviral therapies that allow many people to live for significantly longer periods of time (Manton & Stallard, 1998). The advent of highly active antiretroviral therapies (HAART) in the 1990s has extended life for many persons with HIV disease and will allow, as never before, individuals who were infected in middle age to live into "old age." These recent trends have created two distinct populations of older persons with HIV/AIDS; those who where infected later in life and those infected earlier and now aging with HIV disease. People who were diagnosed with HIV before age 50 but have aged into the older adult category, considered "long-term survivors," will continue to increase as the treatments for HIV improve (Mack & Ory, 2003). As increasing numbers of older adults with HIV live longer lives, it is incumbent upon social workers, AIDS service providers and the health care system in general, to better understand the factors that contribute, either positively or negatively, to their quality of life. It is now time to systematically improve our understanding of effective psychosocial intervention strategies for older persons.

In examining race, gender and sexual orientation characteristics, the majority of individuals diagnosed with HIV/AIDS in the U.S across all age groups continue to be men. As of the end of 2004, however, 26.6% of the estimated 462,792 individuals living with HIV/AIDS in the U.S. were women (CDC, 2005). In older age groups, the proportion of women with AIDS is on the rise. Recently, Zablotsky and Kennedy (2004) reported that between 1988 and 2000 the percentage of women 50 + with AIDS rose from 8.9 to 15%. HIV/AIDS has increasingly been seen as a disease that impacts women, and the data on older adults confirm that this holds true for older women as well.

As with younger adults, HIV/AIDS among older persons is disproportionately affecting elders of color. Mack and Ory (2003) compared characteristics of older adults with AIDS between 1990 and 1999, and found that within that nine-year period, the proportion of whites with AIDS diagnosed at age 60 or later decreased from 60.4 to 30%. The most dramatic increase appears to be in older, African American men where the percentage in that age group increased from 25.2 to 48.6% of all AIDS cases, During that same period, the percentage of AIDS cases in older Hispanic men also increased from 13.4 to 20.2%.

As with other aspects of the epidemic, changing modes of transmission represent a dynamic element of the impact of HIV/AIDS on older adults (Zablotaky & Kennedy, 2004). In particular, changes in the modes of transmission of HIV among both older men and women have taken place. The analysis of HIV trends by Mack and Ory (2003) included transmission routes. In their analysis of surveillance data, those men exposed through men having sex with men (MSM) in older age groups decreased between 1990 and 1999. Among men 50-59 years, for example, the proportion exposed from MSM decreased from 35.8 to 35.6%. Injection drug use, heterosexual exposure and unreported exposure all increased during that time. Within the same period, modes of transmission for older women also changed somewhat. Injection drug use had decreased among older women and heterosexual contact had become the primary exposure route for this group (Mack & Ory, 2003).

NATURE OF THE PROBLEM

For all age groups, HIV/AIDS represents a convergence of physical, psychosocial, spiritual and service issues. Because of the focus on evidence-based practice related to social work, the authors have identified three significant psychosocial issues pertinent to older adults and HIV disease for examination. These three issues are stigma, social support and coping. These entities represent issues that are both interrelated and can be addressed through intervention processes.

HIV-Related Stigma

HIV stigma is a ubiquitous phenomenon which the Joint United Nations Programme on HIV/AIDS suggests is "universal, occurring in every country and region of the world" (UNAIDS, 2004, p. 5). Based on the work of Goffman (1963), HIV-related stigma has been defined as prejudice, discounting, discrediting and discrimination directed at people perceived to have HIV or AIDS (Herek, Mitnick & Burris, 1998). Numerous studies have found HIV stigma to be associated with various interpersonal and psychosocial issues such as feelings of shame, guilt, fear and anger (Bennett, 1990; Laryea & Gien, 1993), mental strain (Green & Platt, 1997) and feelings of self-loathing (Bennett, 1990; Herek, 1999; Herek et al., 1998). HIV stigma has also been associated with clinical symptoms of depression and with decreased initiation and continuation of antiretroviral therapy in a variety of HIV infected populations (Crandall & Coleman, 1992; Hall, 1992; Heckman, Kochman & Sikkema, 2002; Laryea & Gien, 1993; Siminoff, Erlen & Lidz, 1991; Swendeman, Comulada, Lee & Rotheram-Borus, 2002). Antidotal reports and case studies have suggested that older adults face increased risk of HIV stigma compared to their younger counterparts (Anderson, 1998; Lavick, 1994; Marr, 1994). Solomon (1996) suggests that older adults may experience stigma more intensely than younger adults due to the fact their contemporaries continue to judge behaviors related to HIV risk as morally wrong. Overall, however, the position of increased stigma with age has been difficult to substantiate empirically as a review of the literature reveals a paucity of stigma-related research including older adults. For example, in studies of HIV stigma done by numerous researchers, older adults were not included (Bennett, 1990; Laryea & Gien, 1993; Green & Platt 1997). Studies that have recruited older persons have, in some instances, eliminated them from the analysis as they were viewed as outliers in the distribution of the sample (McCain & Gramling, 1992).

In a recently completed study, Emlet (in press) compared 44 adults, age 50 and over, living with HIV/AIDS with 44 matched younger adults. The study found a substantial proportion of older adults had significant experiences with HIV stigma. For example, 50% of older adults felt ashamed of their illness or felt people were uncomfortable being with them due to their illness "sometimes" or "often." Nearly 40% of those 50 + reported losing friends due to their HIV, while 34.1% felt people avoided them sometimes or often because of HIV/AIDS. While these percentages are high, the study found no significant differences between younger and older age groups in these domains. In their study of internalized stigma, Lee, Kochman and Sikkema (2002) studied 268 HIV-positive individuals and not only included older adults, but used age as an independent variable in the study. While the number of older people in the sample was not stated, these researchers found no significant difference in internalized HIV stigma. HIV-related stigma is, in fact, a formative psychosocial issue, but the question of older adults experiencing greater stigma than their younger counterparts remains unclear and requires further research.

Social Support

Previous research has consistently demonstrated the importance of social support as a critical resource for older adults adjusting to chronic illness. This protective factor may be true for HIV-infected elders. Heckman and colleagues (2002) suggest that older adults with social support are more likely to receive messages of empathy, encouragement and validation related to their illness and are less likely to engage in unhealthy behaviors such as excessive alcohol use, overeating and high-risk sexual behaviors. Emlet (2005) found the availability of a confidant (affective support) and the availability of instrumental social support to be negatively correlated with HIV stigma in a population of 88 older and younger HIV-infected individuals. Lee and Rotheram-Borus (2001) found that seeking out social support was associated with improved coping and longer survival in a sample of 307 adults (including older adults) in New York City. The growing population of older adults with HIV may not, however, have available the protective effects of support from family members and friends. Studies of older HIV-positive adults found significant levels of unmet need for instrumental and emotional assistance, regardless of the number of people in an individual's social network (Schrimshaw & Siegel, 2003; Shippy & Karpiak, 2005). Nichols' et al. (2002) meta-analysis of survey studies showed that support services are not aimed at the aging HIV population and those who receive marginal social support feel isolated, stigmatized and show a decreased ability to cope with their illness. Heckman and colleagues (2002) reported that older adults with HIV who live alone, receive little support from friends, and have limited access to support services (e.g., therapy, group support, etc.) reported significantly higher rates of anxiety, depression (25% described their depression as "severe") and greater numbers of somatic symptoms than a control group of older adults being treated for psychiatric disorders. In a study of 133 older, HIV-positive adults age 45 and older, Kalichman and colleagues (2000) found decreased social support from friends and family to be associated with thoughts of suicide.

Coping

A third important psychosocial issue for older adults is coping. Lazarus and Folkman's (1984) stress and coping model views stress as a significant person-environment interaction that overwhelms the coping resources of the individual. Various studies have found that those HIV-infected people who engage in active coping strategies report greater quality of life. Fleishman and Fogel (1994) reported that HIV-infected individuals who used positive coping strategies reported fewer depressive symptoms. As mentioned previously, Lee and Rotheram-Borus (2001) found a coping style that involved seeking social support to be associated with increased survival over a period of 28 months in a population of 307 parents living with HIV disease. Simoni and colleagues (2000) found adaptive coping and satisfactory support to be associated with decreased affective symptoms in 103 women of African descent. In their study of 83 older, HIV-infected adults, Heckman et al. (2002) found a significant correlation between engagement coping and social support. In turn, social support was associated with decreased cognitive-affective symptoms.

CONSEQUENCES

If we are to make progress in areas of education, prevention and care of older adults living with HIV/AIDS, we must confront the attitudes and beliefs of the public, service providers and older adults themselves about aging and sexuality. The misconceptions and ageist attitudes infused in our society result in poor prevention efforts, unnecessary infections, delayed diagnoses, misdiagnosis and ultimately, unnecessary deaths. The "invisibility" of this older group, referred to as a hidden population (Emlet, 1997), is illustrated by the perception that older persons are neither "at-risk" for HIV infection nor HIV-infected. Nearly all HIV/AIDS prevention messages and public education programs are targeted toward younger adults, adolescents and children, while older adults are often neglected (Linsk, 2000). It is not surprising that empirical evidence suggests that older persons have more misconceptions about HIV/AIDS and know less about prevention of the disease than their younger counterparts. In a study in Central Florida, Nichols and colleagues (2002) found that over 60% of older respondents had minimal knowledge of behaviors that are associated with risk for HIV exposure. Zablotsky (1998) reported that many older women are completely uninformed about their HIV/AIDS risk. Since many older women associate condom use with birth control, they may not use barrier protection during sex. Condom use in sexually active individuals age 35-59 is markedly less frequent than their younger counterparts, and sexually active individuals over the age of 60 have been found even less likely to use a condom (Anderson, 2003). Linsk (2000) reported that older men, like younger men, often intentionally conceal or deny their sexual orientation, particularly with health-care providers. Consequently, many older adults are more likely to avoid or delay HIV testing, even if they are engaging in high-risk behaviors (Mack & Bland, 1999).

The lack of HIV-related knowledge among older adults is particularly perilous for older adults because HIV-related illnesses mimic symptom profiles of common age-related health problems. The result is often a delayed HIV diagnosis that creates a critical lag in beginning HAART (Highly Active Antiretroviral Therapy) treatment. Older adults who are concurrently diagnosed with HIV/AIDS have a significantly shorter survival rate than younger individuals with the same diagnosis (Inungu, Mokotoff & Kent, 2001). Thus, age-specific information, education and counseling programs are needed to promote physical and mental health among older adults living with HIV/AIDS. Unlike other psychosocial problems faced by older adults, the issue of HIV/AIDS is relatively new and only in the past few years has it become more widely recognized. Since 1986, only five books have been published on the topic of HIV and aging. In addition to these five books, approximately six special issues of peer-reviewed journals devoted solely to the topic have been produced in the past 20 years (Poindexter & Keigher, 2004). Comparatively, a recent search of books in print on the general topic of HIV/AIDS yielded over 2600 hits. While the literature on aging and HIV has grown many times over during this period, it pales compared to the vast literature on this disease in general.

In addition to prevention messages and medical treatment, aging with HIV/AIDS presents unique psychosocial challenges that may be exacerbated by the aging process. Three important areas of psychosocial functioning that this paper will address are: HIV-related stigma, social support and coping.

INTERVENTION RESEARCH
IN OLDER ADULTS WITH HIV DISEASE

The review of the literature that follows suggests a relatively underdeveloped body of research with regard to intervention studies among older adults and HIV disease. It is important to put a context to the topic at hand. Compared to many of the issues aging research has focused on in the past, HIV/AIDS is a relatively new phenomenon. The CDC first published reports of a rare pneumonia affecting gay men in Los Angeles in 1981 and it was not until mid-1982 that this syndrome was named AIDS (Wolf, 2002). The first case of AIDS in an older adult was not documented in the literature until 1986 (Mirra, Anand & Spira, 1986). Because AIDS research often involves recruitment of individuals engaging in hidden, illegal or stigmatized behavior, recruitment can be difficult and may be made more difficult when attempting to include people at the end of the life course (Levy, Holmes & Smith, 2003). It is not surprising that Coon and colleagues (2003) recently reported that the Center for Disease Control and Prevention's Prevention Research Synthesis Project had no study populations with a mean age over 40 years.

REVIEW OF EMPIRICAL STUDIES

The literature review on the topic of psychosocial treatments for older adults living with HIV/AIDS was conducted using specific parameters. Initially, the review was done examining empirical, intervention studies related to HIV stigma, social support or coping in a population of adults age 50 and over with HIV/AIDS. The search was then expanded to include all empirical HIV/AIDS psychosocial intervention studies that focused on, or specifically included, older adults. Those studies that contained older subjects but did not specifically analyze results for this age group were excluded. Whenever possible, older adults were defined as those age 50 years or older. The following databases were surveyed for this literature review: Psycinfo, Pubmed, Cumulative Index of Nursing and Allied Health Literature (CINAHL) and Social Work Abstracts. Articles published between 1990 and 2005 dealing with HIV/AIDS and older adults related to stigma, social support or coping were examined. In addition, personal communication was conducted with one researcher whose research was completed and in press, but not yet published. The vast majority of published articles fell short of the criteria used for inclusion in this review. Many of the published articles consisted of an overview of the topic.

The choice to define "older" or "aging" as 50 or older in HIV/AIDS research has an historical precedent. As previously mentioned, AIDS in an older individual was first documented as a case study in 1986 when a 57-year-old man, diagnosed with Alzheimer's Disease (AD), was found on autopsy to have progressive dementia caused by HTLV-III (the term used at that time for HIV) (Mirra et al., 1986). At that time, the Center for Disease Control (CDC) did not stratify age categories past 50 years in reporting AIDS cases. All individuals who were 50 years or older and diagnosed with AIDS were, thus, categorized together.

While many articles provided empirical data, they did not qualify for review either because they were not intervention studies, they did not include older persons, or provided no specific information on how age impacted the intervention. While numerous empirical studies do exist on older adults and HIV/AIDS, most were not intervention studies and, thus, not appropriate for this review. After all criteria were applied, the literature review yielded three intervention studies related to the three psychosocial issues being examined (see Table 1). Two studies focused on a group intervention for improvement in coping strategies for adults 50 + with HIV/AIDS. The third study described a telephone support group aimed at improving the social support networks of individuals in this same population.

Heckman and his colleagues (2001) reported on a coping improvement group intervention that consisted of 10 face-to-face group sessions, each lasting approximately 75 minutes. Groups consisted of four

TABLE 1. Psychosocial Treatment Studies for Older Adults Living with HIV/AIDS

Author	Population	Psychosocial Focus	N	Treatment	Outcome
Heckman, Kochman, Sikkema, Kalichman, Masten, Bergholte & Catz (2001).	HIV-infected older adults (Mean age 55.4 yrs)	Coping improvement intervention	16	10 face-to-face closed group sessions	Marginally significant changes in ways of coping, including confrontive problem solving and future optimism. Marginal increase in social support and quality of life. Statistically significant increase in social well-being.
Nokes, Chew & Altman (2003)	HIV-infected adults 50 years and older (Mean age 67 yrs)	Increase social support and improve health-related knowledge	5	2 sets of 10 telephone-based open group sessions	Sharing of coping strategies and increased sense of community. All results reported in qualitative terms.
Heckman, Barcikowski, Ogles, Suhr, Carlson, Holroyd & Garske (in press)	HIV-infected adults 50 years and older (Mean age 53.5 and 54.7)	Coping improvement group intervention	90	12 session coping improvement group delivered via teleconference	Decreased psychological symptoms, lower levels of life stress burden and healthier coping. Immediate treatment group reported reduced depressive symptoms from pre-intervention levels.

to six people and were homogenous according to gender and sexual orientation, in order to promote cohesiveness. The groups were kept small to facilitate intervention-related activities, including role-play exercises and sharing personal histories. A closed-group format was chosen, so that once a group was formed, no new members could join. The intervention emphasized the following: the identification of stressors and the decomposition of stressors into more specific issues; the development of problem-focused and emotion-focused coping strategies appropriate for older adults living with HIV; the determination of the fit between the changeability of a stressor and the appropriateness of coping strategies; the optimization of social support; and a focus on stressors particular to HIV-infected older adults, such as longer periods of hospitalization and the presence of comorbid health conditions.

These goals were addressed through the 10 sessions as follows: (1) an introduction intended to build rapport and establish trust; (2) identification of stressors and cognitive appraisal training (participants work through changeable and unchangeable aspects of stressors common to HIV-infected older adults); (3) and (4) problem-focused coping (for example, for individuals with health concerns, a potential coping strategy includes the differentiation of health changes associated with normal aging from those that are AIDS-related); (5) and (6) emotion-focused coping; (7) social support and living with HIV as an older adult (participants discuss ways to expand current social networks using group exercises); (8) obtaining and maintaining social support through HIV serostatus disclosure (participants decide if, how, with whom and under what circumstances to disclose serostatus); (9) hospitalization, treatment concerns and planning of adequate home health-care environments (this training is focused on the development of a specific plan in the event that participants are hospitalized); and (10) a review and group closure. Twelve men and four women living with HIV (with a mean age of 55.4 years of age) were recruited for the study. Participants completed a baseline survey prior to the group sessions and completed an identical one immediately after the last session. The surveys included several measures of coping, stressful life events, quality of life, and social support.

The researchers found that participating in this type of cognitive-behavioral, coping improvement group intervention may enhance coping and adjustment among older adults with HIV. After the 10-session intervention, participants reported higher rates of planful problem-solving, confrontive coping and future optimism. In addition, participants completing CET reported having more support from friends, higher perceptions of social well-being and less stress as a result of AIDS-related loss and health worries.

In the other intervention study, Nokes, Chew and Altman (2003) report on a telephone psychoeducational support group for older, HIV-positive individuals in New York City. This telephone-based intervention was co-facilitated by a social worker and registered nurse. The sessions were 10 weeks in duration and each session was approximately 50-60 minutes long. Participation ranged from one to five clients, with an average participation rate of three individuals. Unlike the previously reported intervention, the group was open and "although regular attendance was encouraged, it was not required" (p. 346). The support group addressed multiple issues including: (1) staying healthy, (2) symptom management, (3) understanding other chronic illnesses, (4) strategies for effective interactions with health-care providers, (5) understanding diagnostic tests, (6) optimizing HIV/AIDS medication use, (7) coping with losses and (8) finding community. A call was made to each participant and once all group members were connected by telephone, the co-facilitators would initiate the session. Group members were encouraged to share phone numbers with each other in order to facilitate contact outside the group.

In the first 10-week session, all five participants were gay men between 62-71 years of age (mean was 67). All men in this group lived alone. The second 10-week group included five older, gay men and one heterosexual female.

The findings from this psychoeducational intervention were reported in qualitative terms. Of particular relevance to the topics discussed in this review, participants voiced the importance of sharing multiple losses. Participants reported that sharing strategies for coping with loss created feelings of connection between them. The researchers indicated that the use of the telephone created some unique challenges as compared to a more traditional support group. For example, nonverbal cues were missing from the interaction and boundaries of respect were more difficult to maintain. Additionally, some group members with hearing impairments did not continue due to those sensory restrictions.

The most recent intervention study was conducted by Heckman and colleagues (in press) and involved a 12-session coping improvement group intervention delivered by teleconference (N = 90). Criteria for inclusion in the study included: (1) being 50 years of age or older; (2) a self-reported diagnosis of HIV infection or AIDS; and (3) a history of a depressive disorder. Subjects were assigned to one of two treatment conditions: the immediate treatment group (n = 44) and the delayed treatment group (n = 46). Each of the group sessions were held weekly and lasted approximately 90 minutes. Separate intervention groups were conducted for men who have sex with men, heterosexual men, and women.

The first two sessions were introductory and designed to develop group cohesion. Session 3 involved the identification of life stressors and sessions 4-6 focused on adaptive problem-focused coping, while sessions 7-9 introduced emotion-focused coping. Sessions 10 and 11 included a discussion of how older adults with HIV/AIDS can increase their social support. Finally, session 12 covered group termination (Heckman et al., in press).

The researchers found that the immediate treatment group reported fewer psychological symptoms, less life stress burden and healthier coping strategies. The same group reported reduced depression symptoms from pre-intervention levels. The delayed treatment group also reported significant reductions in psychological symptoms, life stress and improved coping after treatment was initiated.

TREATMENT SUMMARY AND CONCLUSION

In January of 2006, the first wave of the baby boom generation turned 60. We will begin to "live" the well-documented demographic imperative that has been described for years. Short of the development and wide distribution of an HIV vaccine, older adults and people of all ages will continue to become infected with HIV, and many, regardless of emerging advances in medical technology, will live their later years with HIV disease. Studies have documented that older persons with HIV face unique disadvantages including physical issues of comorbidity and the natural senescence of the immune system (Skeist & Keiser, 1997; Wutoh et al., 2003). Thus, we can expect, for the foreseeable future, growing numbers of older adults living with HIV/AIDS. Social workers and other health professionals must have an increased understanding of the impact of this disease and they also have the opportunity (if not the obligation) to move research to the level of applicable and appropriate interventions.

The literature review conducted for this paper shows the embryonic nature of psychosocial intervention research with older adults related to HIV/AIDS. In planning for the future of this important research agenda, there are a number of considerations of which we must remain mindful. First, ageist assumptions that have contributed to the lack of recruitment of older individuals in HIV intervention studies must be challenged.

Coon and colleagues (2003) remind us that older cohorts have been successfully recruited into health promotion programs, and other papers in this volume speak to the varied success of involving older persons in evidence-based research. Second, at the same time we challenge our own ageist assumptions, it is important to recognize the enormous stigma associated with this disease. Many vulnerable populations, including older people, may identify greater incentives for remaining hidden than risking disclosure and gaining any potential rewards of involvement in research (Levy et al., 2003). Levy and colleagues go on to suggest the importance of designing studies specifically with older adults in mind in order to "recognize the special challenges of conducting AIDS research within the context of human aging" (p. S206). Challenges may include a decreased willingness to disclose (Nokes, Holzemer & Corless, 2000; Emlet, in press), an unwillingness to participate in mental health oriented psychosocial treatments (Coon, Lipman & Ory, 2003) and the potential for physiological impairments such as memory loss and aging or HIV-related cognitive decline (Levy, Holmes & Smith, 2003). Third, two separate groups need to be considered when developing education and intervention strategies: those older persons contracting HIV in old age and those who are aging with HIV (Zablotsky & Kennedy, 2004). Research outcomes, intervention approaches and recruitment efforts will differ dramatically between these two distinct groups.

As we consider developing intervention studies with older persons at-risk for or living with HIV/AIDS, we must not lose sight of the driving purpose. McNeece and Thyer (2004) define evidence-based practice as the "integration of the best research evidence with clinical expertise and client values in making practice decisions" (p. 9). If the underlying purpose is to improve available treatments and services, we must work toward closing gaps between research and practice. This may mean considering alternative ways to disseminate research findings to professional providers and policymakers (Levy et al., 2003).

In conclusion, social work researchers will need to carefully consider how best to integrate older adults into HIV-intervention research, or design age-specific studies in order to create a climate conducive to evidence-based HIV research. At this point in time, there is no indication that the traumatic and devastating physical and psychosocial consequences of HIV/AIDS will change markedly in the near future. We can no longer accept ageist assumptions that older persons are not sexually active, engaging in risky sexual and drug use behaviors, or are immune from being infected with the HIV virus.

TREATMENT RESOURCE APPENDIX

BOOKS

Emlet, C. A. (Ed.). *HIV/AIDS and older adults: Challenges for individuals, families and communities*. New York: Springer Publishers.

Nichols, J. E., Speer, D. C., Watson, B. J., Watson, M. R., Vergon, T. L., Vallee, C. M. & Meah, J. M. (2002). *Aging with HIV: Psychological, social and health issues*. Boston: Academic Press.

Nokes, K. M. (Ed.) (1996). *HIV/AIDS and the older adult*. Bristol, PA: Taylor and Francis.

Poindexter, C. P. & Keigher, S. (Eds.) (2004). *Midlife and older adults and HIV: Implications for social service research, practice and policy*. New York: The Haworth Press.

Riley, M. W., Ory, M. G. & Zablotsky, D. (Eds.) (1989). *AIDS in an aging society: What we need to know*. New York: Springer Publishers.

THEMATIC JOURNAL ISSUES
(in chronological order)

Ory, M. G., Zablotsky, D. & Crystal, S. (Eds.) (1998). HIV/AIDS and aging. Special issue of *Research on Aging, 20*(6).

Emlet, C. A. & Valee, C. (Eds.) (2002). HIV/AIDS in adults 50 and over. Special issue of the *Journal of Mental Health and Aging, 8*(4).

Levy, J. A., Ory, M. G. & Crystal, S. (Eds.) (2003). The graying of the AIDS epidemic: HIV/AIDS and people age 50 and older. Special issues of *Journal of Acquired Immune Deficiency Syndrome, 33*(Supplement 2).

Poindexter, C. C. & Keigher, S. M. (Eds.) (2004). Midlife and older adults and HIV: Implications for social service research, practice and policy. Special issue of *Journal of HIV/AIDS & Social Services, 3*(1).

Stoff, D. M., Khalsa, J., Monjan, A. & Portegies, P. (Eds.) (2004). HIV/AIDS and aging. Special issue of *AIDS, 18*(Supplement 1).

ORGANIZATIONS

***National Association on HIV Over Fifty* (NAHOF)** is an organization whose mission is to promote the availability of a full range of educational, prevention, service and health-care programs for persons over age fifty affected by HIV. Activities include a biannual conference. Information available at: www.hivoverfifty.org

HIV Wisdom for Older Women is an organization dedicated to the prevention of HIV in older women and to life enrichment for those who are infected. Information is available at www.hivwisdom.org

New York Association on HIV Over Fifty is an organization whose purpose is to ensure that the concerns of persons over the age of fifty and their support networks are addressed, and to generate educational, programmatic, and policy initiatives in the field of aging. Information is available at http://www.nyahof.org/mission.htm

OTHER WEB SITES

Senior Action in a Gay Environment (SAGE) provides counseling, support groups and other services to older GLBT individuals including those impacted by HIV/AIDS. Information available at www. sageusa.org

Senior HIV Intervention Project (SHIP) administered through the Broward County Health Department. Broward County, Florida provides peer education and other services to older adults related to HIV/AIDS. Information available at: http://www.browardchd.org/ Services/AIDS/ship.htm

WebMD. This online health information resource provides information specific to older adults who have contracted HIV. Included is information about transmission, infection, and uniqueness in the older population. http://www.webmd.com/content/article/8/1680_50190

REFERENCES

Anderson, G. (1998). Providing services to elderly people with HIV. In Aronstein D.M., Thompson, B.J., eds. *HIV and social work: A practitioner's guide* (pp. 443-450). New York, NY: The Harrington Park Press.

Anderson, J. E. (2003). Condom use and HIV risk among US adults. *American Journal of Public Health, 93*(6), 912-914.

Bennett, M. J. (1990). Stigmatization: Experiences of persons with Acquired Immune Deficiency Syndrome. *Issues in Mental Health Nursing, 11*, 141-154.

Centers for Disease Control and Prevention (2005). *HIV/AIDS Surveillance report 2004*. Vol. 16. Atlanta: Author.

Centers for Disease Control and Prevention (2003b). AIDS cases in adolescents and adults by age–United States, 1994-2000. *HIV/AIDS Surveillance Supplemental Report, 9*(1). Available at: http://www.cdc.gov/hiv/stats/hasrsuppVol9No1.htm .

Coon, D. W., Lipman, P. D. & Ory, M. G. (2003). Designing effective HIV/AIDS social and behavioral interventions for the population of those age 50 and older. *Journal of Acquired Immune Deficiency Syndromes, 33* (Supplement 2), S194-S205.

Crandall, C. S. & Coleman, R. (1992). AIDS-related stigmatization and the disruption of social relationships. *Journal of Social and Personal Relationships, 9*, 163-177.

Emlet, C. A. (in press). A comparison of HIV-stigma and disclosure patterns between older and younger adults living with HIV/AIDS. *AIDS Patient Care and STDs.*

Emlet, C. A. (1997). HIV/AIDS in the elderly: A hidden population. *Home Care Provider, 2*, 69-75.

Emlet, C. A. (2005). Measuring stigma in older and younger adults with HIV/AIDS: An analysis of an HIV stigma scale and initial exploration of subscales. *Research on Social Work Practice, 15*, 291-300.

Fleishman, J. A. & Fogel, B. (1994). Coping and depressive symptoms among people with AIDS. *Health Psychology, 13*, 156-169.

Goffman, E. (1963). *Stigma: Notes on the management of spoiled identity.* Prentice-Hall: Englewood Cliffs.

Green, G. & Platt, S. (1997). Fear and loathing in health care settings reported by people with HIV. *Sociology of Health and Illness, 19*(1), 70-92.

Hall, B. A. (1992). Overcoming stigmatization: Social and personal implications of the Human Immunodeficiency Virus diagnosis. *Archives of Psychiatric Nursing, VI*(3), 189-194.

Heckman, T., Barcikowski, R., Ogles, B., Suhr, J., Carlson, B., Holroyd, K. & Garske, J. (in press). A telephone-delivered coping improvement group intervention for middle-aged and older adults living with HIV/AIDS. *Annals of Behavioral Medicine.*

Heckman, T., Kochman, A., & Sikkema, K. (2002). Depressive symptoms in older adults living with HIV disease: Application of the chronic illness quality of life model. *Journal of Mental Health & Aging, 8*(4), 267-279.

Heckman, T. G., Kochman, A., Sikkema, K. J., Kalichman, S. C., Masten, J. Bergholte, J., & Catz, S. (2001). A pilot coping improvement intervention for late middle-aged and older adults living with HIV/AIDS in the USA. *AIDS Care, 13*(1), 129-139.

Herek, G. M. (1999). AIDS and stigma. *American Behavioral Scientist, 42*(7), 1106-1116.

Herek, G. M., Mitnick, L. & Burris, S. (1998). Workshop report. AIDS and stigma: A conceptual framework and research agenda. *AIDS Public Policy Journal, 13*(1): 36-47.

Inungu, J. N., Mokotoff, E. D. & Kent, J. B. (2001). Characteristics of HIV infection in patients fifty years or older in Michigan. *AIDS Patient Care & STDs, 15*(11), 567-573.

Kalichman, S. C., Heckman, T., Kochman, A., Sikkema, K. & Bergholte, J. (2000). Depression and thoughts of suicide among middle-aged and older persons living with HIV-AIDS. *Psychiatric Services, 51*, 903-907.

Laryea, M. & Gien, L. (1993). The impact of HIV-positive diagnosis on the individual, part 1: Stigma, rejection, and loneliness. *Clinical Nursing Research, 2*(3), 245-266.

Lavick, J. (1994). Psychosocial considerations of HIV infection in the older adult. *AIDS Patient Care* (June), 127-129.

Lazarus, R. S. & Folkman, S. (1984). *Stress, appraisal and coping.* New York: Springer.

Lee, M. & Rotheram-Borus, M. J. (2001). Challenges associated with increased survival among parents living with HIV. *American Journal of Public Health, 91*, 1303-1309.

Lee, R. S., Kochman, A. & Sikkema, K. J. (2002). Internalized stigma among people living with HIV-AIDS. *AIDS and Behavior, 6*, 309-319.

Levy, J. A., Holmes, D. & Smith, M. (2003). Conceptual and methodological issues in research on age and aging. *Journal of Acquired Immune Deficiency Syndromes, 33* (Supplement 2), S206-S217.

Linsk, N. L. (2000). HIV among older adults: Age-specific issues in prevention and treatment. *AIDS Reader, 10*(7), 430-440.

Mack, K. A., & Bland, S.D. (1999). HIV testing behaviors and attitudes regarding HIV/AIDS of adults aged 50-64. *The Gerontologist, 39*, 687-694.

Mack, K.A. & Ory, M. G. (2003). AIDS and older Americans at the end of the 20th century. *Journal of Acquired Immune Deficiency Syndromes, 33*, S68-S75.

Manton, K. G., & Stallard, E. (1998). Forecasting methods for HIV/AIDS and aging. *Research on Aging, 20*, 846-864.

Marr, J. (1994). The impact of HIV on older people: Part 2. *Nursing Standard. 8*(47): 25-27.

McCain, N.L. & Gramling, L. F. (1992). Living with dying: Coping with HIV disease. *Issues in Mental Health Nursing, 13*, 271-284.

McNeese, C. A. & Thyer, B. A. (2004). Evidence-based practice and social work. *Journal of Evidence-Based Social Work, 1*(1), 7-25.

Mirra, S. S., Anand, R. & Spira, T. J. (1986). HTLV-III/LAV infection of the central nervous system in a 57-year-old man with progressive dementia of unknown cause. *The New England Journal of Medicine, 314*(18), 1191-1192.

New York City Department of Health and Mental Hygiene (2005). *HIV Surveillance and Epidemiology Program Quarterly Report, 3*(1). New York: New York City Department of Health and Mental Hygiene. Retrieved March 30, 2005 (http://www.nyc.gov/html/doh/html/pub/pub.html).

Nichols, J. E. (2004). Prevention of HIV disease in older adults. In Emlet C.A. ed. *HIV/AIDS and older adults: Challenges for individuals, families and communities* (pp. 21-35). New York, NY: Springer.

Nichols, J. E., Speer, D., Watson, B., Watson, M., Vergon, T., Vallee, C. & Meah, J. (2002). *Aging with HIV: Psychological, social, and health issues.* San Diego, CA: Academic Press.

Nokes,, K. M., Chew, L. & Altman, C. (2003). Using a telephone support group for HIV-positive persons aged 50 + to increase social support and health-related knowledge. *AIDS Patient Care and STDs, 17*(7), 345-351.

Nokes, K. M., Holzemer, W. L., & Corless, I.B. (2000). Health-related quality of life in persons younger and older than 50 who are living with HIV/AIDS. *Research on Aging, 22*: 290-310.

Ory, M. G. & Mack, K. A. (1998). Middle-aged and older people with AIDS. *Research on Aging, 20*, 653-664.

Poindexter, C. C. & Keigher, S. M. (2004). Inclusion of "older" adults with HIV. *Journal of HIV/AIDS & Social Services, 3*(1), 3-8.

Schrimshaw, E. W. & Siegel, K. (2003). Perceived barriers to social support from family and friends among older adults with HIV/AIDS. *Journal of Health Psychology, 8*, 738-752.

Shippy, R. A. & Karpiak, S. E. (2005). Perceptions of support among older adults with HIV. *Research on Aging, 27*(3), 290-306.

Siminoff, L. A., Erlen, J. A. & Lidz, C. W. (1991). Stigma, AIDS and quality of nursing care: State of the science. *Journal of Advanced Nursing, 16*, 262-269.

Simoni, J. M., Demas, P., Mason, H. R. C., Drossman, J. A. & Davis, M. L. (2000). HIV disclosure among women of African descent: Associations with coping, social support and psychological adaptation. *AIDS and Behavior, 4*, 147-158.

Swendeman, D. T., Comulada, W. S., Lee, M. & Rotheram-Borus, M. J. (2002). *The impact of stigma on the adjustment of young HIV + persons.* Abstract ThPeE7916. Paper presented at the XIV International AIDS Conference, Barcelona Spain. Retrieved December 9, 2002 from http://www.aids2002.com/Home.asp.

Solomon, K. (1996). Psychosocial Issues. In Nokes, K.M., ed. *HIV/AIDS and the older adult* (pp. 33-46). Bristol, PA: Taylor & Francis.

UNAIDS/WHO (December, 2005). *AIDS epidemic update.* Available on: http://www. unaids.org/Epi2005/doc/report.html

Wolf, E. (2002). The HIV time line: 1980-2001. *Journal of HIV/AIDS & Social Services, 1*(1), 11-23.

Wutoh, A. K., Elekwachi, O., Clarke-Tasker, V., Daftary, M., Powell, N. J. & Campusano, G. (2003). Assessment and predictors of antiretroviral adherence in older HIV-infected patients. *Journal of Acquired Immune Deficiency Syndromes, 33*(Supp 2), S106-S114.

Zablotsky, D. L. (1998). Overlooked, ignored and forgotten: Older women at risk for HIV infection and AIDS. *Research on Aging, 20*, 760-766.

Zablotsky, D. & Kennedy, M. (2004). Assessing the progress and promise of research on midlife and older adults and HIV/AIDS. In Emlet, C.A., ed. *HIV/AIDS and older adults: Challenges for individuals, families and communities* (pp. 1-20). New York, NY: Springer.

EVIDENCE-BASED INTERVENTIONS FOR COGNITIVE AND MENTAL HEALTH ISSUES

The following three chapters summarize effective interventions for older adults who are experiencing cognitive or mental health issues in later life. While there are some normative alterations in cognitive functioning (e.g., slowing of reaction time) that occur with age, dementia, depression/anxiety, and substance abuse are not among these. Rather, such conditions represent disease processes that warrant professional intervention. Some of the intervention approaches summarized in these chapters target the older person himself/herself, while others focus on the needs of family members who occupy caregiving roles.

Similar to these conditions in early age periods, late life depression, anxiety, and substance abuse addiction are treatable disorders for older adults. Unfortunately, many older people suffer needlessly from debilitating mental health and addiction disorders because they are undiagnosed or misdiagnosed. Mental health and addiction screening in reasonable contexts (e.g., primary health care, emergency rooms) are important initial steps in helping people receive the support and treatment that they need. A variety of treatments tailored toward the particular needs of older adults have been found effective for reducing the deleterious effects of these illnesses.

Because of the lack of both precise understanding about the cause and effective treatments to stop the disease, Alzheimer's Disease (AD) is one of the most difficult challenges of later life for older adults and their families. The high profile case of Ronald Reagan's progression of the disease has raised awareness of the length of time and the emotional impact that AD renders on individuals and families. While family caregiving is the topic of another chapter in this volume (Chapter 12), effective interventions for the older AD patient himself or herself are reported in this section.

Several types of interventions have demonstrated efficacy for mental health and cognitive issues of later life. Group approaches have been employed for older depressed individuals and those with alcohol addictions. The positive outcomes found include enhanced social support, adherence to treatment protocols for those with addictions, and enhanced communication and behavior for persons with dementia. Similar to earlier life treatment, cognitive behavior therapy has positive outcomes in reducing depression and anxiety, enhancing social participation, and increasing treatment adherence.

Similar to the treatment contexts in the Health Section, social workers and other practitioners employ interventions in a variety of settings. Interventions with persons who have AD can be in community settings, and within long-term care such as nursing homes. Depression and anxiety are mental health challenges that affect both the community-based population, and those who are in long-term care settings. Interventions to decrease these mental health problems should be considered for both of these populations. Substance abuse treatment may also be in a community-based or residential setting. While few addiction facilities currently exist for older adults, treatment programs may have specific groups for people who are in later life.

In summary, three mental health and cognitive issues of later life are presented within this section. While none of these conditions are a normal part of aging, significant numbers of older adults suffer from these conditions. As with younger cohorts, the first step is comprehensive screening and diagnostic process to determine if an older adult is dealing with depression, anxiety, addiction, or dementia. Effective treatment can help affected individuals adhere to their protocols, maintain and enhance a social support network, and improve overall quality of life and functioning.

Chapter 7

Depression and Anxiety

Margaret E. Adamek, PhD
Greta Yoder Slater, PhD

Depression and anxiety are the most common psychiatric conditions in late life. Despite their prevalence, we know relatively little about their unique manifestation in older adults. And, although the most common intervention for late-life depression and anxiety continues to be medication, research on psychosocial interventions for late-life depression and anxiety has burgeoned in the past several years. Unfortunately, this growing body of intervention research has yet to be widely translated into improved systems of care for late-life depression (Callahan, 2001). This chapter is one step toward synthesizing the knowledge in this growing area of research.

PREVALENCE OF LATE-LIFE DEPRESSION AND ANXIETY

According to the U.S. Department of Health and Human Services (USDHHS, 1999), anxiety and depression are the most common mental health diagnoses among older adults (see Table 1). As many as one in five older adults experience mental health problems that are not associated with normal aging (USDHHS, 1999). Estimates of the prevalence of depression and anxiety among older adults vary according to definitions of "older adults," "depression," and "anxiety disorder." Given the varying definitions that have been used, prevalence estimates for late-life depression range from 8-20% of older adults in the community (American Association of Geriatric Psychiatry, 2005, Depression section) and up to 37% of geriatric primary care patients (Garrard et al., 1998; Glasser & Gravdal, 1997). The highest rates–up to 50%–are found among older adults living in long-term care facilities (Adamek,

TABLE 1. Best Estimates of 1 Year Prevalence Rates Based on Epidemiologic Catchment Areas (Ages 55+)

	Prevalence %
Any Anxiety Disorder	11.4
Simple Phobia	7.3
Social Phobia	1.0
Agoraphobia	4.1
Panic Disorder	0.5
Obsessive-Compulsive Disorder	1.5
Any Mood Disorder	4.4
Major Depressive Episode	3.8
Unipolar Major Depression	3.7
Dysthymia	1.6
Bipolar I	0.2
Bipolar II	0.1
Schizophrenia	0.6
Somatization	0.3
Severe Cognitive Impairment	6.6
Any Disorder	19.8

Based on data from DHHS, 1999

2003). The Surgeon General's report on older adult mental health suggests that the prevalence and incidence of major depression tend to decline with age when based on DSM-IV diagnostic criteria, whereas symptom-based assessment studies show increased rates of depression among older adults (USDHHS, 1999). Alexopoulos (2005) reports that both the prevalence and incidence of depression double after age 70-85. In addition to age differences, gender differences are evident: twice as many older women as older men are affected by depression (Alexopoulos, 2005). According to the American Psychiatric Association (2000), the prevalence rates for major depression appear to be unrelated to ethnicity, education, income, or marital status.

Anxiety disorders affect at least one in 10 older adults (USDHHS, 1999), with some estimates reaching 20% (Alwahhabi, 2003). Anxiety disorders involving simple phobias are the most common in late life (AAGP, 2005, Anxiety section). Simple phobia may also be referred to as Generalized Anxiety Disorder (GAD). When anxiety symptoms that do not reach the DSM-IV criteria for a specific disorder are taken into account, prevalence rates among older adults in the community may reach 25% (Wetherell, 1998). As with depression, anxiety disorders tend to affect more women than men (APA, 2000). While one study found no racial differences in prevalence of anxiety disorders in primary care patients ages 18-64 (Brown, Shear, Schulberg, & Madonia, 1999), relatively little is known about racial/ethnic differences in the prevalence of anxiety disorders among older adults. Though not necessarily tied to prevalence rates, Husaini and colleagues (2002) did find some race and gender differences in health-care utilization and costs among older adults with psychiatric diagnoses.

Estimates of the prevalence of depression and anxiety in older adults are complicated not only by definitional issues but also by the fact that these two diagnoses frequently co-occur. Older adults suffering from depression may become anxious; those experiencing anxiety may become depressed. Differential diagnosis is often difficult. Disentangling these symptoms requires the careful attention of professionals with specialized geriatric mental health training. Unfortunately, the supply of well-trained geriatric mental health specialists is not sufficient to meet current needs, let alone the projected demand (Jeste et al., 1999).

A clear understanding of late-life depression and anxiety requires agreement on diagnostic issues. A variety of terms are used in relation to late life depression including *major depressive disorder, geriatric depression, subsyndromal* or *subthreshold depression, minor depression, dysthymia, mixed anxiety and depression, depressed mood, mood disorder*, and *clinical depression*. As specified in the *Diagnostic and Statistical Manual* [DSM-IV (TR)] [American Psychiatric Association (APA), 2000], symptoms of major depressive disorder (MDD) include: depressed mood, loss of interest or pleasure in activities, weight or appetite changes, sleeping disturbances, psychomotor agitation or retardation, low energy level, feelings of worthlessness, difficulty concentrating, and suicidal ideation. Depressed mood and lack of interest are the two core symptoms in late life. One or both of these symptoms and four or more other symptoms must be present for a minimum of two weeks to meet the diagnostic criteria for MDD (Blazer, 2003).

While the DSM-IV criteria for major depression are fairly explicit, there is less clarity in the language describing other, more prevalent, mood disorders (Charney et al., 2003). Most of the depression experienced by older adults is of the minor or subthreshold type. While subthreshold disorders such as minor depression do not meet the full criteria to be listed as mental disorders, they nevertheless may produce clinically significant impairment (Hegel, Stanley, & Areán, 2002). According to Blazer (2003), minor depression in older adults "has been associated with impairment similar to that of major depression including impaired physical functioning, disability days, poorer self-rated health, use of psychotropic drugs, perceived low social support, female gender, and being unmarried" (p. 250). Despite its label, minor depression can be serious for older adults and produce negative outcomes for health and well-being.

As with depression, there are several forms of anxiety disorder that may affect older adults. These include generalized anxiety disorder (GAD), post-traumatic stress disorder (PSTD), social phobia, agoraphobia, panic disorder, and obsessive-compulsive disorder. GAD is the most common type of anxiety disorder (Stanley & Novy, 2000) with prevalence rates ranging from .71% to 7.10% (Mohlman, 2004). Using catchment area data, Blazer et al. (1991 cited in Stanley & Novy, 2000) estimated one month and lifetime prevalence rates for GAD in older adults of 1.9% and 4.6%, respectively, making GAD a significant public health concern (Stanley & Novy, 2000). This chapter focuses on GAD, the most common form of anxiety disorder in late life. A diagnosis of generalized anxiety disorder, according to the DSM-IV (TR) requires:

> excessive anxiety and worry (apprehensive expectation), occurring more days than not for at least 6 months, about a number of events or activities. The person finds it difficult to control the worry. The anxiety and worry are associated with three (or more) of the following six symptoms–restlessness or feeling keyed up or on edge, being easily fatigued, difficulty concentrating or mind going blank, irritability, muscle tension, sleep disturbance. The focus of the anxiety and worry is not confined to features of an Axis I disorder . . . and must cause clinically significant distress or impairment. (APA, 2000)

While there is some similarity in the expression of GAD in younger and older adults, Stanley and Novy (2000) highlight three unique manifestations of GAD in older adults: (1) worry content varies with older adults expressing more worries about health and less about work issues, (2) older adults tend to have a different affective expression of worry, or at least, seem to prefer avoiding terms with psychiatric associations, (3) older adults are more likely to express somatic symptoms rather than cognitive or psychic stressors. An increased likelihood of cognitive de-

TABLE 2. Commonalities Between Late-Life Anxiety and Depression

The following descriptions have been separately stated in the literature about both anxiety and depression in late life:

- Is the most common psychiatric condition in late life
- Is a major public health problem for older adults
- Often goes undetected
- Can be pervasive and chronic in nature
- Often viewed as a normal part of aging so there is a tendency to discount the disorder
- Has a negative impact on quality of life and daily functioning
- Commonly co-occurs with physical illness
- More likely to be presented in primary care than in mental health settings
- Affected older adults tend to emphasize somatic experiences
- An understanding of the disorder as it impacts older adults is lacking
- Most intervention studies are based on younger adults
- Is most often treated with medication
- Psychosocial interventions are underutilized and under-studied
- Rigorous studies of psychosocial interventions are lacking
- Available studies indicate that psychosocial treatment holds promise

cline in older adults and the possibility of attendant depressive symptoms further complicate the diagnosis of GAD in older adults (Stanley & Novy, 2000). Other barriers to successful diagnosis and treatment of late-life anxiety include: a limited understanding of its expression in older adults, the lack of diagnostic tools specifically geared to older adults, and the lack of intervention research focusing on the treatment of GAD in older adults (Alwahhabi, 2003).

THEMES AND NATURE OF THE PROBLEM

Even a cursory review of both literatures, geriatric depression and anxiety disorders in late life, reveals the significant overlap in how these two conditions are described, evaluated, treated, and studied (see Table 2). Both conditions are described as relatively common psychiatric conditions in late life, are frequently misdiagnosed or under-diagnosed and therefore left untreated with significant consequences to older adults, and are most often treated with medication.

Older adults with chronic, disabling illnesses are at particular risk for developing depression and/or anxiety (Hocking & Koenig, 1995; Lenze et al., 2001). For example, elevated rates of depression and/or anxiety have been found in older adults with arthritis (Nadal, 2000), Alzheimer's disease (Lyketsos & Olin, 2002), chronic obstructive pulmonary disease (Rose et al., 2002), dementia (Raicu & Workman, 2000), diabetes (Ciechanowski, Katon, & Russo, 2000), and Parkinson's disease (Cummings & Masterman, 1999; Erickson & Muramatsu, 2004; Zesiewicz, Gold, Chari, & Hauser, 1999). Although the disability and pain often accompanying chronic illnesses may contribute to depression or anxiety, sometimes it is the treatment for the physical ailment that leads to depression or anxiety (Kim, Braun, & Kunik, 2001). Treatments that are invasive, repetitive, time-consuming or painful may exacerbate depression and anxiety symptoms.

Too often, depression is accepted as a natural consequence of the debilitating physical condition rather than as a condition that is amenable to treatment. To the extent that depression and anxiety are consequences of chronic physical illnesses and/or their treatment, it follows that treatments which improve medical outcomes of older adults would, in turn, improve mental health outcomes. Empirical support exists for interventions in the area of physical health. For example, Lenze and colleagues (2001) found that physical disability improved with successful treatment of late-life depression.

A major challenge in addressing late-life anxiety and depression is the tendency to dismiss these conditions as an expected part of growing older. Through "gray-colored lenses" (i.e., viewing late life as full of decline and disability), we too readily accept or tolerate depression and anxiety as a normal part of aging. Unfortunately, health-care professionals often subscribe to this assumption as well. For example, physicians are less likely to offer treatment for depression to older patients and are more likely to consider suicidal thoughts in late life as rational and normal (Uncapher, 2000; Uncapher & Areán, 2000).

CONSEQUENCES OF DEPRESSION AND ANXIETY

The consequences of untreated depression and anxiety for older adults are significant and include: decreased quality of life, increased morbidity, and a shorter life span (Freudenstein et al., 2001). Simply put, older adults with untreated depression and anxiety are less happy, more likely to become ill, and more likely to die prematurely. Creed and colleagues (2002) found a reduced health-related quality of life (HRQoL) among medical inpatients with anxiety and depression. Similarly, in a study involving over 1,300 community-dwelling older adults, Stein and Barrett-Conner (2002) found an association between taking medications for anxiety or depression and a reduced HRQoL. There are also consequences of depression for older adults as a result of excess medical disability and increased use of health services (Karel & Hinrichsen, 2000). In a community-based study of 3,767 older primary care patients, depressive symptoms were associated with twice the level of functional impairment (Callahan et al., 1998). Alexopoulos and colleagues (1996) found that both depression and anxiety in adults 60 and over were significantly associated with instrumental activities of daily living (IADL) impairment. In addition to the diminished quality of life experienced by depressed older adults, studies have demonstrated increased costs associated with the care of patients who also have mood disorders (Creed et al., 2002; Enguidanos & Gibbs, 2005). The direct and indirect costs of depression have been estimated at $43 billion annually (American Association of Geriatric Psychiatry, 2005, Depression section).

Many older adults suffering from untreated depression become suicidal. In fact, over 5,000 adults age 65 and over commit suicide every year in the United States, making them the age group with the highest suicide rates (Adamek & Slater, 2005). Much of the elderly suicide phenomenon is attributed to untreated depression (NIMH, 2006). The good news, according to Steffens (2004), is that "most primary care physicians have come to recognize that depression is highly prevalent, diminishes overall quality of life, and adversely impacts functional status" (p. 30). Unfortunately, the growing recognition of the prevalence and consequences of late-life depression has not been met with the provision of the level of efficacious interventions needed to avoid these consequences. Empirical study of interventions for late-life anxiety and depression is a critical step in promoting efficacious interventions.

REVIEW OF EMPIRICAL LITERATURE

The majority of published studies on interventions for late-life depression and anxiety examine the efficacy of pharmacologic treatments; however, the literature on the effectiveness of psychosocial interventions has grown as well. The empirical literature on interventions for geriatric depression, in particular, has grown enormously in the past several years (Blazer, 2003). Although it is a crude measure, it is interesting to consider the extent of published research on pharmacologic versus psychosocial interventions for late-life depression and anxiety. A search of the entire PubMed database conducted in March 2006 using the search terms "geriatric, depression, clinical trial, and psychotherapy" resulted in 431 hits; a search using "geriatric, depression, clinical trial, and pharmacology" produced 3,306 hits—nearly eight times as many. A similar search replacing "depression" with "anxiety" found 304 hits for psychotherapy and 1,226 hits for pharmacology—over four times as many. Clearly, more research has focused on pharmacologic interventions for late-life depression and anxiety than on psychosocial interventions. Given the increase in the number of studies assessing psychosocial interventions for late-life mental disorders, the research reviewed here focused primarily on meta-analyses that have attempted to characterize the evidence base for psychosocial interventions. Meta-analyses are useful because they summarize key findings across multiple intervention studies. After examining the outcomes of these meta-analyses, a review of individual studies focusing on specific therapeutic approaches for depressed and anxious older adults is provided.

Before proceeding, it is useful to distinguish "efficacy" and "effectiveness" research. According to Fishman (2000), efficacy research involves empirical testing of clinical practice that follows a manualized treatment protocol in which all of the therapeutic goals are clearly defined—preferably based on best practice guidelines for a particular diagnosis—then measured and systematically evaluated. Efficacy research attempts to be as close to laboratory testing as possible with the goal of being a clearly controlled social experiment. Effectiveness research is a practical, patient-centered treatment and research approach that has a more fluid definition of fidelity to the treatment protocol. Fishman asserts that manualized treatment protocols in the strict sense of empirically supported treatments (EST) are designed for high internal validity but may have little generalization to diverse populations or multiple presenting problems and diagnoses. Effectiveness research, by contrast, has high external validity, but low internal validity due to multiple confounding factors, such as patient-chosen goals. Both types of research have their place and can inform our understanding of evidence-based psychosocial interventions for depressed and anxious older adults.

Meta-Analyses Examining Depression Interventions

The meta-analyses selected for inclusion in Tables 3 and 4 were limited to those focused on psychosocial or psychological interventions for older adults (age 50+). The 10 meta-analyses displayed in Table 3 examined dozens of studies of psychosocial interventions for depressed elders. The types of therapies examined included behavioral, cognitive-behavioral, psychodynamic, reminiscence, bibliotherapy, and problem-

TABLE 3. Meta-Analyses of Psychosocial Interventions for Late-Life Depression

AUTHORS	# STUDIES	POPULATION	TYPE OF INTERVENTION	EFFECT SIZE	RESULTS
Scogin & McElreath, 1994	17	Mean age 60+	Behavioral, CBT, psychodynamic, reminiscence, & eclectic	.78	Psychosocial interventions were more effective than no-treatment or placebo in decreasing depressive symptoms in older adults
Koder, Brodaty, & Anstey, 1996	7	Age 65+	CT and CBT	NR	CT is clearly more effective than therapy or placebo; outcomes for younger and older depressives were comparable
Engels & Vermey, 1997	17	"elderly"	CBT, CT, RT, anger expression	.74	Psychological treatment for depression was more effective than placebo or no treatment
Cuijpers, 1998	14	Community elders age 55+	CBT, PST, RT, PDP, and bibliotherapy	.77	CBT was more effective than other psychological treatments
Gerson, Belin, Kaufman, Mintz & Jarvik, 1999	4	Age 55+	CBT, Behavioral, psychodynamic	NR	CBT, behavioral, and psychodynamic therapies are significantly better than placebo
Freudenstein, Jagger, Arthur, & Donner-Banzhoff, 2001	15	Age 60+	CBT, IPT, counseling, social support, drug treatment	NR	Using a flexible treatment approach, a community psychiatric team can lead to considerable improvement in 40-50% of older adults treated
Pinquart & Sorenson, 2001	122	Age 55+ (median)	CBT, control enhancing interventions	NR	CBT had above average effects on depression
Bohlmeijer, Smit, & Cuijpers, 2003	20	"elderly"	RT & Life Review	.84	RT and Life Review are effective treatments for depressive symptoms in older adults
Hsieh & Wang, 2003	9	Age 55+, outside of primary care	RT (individual and group)	NR	RT significantly decreased depression in both individual and group treatment
Frazer, Christensen, & Griffiths, 2005	48	Age 60+	CBT, IT, DBT, RT, PST, PDP, and bibliotherapy	NR	The psychological treatments with the best evidence of effectiveness are CBT, PDP, RT, PST, and bibliotherapy

Note: CT= Cognitive Therapy, CBT= Cognitive Behavioral Therapy, RT= Reminiscence Therapy, DBT= Dialectical Behavior Therapy, PST= Problem-Solving Therapy, PDP= Psychodynamic Psychotherapy, NR= Not reported

TABLE 4. Meta-Analyses of Psychosocial Interventions for Late-Life Anxiety

AUTHORS	# STUDIES	POPULATION	TYPE OF INTERVENTION	RESULTS
Stanley & Novy, 2000	6	N = 246 Age 60+	CBT	CBT, especially relaxation training, is potentially useful for reducing both anxiety and affective symptoms for community older adults
Alwahhabi, 2003	3*	N = 54	CBT	Psychosocial interventions such as CBT should be considered first-line treatments
Nordus & Pallesen, 2003	15	N = 495 X = 69.5 yrs	CBT (individual and group) (4-20 sessions)	Psychosocial interventions were reliably more effective than no treatment
Mohlman, 2004	8	N = 322 Age 55+	CBT (individual and group) ST, Supportive Therapy Discussion Groups	Both individual and group CBT are somewhat effective for treating late-life GAD

Note: *This review included 3 studies of CBT as a treatment for anxiety in older adults; several additional studies were reviewed that evaluated various pharmacologic treatments.

solving therapy. Studies involving both individual and group modalities were investigated.

Four of the meta-analyses on depression interventions reported effect sizes which ranged from .74 to .84, indicating that the interventions had a high degree of success. An effect size of .5 to .7 is considered a medium effect (Becker, 2005). As Becker (2005) explains, an effect size of .8 indicates a non-overlap of 47% in the distributions of the intervention and control groups. An effect size indicates the difference between the progress made by the intervention participants and the control participants. Effect sizes, the "common currency" of meta-analyses, are useful for making comparisons among studies because they provide a measure of the magnitude of the treatment effect that is independent of sample size (Becker, 2005). A brief description of the 10 meta-analyses presented in Table 3 follows.

Scogin and McElreath (1994) examined 17 studies that included both individual and group interventions using cognitive behavioral therapy, behavioral therapy, and psychodynamic therapy. Sample sizes ranged from 16 to 162 and the mean age of study participants ranged from 61.8

to 82.3 years. Based on an effect size of .78, Scogin and McElreath (1994) concluded that all three therapies produced outcomes that were reliably better than no treatment or placebo. They reported equivalent results for all three therapeutic approaches. Meta-analyses conducted by Koder, Brodaty and Anstey (1996) and by Engels and Vermey (1997) similarly reported that cognitive therapies produced outcomes that were reliably better than no treatment or placebo. Koder, Brodaty and Anstey (1996) further reported that the outcomes for older adults with depression were comparable to outcomes with younger adults.

Cuijpers (1998) conducted a meta-analysis of outreach programs offering a variety of psychosocial interventions to depressed older adults in the community. The reported effect size of .77 was taken as an indication of greater efficacy of CBT compared to the seven other types of psychosocial interventions examined. Freudenstein and colleagues (2001) searched for studies published in English, French or German between 1980 and 1999. They were specifically interested in RCTs that examined the effectiveness of psychiatric team care. While they examined 15 studies, only two met all of their inclusion criteria for content and quality. Based on their limited analysis, they concluded, "a flexible approach to the treatment of depression in older people led by a community psychiatric team can lead to the considerable improvement of 40-50% of those treated" (p. 322). Of the 45 studies analyzed by Gerson and colleagues (1999), only four involved psychosocial or "non-drug" therapies. Three of the four studies compared cognitive, behavioral, and psychodynamic therapies, and the fourth compared cognitive and psychodynamic therapies. Gerson et al. limited their review to studies that reported outcomes using the Hamilton Rating Scale for Depression (HAM-D). They found that the groups receiving psychosocial treatment showed significantly greater improvement in HAM-D scores than did the placebo group ($t = .7.94$, df 21, $p = .0001$). There were no significant differences between cognitive behavioral and psychodynamic treatment groups as measured by the HAM-D.

Pinquart and Sorenson (2001) conducted the largest meta-analysis covering 122 studies and reported "above average" effects for CBT on depression. Bohlmeijer, Smit and Cuijpers (2003) focused on interventions that used reminiscence and life review. Their analysis of 20 studies published between 1993 and 2000 resulted in an overall mean effect size of .84, the largest effect size reported by any of the meta-analyses reviewed. Bohlmeijer and colleagues noted that this effect size is comparable to those found for well-established treatments such as CBT and anti-depressants.

Hsieh and Wang (2003) similarly examined studies that evaluated reminiscence therapy as a treatment for depression in older adults. Of the nine RCTs they identified, about half demonstrated statistically significant declines in depression. Finally, Frazer, Christensen and Griffiths (2005) analyzed 48 studies that included seven different psychosocial interventions for late life depression. Using Australia's National Health and Medical Research Council's levels of evidence, they found "sound evidence" of effectiveness for cognitive behavioral therapy, psychodynamic therapy, reminiscence and life review, and bibliotherapy, "some evidence" of effectiveness for interpersonal therapy and problem-solving therapy, and evidence of effectiveness for dialectical behavior therapy when used as an adjunct to drug therapy.

Though not featured in Table 3, two other meta-analyses focused on interventions to *prevent* depression (Cole & Dendukuri, 2004; Jane-Llopis, Hosman, Jenkins, & Anderson, 2003). Cole and Dendukuri (2004) identified 10 studies that evaluated brief interventions for preventing depression among adults age 50 and over. Inclusion criteria included controlled trials of psychosocial interventions lasting less than 12 weeks. "Psychosocial intervention" was broadly defined and included cognitive-behavioral therapy, life review, ego support, bereavement counseling, group therapy, mind/body wellness, as well as health education. Cole and Dendukuri (2004) concluded that brief interventions have the potential to prevent depression in older adults. Though not restricted to programs in the U.S. or programs targeting older adults, Jane-Llopis and colleagues (2003) reviewed 69 depression prevention programs and concluded that, overall, the programs achieved an 11% improvement in depressive symptoms with larger effect sizes for programs that were multi-component, of longer duration (60-90 minute sessions), lasted more than eight sessions, included competence techniques, had a rigorous research design, and were delivered by a healthcare provider in targeted programs.

Meta-Analyses Examining Anxiety Interventions

Psychosocial interventions for anxiety among older adults have received less research attention than interventions for depression. Yet, "given that medication is currently the first-line of treatment for late-life anxiety and that older adults are at increased risk for side effects and drug to drug interactions, identification of effective psychosocial interventions should be made a priority" (Mohlman, 2004, p. 150). As recently as

2000, Sheik and Cassidy decried the lack of "definitive studies regarding the best treatments for anxiety disorders" in older adults (p. 173).

Four meta-analyses examining psychosocial interventions for older adults with anxiety disorder were identified (see Table 4). While the depression meta-analyses date back to 1994, the anxiety meta-analyses have all been conducted since 2000. Only Nordus and Pallesen (2003) reported an effect size; they found an effect size of .55 across 15 studies, or a 35% better result than the controls. The four meta-analyses examined 32 studies (with some overlap), all of which investigated the effect of CBT on anxiety symptoms.

Stanley and Novy (2000) conducted the earliest meta-analysis of psychosocial interventions for late-life anxiety. Their analysis examined six efficacy studies conducted between 1975 and 1992. The psychosocial interventions evaluated through controlled trials included rational emotive therapy, relaxation-meditation, cognitive restructuring, and reminiscence therapy. The mean age of study participants ranged from 63-79 for the six studies. Based on their analyses, Stanley and Novy (2000) concluded that cognitive behavioral therapy and, in particular, relaxation training, produced significant reductions in anxiety symptoms of community-dwelling adults age 60 and over. Alwahhabi (2003) analyzed both pharmacologic and psychosocial interventions for late-life anxiety. All three studies of psychosocial interventions were efficacy studies that involved some form of CBT. Alwahhabi (2003) concluded that CBT is a "promising" treatment for GAD in older adults.

Nordus and Pallesen (2003) conducted the most comprehensive meta-analysis of psychosocial interventions for late-life anxiety. They identified and analyzed 15 outcome studies published between 1975-2002 involving 495 older participants (mean age > 55) and involving a wide range of psychosocial treatments, mostly variants of CBT. Six of the studies evaluated individual treatments and nine evaluated group treatments. Nordus and Pallesen (2003) concluded that psychological interventions were reliably more effective than no treatment as indicated by both self-rated and clinician-rated anxiety measures. They also found that group treatments were as effective as individual treatment for older adults with anxiety.

The most recently published meta-analysis on psychosocial treatments for late-life anxiety was conducted by Mohlman (2004). Mohlman's analysis included eight clinical intervention studies involving three types of group intervention (CBT, supportive therapy, discussion groups) and five studies of individual interventions, all involving some variation of CBT. Six of the studies included community-dwelling adults age 60 and over, one study involved 10 participants referred for treatment of anxiety, and one involved 12 adults undergoing medical care. Mohlman (2004) concluded that both individual and group interventions using CBT were "somewhat effective" for treating late-life GAD (p. 160). In sum, the four meta-analyses of interventions for anxiety indicate that both individual and group psychosocial interventions can be effective in relieving anxiety among older adults.

Meta-Analysis Summary

Given our review of 14 meta-analyses examining dozens of clinical intervention studies with older adults, we affirm that empirical support for psychosocial interventions for late-life anxiety and depression is solid. Other comprehensive reviews of the empirical literature have reached a similar conclusion. Bartels et al. (2002) conducted a thorough review of the literature to determine whether there is an evidence base for treatments in geriatric mental health, covering both pharmacologic and psychosocial interventions. Their review uncovered 26 meta-analyses on geriatric mental health interventions, eight systematic evidence-based reviews, and 12 expert consensus statements. In the area of psychosocial treatment, they concluded that there is a robust literature that shows that CBT works for older adults. Based on their comprehensive review of 45 intervention studies covering both pharmacological and psychological treatments for depression, Gerson and colleagues (1999) concluded:

> Effective psychological interventions constitute a much-needed addition to antidepressant medications for depressed older patients, particularly in light of these patients' high prevalence of medical problems, their use of multiple medications, their increased sensitivity to adverse drug effects, and the many psychological stresses to which they are exposed. (p. 20)

Similarly, Scogin, Welsh, Hanson, Stump, and Coates (2005) reported on 28 studies in their review of psychosocial treatments for late-life depression. While they identified six treatments that met the criteria for being evidence-based (behavioral therapy, cognitive-behavioral therapy, cognitive bibliotherapy, problem-solving therapy, brief psychodynamic therapy, and reminiscence therapy), they also note the lack of studies that match treatment type to client characteristics.

After completing this review of meta-analyses, attention is now turned to a brief discussion of individual studies that examine the effectiveness of specific types of interventions for depressed and anxious older adults. The types of therapeutic approaches reviewed below are those that have received considerable research attention and have garnered a base of evidence-based support.

Cognitive-Behavioral Therapy

The CBT model of intervention has demonstrated effectiveness with depressed elders (Bartels et al., 2002; Dick-Siskin, 2002; Floyd & Scogin, 1998; Gatz et al., 1998; Hawton et al., 1998; Knight & Satre, 1999; Pinquart & Sorenson, 2001; Walker & Clarke, 2001; Wampold et al., 2002) and with depressed family caregivers (Gallagher-Thompson & Steffen, 1994). Using criteria developed by the American Psychological Association, Gatz and colleagues (1998) determined which types of psychological treatments for older adults could be considered empirically validated. They concluded that cognitive and behavioral therapy with depressed elders met the criteria at the level of "probably efficacious." Brief CBT has demonstrated effectiveness with depressed elders as well (Cappeliez, 2001; Leung & Orrell, 1993).

Several studies have established the effectiveness of CBT for clinically anxious elders (Barrowclough et al., 2001; Stanley, Beck, & Glassco, 1996; Walker & Clarke, 2001; Wetherell, 1998). For example, in a study conducted by Barrowclough and colleagues (2001), a CBT treatment group rated themselves significantly less anxious during each of three-, six-, and 12-month follow-up periods than did supportive counseling groups. Stanley and colleagues (1996) administered CBT to small groups of elders for 14 weeks and effects were measured at post-treatment and six-month follow-up periods. They found large reductions in worry and anxiety at both measurement periods. The treatment effects were large and maintained through the six-month follow-up period (Stanley, Beck, & Glassco, 1996). Walker and Clarke (2001) administered CBT for clients with a wide range of mixed anxiety and depression disorders. CBT had demonstrated effectiveness with both groups, but they found a significantly shorter treatment time for elders, due in part to higher attendance rates.

Interpersonal Therapy/Brief Intervention

While there have been fewer clinical studies assessing IPT as a treatment for depression, the available evidence suggests that IPT is effective in reducing depression in older adults, either alone or in combination with medication (Frazer et al., 2005; Hinrichsen, 1999; Mossey, Knott, Higgins, & Talerico, 1996). Areán (2004) provides a description of IPT for late-life depression along with case illustrations, and points out that most of the research on IPT focuses on its use in combination with medication.

Reminiscence Therapy/Life Review

We identified 23 separate clinical studies spanning the past 25 years that examined the impact of RT on late-life depression–nine studies reviewed by Hseih and Wang (2003), 20 studies reviewed by Bohlmeijer, Smit, and Cuijpers (2003) and a recent clinical trial by Wang (2005). All nine studies reviewed by Hsieh and Wang (2003) and 15 of the 20 reviewed by Bohlmeijet et al. (2003) were randomized controlled trials as was the recent Wang (2005) study. While the diversity in study methods in these 23 studies contributed to a range of study outcomes, the overall conclusion from the two meta-analyses and the recent Wang (2005) study was that RT can be effective in decreasing depression among older adults. In a study involving 256 newly relocated nursing home residents, Haight, Michel, and Hendrix (1998) found a life review intervention to be effective at preventing depression. Long-term effects at one year also showed significant decreases in residents' depression.

Combined Intervention

Though the focus of this chapter is on psychosocial interventions, it should be acknowledged that the *Consensus Panel on the Diagnosis and Treatment of Geriatric Depression* (Lebowitz et al., 1997) recommended that the "best practice" is a combined pharmacologic/ psychosocial approach to treatment. Several studies have examined the efficacy of combined pharmacologic and psychosocial interventions. Hollon and colleagues (2005) conducted a meta-analysis to examine the relative efficacy of medication, psychosocial intervention, or a combination of the two approaches for treating adult depression. Their analysis determined that both CBT and IPT can be as effective as pharmacologic intervention in treating depressed outpatients. This finding supports Thompson and colleagues' (2001) conclusion that combined therapies and CBT alone had similar levels of improvement for clients suffering from late-life depression. These therapies demonstrated significant improvement in symptoms when compared to the medication-only treatment group. They concluded that the combination of CBT and medication therapy was the most effective in treating late-life depression, but that CBT could be an effective alternative if the older client does not wish to be medicated. According to Bartels et al. (2002), combined pharmacologic and psychosocial interventions have a synergistic effect in preventing relapse of geriatric mental health conditions.

Other Non-Pharmacologic Treatments

Though the research on other non-pharmacologic interventions for late-life anxiety and depression is less extensive, these approaches deserve mention because they offer another alternative to conventional drug treatment. Christensen, Giffiths and colleagues conducted two meta-analyses that included alternative treatments for depression (Frazer, Christensen, & Griffiths, 2005; Jorm, Christensen, Griffiths, & Rodgers, 2002). They found that the alternative treatments with the best evidence of effectiveness for treating depression in older adults included *bibliotherapy* and *exercise*. Buschmann, Hollinger-Smith, and Peterson-Kokkas (1999) found that *expressive physical touch* was effective in reducing depression among institutionalized older adults. The literature on the role of *activity/exercise* in reducing late-life depression and anxiety has consistently demonstrated a positive impact of exercise on mental health outcomes (e.g., Bragin et al., 2005; Frazer et al., 2005; Herman et al., 2002; McWha, Pachana, & Alpass, 2003; Singh et al., 2005). Physical activity can help in the management of mild-to-moderate mental health conditions, especially depression and anxiety (Paluska & Schwenk, 2000). *Qigong,* a form of Chinese therapeutics involving breathing and mind control exercise, has been found to alleviate older adults' depression (Tsang, Cheung, & Lak, 2002). Taking advantage of today's information superhighway, White and colleagues (2002) at Duke University demonstrated that offering *internet training and access* to older adults can help avoid social isolation and thus reduce depression. The *Eden Alternative*, a paradigm change in the delivery of long-term care, aims to transform institutional settings to make them more homelike by incorporating animals, plants, and children (Thomas, 1996). Numerous studies have demonstrated a reduction in depression among residents of "edenized" facilities (e.g., Bergman-Evans, 2004). Mosher-Ashley and Barrett (1997) provide a description of 11 "alternative therapies" for late-life depression including *horticulture therapy, drama therapy, music therapy, animal-assisted therapy, bibliotherapy,* and *art therapy*. Not surprisingly, many, if not all, of the alternative approaches to depression and anxiety reduction or prevention have a social component. It would be interesting to determine whether the therapeutic approach (e.g., art, drama, music) is the critical element leading to improved mental health or, rather, the social relationships that it takes to deliver the therapy.

Some experts have begun to question whether it is the social aspect of depression interventions that is the key factor in reducing older adults' depression. Wernert (2005) questions the extent to which geriatric depression is a biochemical abnormality versus a lack of psychosocial stimulation. He cites an RCT of 174 patients over age 75 who were treated with anti-depressants for unipolar depression at 15 sites (Roose et al., 2004). The group receiving anti-depressants had a 35% remission rate. Interestingly, the placebo group who received only office visits had a similar remission rate–33%. In explaining why the medication was not more effective than a placebo for treatment of depression among very old patients, Roose et al. (2004) acknowledged that all the patients received considerable psychosocial support through office visits, suggesting that lack of social stimulation was a primary factor in these older adults' depression. In their review of 69 depression prevention programs, Jane-Llopis and colleagues (2003) similarly reported that older adults benefited from social support and not particularly from behavioral interventions. Before summarizing the evidence base for psychosocial interventions for late-life depression and anxiety, it is useful to consider the challenge posed by treatment resistance.

Treatment Resistance

Treatment resistance has been identified as an important factor impacting the effectiveness of treatments for mental health conditions of older adults. Treatment resistance is the tendency of older adults to be fearful, suspicious or disparaging about seeking care for mental health issues (Sirey, Bruce, & Alexopolous, 2005). In recognition of older adults' resistance to treatment, Sirey, Bruce, and Alexopolous (2005) offered an individualized, early intervention program to older adults with major depression to address their attitudes about depression and treatment. They found that older adults participating in the Treatment Initiation Program (TIP) stayed in treatment longer and had better depression outcomes than patients receiving usual care. Yang and Jackson (1998) offer strategies for overcoming barriers to mental health treatment for elders. Their research has found physical, financial, cognitive, emotional, and attitudinal barriers that impede mental health service delivery. They offer many adaptations that can improve use and adherence issues (Yang & Jackson, 1998).

While our understanding of patient resistance issues is growing, there has been little investigation of professionals' resistance to using psycho-social interventions to treat late-life depression and anxiety. Callahan, Dittus and Tierney (1996) point to physician doubts about the potential benefits of treatment for late-life depression as a barrier. In their clinical trial involving 111 primary care physicians, less than half of the patients who had been diagnosed as depressed actually received treatment of any kind. Uncapher and Areán (2000) found that physicians were less likely than psychologists or psychiatrists to offer treatment for depression to older adults, were less optimistic about the recovery of older clients with depression, and were more likely to think of a suicidal elder's hopeless thoughts as rational and logical than the same statement made by a young person. Just over one-quarter (27%) of internists in one study said they would refer a depressed older patient for psychotherapy (Alvidrez & Areán, 2002). These findings are particularly discouraging considering that elders are more likely to seek treatment for medical rather than emotional symptoms (Simon, Von Korff, Piccinelli, Fullerton, & Ormel, 1999; Kroenke, 1997) and are, therefore, more likely to visit a physician than a psychiatrist, psychologist, or social worker.

To better address geriatric mental health concerns presented in primary care settings, Oxman, Dietrich, and Schulberg (2003) recommend having a designated "Depression Care Manager" and a mental health specialist working in collaboration with primary care physicians. The challenge for delivery systems is to find ways to offer a coordinated approach to effectively treat both the physical and mental conditions of older adults with a blend of medical and psychosocial interventions. As part of the IMPACT study, a national randomized controlled trial (RCT) involving 1,801 depressed older adults treated in 18 primary care clinics in five states, Harpole and colleagues (2005) investigated whether the presence of medical illness affected treatment for depression. They found that older adults receiving collaborative care–a multidisciplinary depression intervention–showed a reduction in depression regardless of the presence of medical illnesses (Harpole et al., 2005). Another RCT associated with Project IMPACT likewise demonstrated that a geriatric care management approach that integrated treatment for depression with medical care resulted in improved patient satisfaction, reduced depression, and fewer visits to the hospital or emergency room (Enguidanos & Gibbs, 2005). Though integrated models of geriatric care management are not widespread, these experimental studies demonstrate that successful treatment of both physical illness and accompanying mood disorders is possible. Acknowledging the frequency of depression co-occurring with chronic illness, Hartman-Stein (2005) calls for the routine treatment of geriatric depression as a comorbid condition within geriatric health care.

TREATMENT SUMMARY

As indicated by the review of literature, a variety of psychosocial approaches have been empirically tested for intervention with depressed or anxious elders. These include cognitive-behavioral therapy (CBT), interpersonal therapy (IPT), and reminiscence therapy (RT). According to Areán (2004), two of these psychotherapies meet the APA standard for evidence-based practice: CBT and IPT. The basic premise of each approach is briefly described followed by a summary of the evidence of their effectiveness or efficacy. Readers are referred to the Appendix for resources that provide a full description of treatment protocols.

CBT is the most studied psychosocial intervention for late-life anxiety and depression, and thus the evidence base for this approach is the strongest. There is evidence of CBT's efficacy in relieving late-life anxiety and depression in both individual and group modalities. While there are several variations of cognitive and cognitive-behavioral therapies, the basic premise of this therapeutic strategy is to identify *cognitive distortions* and formulate more realistic alternative thoughts (which then lead to changes in behavior). In short, this approach assumes that thinking and behavior are learned and can be relearned as well. Several prominent experts have written about CBT and the ways that thinking affects behavioral outcomes (Adler, 1963; Beck, 1995; Ellis, 1962). For example, when a person is depressed, frequent thoughts like "I am worthless" come to mind. In reality, the person has worth, so the thinking is considered irrational and the person can work on replacing those negative thoughts with positive, more realistic ones like "I make mistakes sometimes." This process takes training and so CBT therapy often requires exercises outside of the therapy setting to "cognitively restructure" the thinking process.

There are some disagreements among clinicians about whether CBT with elders requires adaptation from the common factors of psychotherapy. For example, Laidlaw (2001) asserts that there is no empirical evidence that substantiates that CBT needs any adaptation to be appropriate for older adults, at least for those without cognitive impairment or frailty. Others, however, assert that there are differences and provide detailed information about how CBT should be practiced with older adults (Knight & Satre, 1999; McInnis-Dittrich, 2002). Koder and colleagues (1996) similarly provide suggestions for how cognitive techniques can be adapted in ways that may benefit older adult clients. Floyd and Scogin (1998) found that the mediational effect of *depressogenic thinking* (i.e., distorted thinking that leads to depressive feelings), as measured by the Dysfunctional Attitudes Scale [DAS], (Beck et al., 1991) was different among elders. Because of this difference between older and younger adults, Floyd and Scogin (1998) recommend an increased need to specifically treat *hopelessness* in older adults. Knight and McCallum (1998) offer a specific model for therapy with elders–the contextual, cohort-based, maturity, specific-challenge model [CCMSC]–in which concepts from gerontology and psychotherapy are intertwined. Knight and Satre (1999) offer particular insights when using CBT with elders who have specific late-life problems such as chronic illness, alcoholism, and insomnia. Their research suggests that although there are important differences between older and younger adults, the similarities often outweigh the differences as the process of psychotherapy unfolds (Knight, 1999; Knight & McCallum, 1998). Knight (1999) also states that the differences are likely due to cohort specifics, context effects, and presenting problems rather than the client's age per se.

Effective practice with depressed and anxious older adults needs to incorporate a manualized treatment approach to CBT in order to reflect the best practices as demonstrated by research and the highest degree of treatment fidelity. While there is not enough evidence regarding practice with older adults, manualized treatment protocols and algorithms will help add to the research knowledge base and help inform our understanding of what works best in treating late-life depression and anxiety. Wetherell (1998) provides a comprehensive list of manuals for psychosocial treatment of anxiety in older adults. It is important that clinicians who work with older adults know what approaches have demonstrated effectiveness and where the gaps are in the treatment literature. Practitioners can help contribute to what is known about the treatment of depression and anxiety in late life.

Less studied psychosocial interventions for late-life depression include Interpersonal Therapy (IPT) and Reminiscence or Life Review Therapy. In Interpersonal Therapy (IPT), the clinician assists the older adult in identifying problems that cause interpersonal or intrapersonal distress. This should not be confused with brief CBT, which focuses on thinking-related distortions and shares the time-limited component of IPT. IPT emphasizes role transitions and conflict, social skills training, and complicated grief (McIntosh et al., 1994). This type of therapy is generally time-limited and focused on tangible, specific problems with current interpersonal relationships. With older adults, four areas are most common: disputes with others, lack of social support, long-term grief following a loss, and difficulty adapting to role changes (Frazer et al., 2005). The evidence base for IPT is not as well-established as that for CBT.

Drawing from Erikson's theory of adult development, reminiscence therapy (RT) aims to assist older adults in reviewing their past as a means to resolving the developmental stage known as ego integrity vs. despair (Hsieh & Wang, 2003). The two meta-analyses that focused on reminiscence interventions for depression found results comparable to the more well-established treatments of CBT and anti-depressant medication. Hsieh and Wang (2003) offer several suggestions for future studies on RT for depressed older adults, including: (1) the use of qualitative approaches to gain a deeper understanding of the impact of RT, (2) analysis of the impact of personal characteristics on the effectiveness of RT, (3) specifying intervention protocols, (4) measuring the impact of RT over time, (5) analyzing the impact on family members, and (6) an investigation of any harmful or negative impacts of RT.

While it is difficult to make comparisons across meta-analyses because of their varying inclusion and exclusion criteria, the overall conclusion of the meta-analyses was that psychosocial interventions are effective in reducing late-life depression and anxiety. Cognitive behavioral therapy is the most often evaluated psychosocial intervention for both depression and anxiety among older adults. Support also exists for the efficacy of other approaches such as reminiscence and psychodynamic therapies in treating depression. Though it is challenging to empirically establish the prevention of negative mental health outcomes, there is some evidence that psychosocial interventions can prevent depression in older adults. No studies were identified that examined the prevention of anxiety symptoms. While the literature on evaluating CBT for late-life anxiety is in a "very early state" (Stanley & Novy, 2000), research evaluating the impact of other psychosocial interventions on late-life anxiety remains sparse.

Given the relative infancy of empirical research on psychosocial interventions in the geriatric mental health arena, few definitive statements about efficacy can be made. There is not yet a sufficient body of comparative empirical literature to conclusively assert which interventions are most efficacious in which settings, using which modalities, with which profile of older adults. Clearly, more research is needed to evaluate and demonstrate the relative efficacy of various psychosocial interventions for the treatment of depression and anxiety in older adults.

CONCLUSION

Empirical evidence has established that psychosocial intervention works with older adults who are depressed or anxious, yet for the most part, psychosocial intervention is not widely used with this population. Is this disconnect simply another instance of the lapse between research being translated into practice, or does the explanation go deeper? Considering that studies demonstrating the efficacy of psychosocial interventions for late-life depression began to appear more than three decades ago, the time lapse explanation does not seem sufficient.

Psychosocial intervention has been thought of as an approach to use when pharmacotherapy does not work (Scogin et al., 2001). Scogin and colleagues (2001) contend that psychosocial treatment can be useful for treating "residual geriatric depression symptoms," meaning those symptoms not relieved by medication. As the barriers to psychosocial intervention are illuminated and better understood, perhaps depression treatment can progress to the point where psychosocial interventions are the primary treatment and psychoactive medications are a second choice strategy. Alwahhabi (2003) makes the same recommendation for the treatment of GAD in older adults.

Despite a growing evidence base demonstrating their efficacy, psychosocial interventions are not often pursued with depressed and anxious older adults. Therefore, future research is needed to elucidate the barriers to implementing psychosocial treatments. Such barriers can be categorized as patient barriers, provider barriers, conceptual barriers, and policy/funding barriers. As discussed earlier, a number of studies have documented treatment resistance among depressed older adults (e.g., Baldwin & Simpson, 1997; Bonner & Howard, 1995; Flint, 1995; Kamholz & Mellow, 1996). Besides patient and provider barriers to using psychosocial interventions, there may also be conceptual barriers as well as barriers stemming from the interrelated issues of policy, funding, and the context of treatment.

In terms of conceptual barriers, the prevailing medical model seems to have inhibited the use of psychosocial interventions. John Wernert

(2005), a geriatrician and President of Indiana Geriatric Associates, suggests that the American health-care system has "a love affair with the disease model." Wernert contends that even dementia is not a disease but more a natural progression of brain aging impacted by such factors as medical illness, genetics, plasticity, and variability. Likewise, much of depression treatment stems from a disease model. Viewing depression primarily as an illness limits our intervention alternatives. A more holistic understanding of the nature of depression in late life is needed.

Many questions remain about the etiology of late-life depression. Undoubtedly, a variety of factors are at play, but which are primary, and which are amenable to intervention? Which interventions are best suited to which older adults? To what extent is diagnosed depression among older adults better identified as apathy? To what extent do medications for physical illness induce apathy? How much of the depression illness burden is created through social neglect? Can social isolation lead to biochemical changes in the brain? These are just a few of the questions yet to be elucidated. While the interplay between physical and mental health has been established, there is much yet to learn. A better understanding of these connections will inform our interventions with depressed and anxious older adults tremendously.

Mohlman (2004) identifies several topics for future research in relation to psychosocial interventions to relieve anxiety among older adults. Those areas include: the impact of spirituality/spiritual interventions, the durability of benefits, the treatment of minority older adults, cognitive versus behavioral treatment, and the effectiveness of interventions with cognitively impaired older adults. These same areas need to be addressed in relation to the treatment of late-life depression. Karel and Hinrichsen (2000) similarly call for additional research on psychological treatment with minority and frail elders. The IMPACT study has demonstrated that an interdisciplinary collaborative care model can effectively treat depression among minority older adults (Areán et al., 2005), and yet relatively few minority elders receive appropriate treatment for depression. Koenig, George, and Peterson (1998) demonstrated an effect of religiosity on remission of depression in hospitalized older adults; few other studies have examined religious belief or spirituality and its impact on mood disorders in late life. Acknowledging the continuing importance of issues of meaning in late life, MacKinlay (2002) suggests that pastoral interventions can alleviate depression and promote mental health.

Clearly, improvements are needed in both the diagnosis and treatment of late-life depression and anxiety. Given the likelihood of anxiety and depression co-occurring in late life–as well as co-morbidity with physical illnesses–a comprehensive assessment of older adults that includes evaluation of physical, cognitive, environmental, and social determinants is critical (Sadavoy & LeClair, 1997). Blazer (1997) calls for differential diagnostic criteria uniquely tailored to older adults' experience of anxiety. The same is needed for accurate assessment of late-life depression. Some conceptual work is being undertaken to better differentiate anxiety and depression in older adults (e.g., Beck et al., 2003). Based on their study of 83 older adults diagnosed with GAD, Beck and colleagues (2003) call for "greater attention to the relative contributions of affect and cognition in differentiating the symptoms of anxiety and depression in older adults" (p. 186). They give several recommendations for future research aimed at differentiating anxiety and depression, including the development of an affect checklist that is specifically geared toward older adults with mood disorders.

Attention must also be paid to older adults' preferences for treatment. Gum and colleagues (2006) demonstrated that a greater proportion of older primary care patients prefer counseling (57%) over medication (43%). Frazer and colleagues (2005) recommend that older adults be offered a range of treatment options including medical, psychological, and life style change/alternative therapies. Bartels similarly (2005) suggests that older adults with mental health disorders be offered a choice between therapy or medication. He further suggests that insurance ought to cover psychosocial interventions. Currently, there is a financial disincentive to offering psychosocial therapy. Medicare recipients have a 20% co-pay for medical interventions including medication, but a 50% co-pay for psychotherapy. To increase the likelihood that psychosocial interventions are available, helping professionals must continue to advocate for mental health parity. Commenting on the fact that public insurance does not cover depression care management strategies in primary care settings despite their reasonable costs, Alexopoulos (2005) contends, "policy needs to catch up with science" (p. 1967).

Policy advocacy is beginning to make some inroads at the national level. In preparation for the 2005 White House Conference on Aging, a Listening Session on Mental Health was held in Washington, DC in January 2005 sponsored by the National Mental Health and Aging Coalition (NCMHA) and hosted by the American Psychological Association (Mays, 2005). NCMHA submitted three broad-ranging resolutions addressing mental health and substance abuse services and interventions, the education and development of the professional mental health work force, and consumer and caregiver issues relevant to mental health and substance abuse among older adults. (For a copy of the entire report, see: http://www.ncmha.org/docs/200501WHCoAresolutions.doc).

The NCMHA was also instrumental in pushing the *President's New Freedom Commission on Mental Health* to address late-life mental health issues. With input from Dr. Steve Bartels, who was invited to be a consultant to the Commission, the Commission has begun an initiative to implement evidence-based practices in geriatric mental health. An expert consensus panel is developing implementation toolkits for geriatric mental health (Bartels, 2005). Also on the national level, the National Institute of Mental Health has established a work group, the *Psychosocial Intervention Development Workgroup*, specifically focused on developing psychosocial interventions for treating depression and bipolar disorder (Hollon et al., 2002). The *Workgroup* recommends the development of new, more effective, and user-friendly interventions that: (1) address functional capacity as well as symptom change, (2) prevent onset and recurrence of clinical episodes, and (3) increase access to evidence-based interventions. These efforts at the policy level must persist in order to be translated into improved delivery systems.

More preventive and creative measures are needed to address the source of older adults' mental distress. While some late-life depression may have medical etiology, we contend that much of late-life depression and anxiety are not diseases but more a logical response to troubling circumstances (e.g., physical disability, loss, social isolation, and institutionalization) affecting some older adults. If we begin to adopt a view of late-life depression and anxiety–at least some proportion–as expressions of older adults' distress stemming from social isolation, multiple losses, and lack of opportunity for meaningful engagement, we will more readily embrace prevention efforts that address these issues.

TREATMENT RESOURCE APPENDIX

Treatment Manuals

Depression in Older Adults: A Guide for Patients and Families
Accessed at:
http://www.psychguides.com/Geriatric%20Depression%20LP%20Guide.pdf.

This publication was drafted by experts in geriatric depression and provides a good overview of late-life depression. It covers symptoms, evaluation protocols, and various treatment modalities. Additional resources and web sites are included.

Barlow, D.H. (2001). *Clinical handbook of psychological disorders: A step-by-step treatment manual* (3rd ed.). New York: Guilford Press.

Dobson, K.S. (Ed.) (2001). *Handbook of cognitive behavioral therapy* (2nd ed.). New York: Guilford Press.

Gorenstein, E.E., Papp, L.A., & Kleber, M.S. (1999). Cognitive behavioral treatment of anxiety in later life. *Cognitive and Behavioral Practice, 6,* 305-319.

Articles/Chapters by Experts

Blazer, D. (2003). Depression in late life: Review and commentary. *Journal of Gerontology, 58A,* 249-265.

Charney, D., Reynolds, C.F., Lewis, L. et al. (2003). Depression and bipolar support alliance concensus statement on the unmet needs in diagnosis and treatment of mood disorders in late life. *Archives of General Psychiatry, 60,* 664-672.

Mohlman, J. (2004). Psychosocial treatment of late-life generalized anxiety disorder: Current status and future directions. *Clinical Psychology Review, 24,* 149-169.

Nordus, I.H., & Pallesen, S. (2003). Psychological treatment of late-life anxiety: An empirical review. *Journal of Consulting and Clinical Psychology, 71,* 643-651.

Websites

American Association for Geriatric Psychiatry
http://www.aagponline.org/programs/default.asp

The association is to promote awareness and provide resources for later-life mental health issues. In addition to information about upcoming conferences and events, there is a section on resources which provides several books and brochures at no cost. Examples are:

- Depression in Late Life: Not a Natural Part of Aging
- Coping with Depression and the Holidays
- A Guide to Mental Wellness in Older Age: Recognizing and Overcoming Depression (A Depression Recovery Toolkit)
- Generalized Anxiety Disorder: Advances in Research and Practice

Mental Health America
http://www.nmha.org

Provides information, resources, and support for people who are experiencing various mental health challenges. Various mental health conditions are presented with information tailored to particular audiences (e.g., families, individuals, professionals). Also included are screenings, links to advocacy and policy issues, and provider contacts.

Geriatric Depression Scale. This site provides an on-line version of the GDS, including scoring.
http://www.psychologynet.org/geriatric.html

National Coalition on Mental Health and Aging

The National Coalition on Mental Health and Aging provides opportunities for professional, consumer and government organizations to work together towards improving the availability and quality of mental health preventive and treatment strategies to older Americans and their families through education, research and increased public awareness. The web site includes a list of members, a directory, and a summary of various political and legislative events that related to aging and mental health. *http://www.ncmha.org/*

National Institute of Aging
http://www.nia.nih.gov

The NIA web site contains a vast array of information on aging. Using the search engine, the latest information on clinical trials and research on depression and anxiety can be accessed.

National Institute of Mental Health
http://www.nimh.nih.gov

The NIMH web site contains information on a variety of mental health issues, treatments, and research studies. Basic information about anxiety and depressive symptoms are included. A link to Pub Med is located on the site and provides a gateway into searching for the latest research on these mental health disorders.

National Mental Health Information Center
http://www.mentalhealth.org/

Provides information and a directory for various mental health conditions, including depression and anxiety.

PsychDirect
www.psychdirect.com

PsychDirect is a public education and information program of the *Department of Psychiatry and Behavioral Neurosciences* at McMaster University in Hamilton, Ontario.
The goals of the program are to: educate about mental health issues, reduce the stigma attached to them, and encourage early detection and early intervention.

REFERENCES

Adamek, M. (2003). Late-life depression in nursing home residents: Social work opportunities to prevent, educate, and alleviate. In B. Berkman & L. Harootyan (Eds.). *Social work and health care in an aging society: Education, policy, practice and research* (pp. 15-47). New York: Springer.

Adamek, M. & Slater, G.Y. (2005). Older adults at risk for suicide. In B. Berkman & S. D'Ambruoso (Eds.). *Handbook of social work in health and aging* (pp. 149-161). New York: Oxford.

Adler, A. (1963). *The practice and theory of individual psychology.* New York: Premier Books.

Alexopoulos, G. (2005). Depression in the elderly. *The Lancet, 365,* 1961-1970.

Alexopoulos, G., Vrontou, C., Kakuma, T., Meyers, B.S., Young, R.C., Klausner, E., & Clarkin, J. (1996). Disability in geriatric depression. *American Journal of Psychiatry, 153,* 877-885.

Alvidrez, J. & Areán, P. (2002). Physician willingness to refer older depressed patients for psychotherapy. *International Journal of Psychiatry in Medicine, 32,* 21-35.

Alwahhabi, F. (2003). Anxiety symptoms and generalized anxiety disorder in the elderly: A review. *Harvard Review of Psychiatry, 11*(4), 180-193.

American Association of Geriatric Psychiatry (2005). *Geriatrics and mental health: The facts.* Retrieved Oct. 30, 2005 from http://www.aagponline.org/prof.facts_mh.asp

American Psychiatric Association (APA) (2000). *Diagnostic & statistical manual of mental disorders (DSM-IV-TR).* Washington, DC: Author.

Areán, P.A. (2004). Psychosocial treatments for depression in the elderly. *Primary Psychiatry, 11*(5), 48-53.

Areán, P.A, Ayalon, L., Hunkeler, E., Lin, E.H., Tang, L., Harpole, B., Hendrie, H., Williams, J.W., & Unutzer, J. (2005). Improving depression care for older minority patients in primary care. *Medical Care, 43,* 381-390.

Areán, P.A. & Cook, B.L. (2002). Psychotherapy and combined psychotherapy/pharmacotherapy for late life depression. *Biological Psychiatry, 52*(3), 293-303.

Baldwin, R.C. & Simpson, S. (1997). Treatment resistant depression in the elderly: A review of its conceptualisation, management and relationship to organic brain disease. *Journal of Affective Disorders. Special Ageing, 46*(3), 163-173.

Barrowclough, C., King, P., Colville, J., Russell, E., Burns, A., & Tarrier, N. (2001). A randomized trial of the effectiveness of cognitive-behavioral therapy and supportive counselling for anxiety symptoms in older adults. *Journal of Consulting and Clinical Psychology, 69*(5), 756-762.

Bartels, S. (2005, June). Toward a comprehensive and effective system of care: Evidence-based mental health services for older adults. *Second Annual Indiana Mental Health and Aging Conference,* Indianapolis, IN.

Bartels, S., Dums, A., Oxman, T., Schneider, L., Areán, P., Alexopoulous, G., & Jeste, D. (2002). Evidence-based practices in geriatric mental health care. *Psychiatric Services, 53*(11), 1419-1431.

Beck, A. (1995). *Cognitive therapy: The basics and beyond.* New York: Guilford Press.

Beck. J.G., Novy, D.M., Diefenbach, G.J., Stanley, M.A., Averill, P.M., & Swann, A.C. (2003). Differentiating anxiety and depression in older adults with Generalized Anxiety Disorder. *Psychological Assessment, 15,* 184-192.

Becker, L. (2005). Effect size. Retrieved 10/30/05 from http://web.uccs.edu/ lbecker/Psy590/es.htm

Bergman-Evans, B. (2004). Beyond the basics: Effects of the Eden Alternative model on quality of life issues. *Journal of Gerontological Nursing, 30,* 27-34.

Blazer, D.G. (1997). Generalized anxiety disorder and panic disorder in the elderly: A review. *Harvard Review of Psychiatry, 5*(1), 18-27.

Blazer, D.G. (2003). Depression in late life: Review and commentary. *Journals of Gerontology: Series A: Biological Sciences and Medical Sciences, 58A*(3), 249-265.

Bohlmeijer, E., Smit, F., & Cuijpers, P. (2003). Effects of reminiscence and life review on late-life depression: A meta-analysis. *International Journal of Geriatric Psychiatry, 18*(12), 1088-1094.

Bonner, D. & Howard, R. (1995). Treatment resistant depression in the elderly. *International Journal of Geriatric Psychiatry, 10*(4), 259-264.

Bragin, V., Chemodanova, M., Dzhafarova, N., Bragin, I., Czerniawski, J., & Aliev, G. (2005). Integrated treatment approach improves cognitive function in demented and clinically depressed patients. *American Journal of Alzheimer's Disease and Other Dementias, 20,* 21-26.

Brown, C., Schear, M.K., Schulberg, H.C., & Madonia, M.J. (1999). Anxiety disorders among African American and White primary medical care patients. *Psychiatric Services, 50,* 407-409.

Buschmann, M.T., Hollinger-Smith, L.M., & Peterson-Kokkas, S.E. (1999). Implementation of expressive physical touch in depressed older adults. *Journal of Clinical Geropsychology, 5,* 291-300.

Callahan, C.M. (2001). Quality improvement research on late life depression in primary care. *Medical Care, 39,* 756-759.

Callahan, C.M., Dittus, R.S., & Tierney, W.M. (1996). Primary care physicians' medical decision making for late-life depression. *Journal of General Internal Medicine, 11,* 218-225.

Callahan, C.M., Wolinsky, F.D., Stump, T.E., Nienaber, N.A., Hui, S.L., & Tierney, W.M. (1998). Mortality, symptoms, and functional impairment in late-life depression. *Journal of General Internal Medicine, 13,* 746-752.

Cappeliez, P. (2001). Presentation of depression and response to group cognitive therapy with older adults. *Journal of Clinical Geropsychology, 6*(3), 165-174.

Charney, D., Reynolds, C.F., Lewis, L. et al. (2003). Depression and bipolar support alliance concensus statement on the unmet needs in diagnosis and treatment of mood disorders in late life. *Archives of General Psychiatry, 60,* 664-672.

Ciechanowski, P.S., Katon, W.J., & Russo, J.E. (2000). Depression and diabetes: Impact of depressive symptoms on adherence, function, and costs. *Archives of Internal Medicine, 160,* 3278-3285.

Cole, M.G. & Dendukuri, N. (2004). Feasibility and effectiveness of brief interventions to prevent depression in older subjects: A systematic review. *International Journal of Geriatric Psychiatry, 19,* 1019-102.

Creed, F., Morgan, R., Fiddler, M., Marshall, S., Guthrie, E., & House, A. (2002). Depression and anxiety impair health-related quality of life and are associated with increased costs in general medical inpatients. *Psychosomatics: Journal of Consultation Liaison Psychiatry, 43,* 302-309.

Cuijpers, P. (1998). Psychological outreach programmes for the depressed elderly: A meta-analysis of effects and dropout. *International Journal of Geriatric Psychiatry, 13,* 41-48.

Cummings, J.L., & Masterman, D.L. (1999). Depression in patients with Parkinson's disease. *International Journal of Geriatric Psychiatry, 14*(9), 711-718.

Dick-Siskin, L.P. (2002). Cognitive-behavioral therapy with older adults. *Behavior Therapist, 25*(1), 3-6.

Ellis, A. (1962). *Reason and emotion in psychotherapy.* New York: Stuart.

Engels, G.I. & Vermey, M. (1997). Efficacy of nonmedical treatments of depression in elders: A quantitative analysis. *Journal of Clinical Geropsychology, 3,* 17-35.

Enguidanos, S. & Gibbs, N. (2005, November). Treating depression among older adults through care management: Results from an evidence-based intervention. *The 58th Annual Scientific Meeting of the Gerontological Society of America,* Orlando, FL.

Erickson, C.L. & Muramatsu, N. (2004). Parkinson's disease, depression, and medication adherence: Current knowledge and social work practice. *Journal of Gerontological Social Work, 42,* 3-18.

Fishman, D. (2000). Transcending the efficacy versus effectiveness debate: Proposal for a new, electronic 'Journal of Pragmatic Case Studies.' *Prevention & Teatment, 3,* 8 (http://journals.apa.org/prevention/volume3/pre0030008a.html retrieved on 6/10/03 from the world wide web).

Flint, A.J. (1995). Augmentation strategies in geriatric depression. *International Journal of Geriatric Psychiatry, 10*(2), 137-146.

Floyd, M. & Scogin, F. (1998). Cognitive-behavior therapy for older adults: How does it work? *Psychotherapy, 35*(4), 459-463.

Frazer, C.J., Christensen, H., & Griffiths, K.M. (2005). Effectiveness of treatments for depression in older people. *Medical Journal of Australia, 182,* 627-632.

Freudenstein, U., Jagger, C., Arthur, A., & Donner-Banzhoff, N. (2001). Treatments for late life depression in primary care–a systematic review. *Family Practice, 18*(3), 321-327.

Gallagher-Thompson, D. & Steffen, A.M. (1994). Comparative effects of cognitive-behavioral and brief psychodynamic therapies for depressed family caregivers. *Journal of Consulting and Clinical Psychology, 62*(3), 543-549.

Garrard, J., Rolnick, S.J., Nitz, N.M., Luepke, L., Jackson, J., Fischer, L.R. et al. (1998). Clinical detection of depression in community-based elderly people with self-reported symptoms of depression. *Journal of Gerontology: Medical Sciences, 53A,* M92-M101.

Gatz, M., Fiske, A., Fox, L.S., Kaskie, B., Kasl-Godley, J.E., McCallum, T.J et al. (1998). Empirically validated psychological treatments for older adults. *Journal of Mental Health & Aging, 4,* 9-46.

Gerson, S., Belin, T.R., Kaufman, A., Mintz, J., & Jarvik, L. (1999). Pharmacological and psychological treatments for depressed older patients: A meta-analysis and overview of recent findings. *Harvard Review of Psychiatry, 7,* 1-28.

Glasser, M. & Gravdal, J.A. (1997). Assessment and treatment of geriatric depression in primary care settings. *Archives of Family Medicine, 6,* 433-438.

Gum, A.M., Areán, P.A., Hunkeler, E., Tang, L., Katon, W., Hitchcock, P., Steffens, D.C., Dickens, J., & Unützer, J. (2006). Depression treatment preferences in older primary care patients. *The Gerontologist, 46,* 14-22.

Haight, B.K., Michel, Y., & Hendrix, S. (1998). Life review: Preventing despair in newly relocated nursing home residents. *International Journal of Aging & Human Development, 47,* 119-142.

Harpole, L.H., Williams, J.W., Olsen, M.K., Stechuchak, K.M., Oddone, E., Callahan, C.M. et al. (2005). Improving depression outcomes in older adults with cormorbid medical illness. *General Hospital Psychiatry, 27,* 4-12.

Hartman-Stein, P.E. (2005). An impressive step in identifying evidence-based psychotherapies for geriatric depression. *Clinical Psychology: Science and Practice, 12,* 283-241.

Hawton, K., Arensman, E., Townsend, E., Bremner, S., Fledman, E., Goldney, R. et al. (1998). Deliberate self-harm: Systematic review of efficacy of psychosocial and pharmacological treatments in preventing repetition. *British Medical Journal, 317,* 441-447.

Hegel, M.T., Stanley, M.A., & Areán, P.E. (2002). Minor depression and 'subthreshold' anxiety symptoms in older adults: Psychosocial therapies and special considerations. *Generations, 26,* 44-49.

Herman, S., Blumenthal, J.A., Babyak, M., Khatri, P., Craighead, W.E., Krishnana, K.R. et al. (2002). Exercise therapy for depression in middle-aged and older adults: Predictors of early dropout and treatment failure. *Health Psychology, 21,* 553-563.

Hinrichsen, G. A. (1999). Treating older adults with interpersonal psychotherapy for depression. *Journal of Clinical Psychology, 55*(8), 949-960.

Hocking, L.B. & Koenig, H.G. (1995). Anxiety in medically ill older patients: A review and update. *International Journal of Psychiatry in Medicine, 25*(3), 221-238.

Hollon, S.D., Jarrett, R.B., Nierenber, A.A., Thase, M.E., Trivedi, M., & Rush, A.J. (2005). Psychotherapy and medication in the treatment of adult and geriatric depression: Which monotherapy or combined treatment? *Journal of Clinical Psychiatry, 66,* 455-468.

Hollon, S.D., Munoz, R.F., Barlow, D.H., Beardslee, W.R., Bell, C.C., Bernal, G. et al. (2002). Psychosocial intervention development for the prevention and treatment of depression: Promoting innovation and increasing access. *Biological Psychiatry, 52,* 610-630.

Hsieh, H. & Wang, J. (2003). Effect of reminiscence therapy on depression in older adults: A systematic review. *International Journal of Nursing Studies, 40,* 335-345.

Husaini, B.A., Sherkat, D.E., Levine, R., Bragg, R., Holzer, C., Anderson, K., Cain, V., & Moten, C. (2002). Race, gender, and health care utilization and costs among Medicare elderly with psychiatric diagnoses. *Journal of Aging & Health, 14,* 79-95.

Jane-Llopis, E., Hosman, C., Jenkins, R., & Anderson, P. (2003). Predictors of efficacy in depression prevention programmes: Meta-analysis. *British Journal of Psychiatry, 183,* 384-397.

Jeste, D.V., Alexopoulos, G.S., Bartels, S.J., Cummings, J.L., Gallo, J.J., Gottlieb, G.L. et al. (1999). Consensus statement on the upcoming crisis in geriatric mental health. *Archives of General Psychiatry, 56,* 848-853.

Jorm, A.F., Christensen, H., Griffiths, K.M., & Rodgers, B. (2002). Effectiveness of complementary and self-help treatment for depression. *Medical Journal of Australia, 176,* 584-596.

Kamholz, B.A., & Mellow, A.M. (1996). Management of treatment resistance in the depressed geriatric patient. *Psychiatric Clinics of North America, 19*(2), 269-286.

Karel, M.J. & Hinrichsen, G. (2000). Treatment of depression in late life: Psychotherapeutic interventions. *Clinical Psychology Review, 23,* 707-729.

Kim, H.F., Braun, U., & Kunik, M.E. (2001). Anxiety and depression in medically ill older adults. *Journal of Clinical Geropsychology, 7,* 117-130.

Knight, B.G. (1999). The scientific basis for psychotherapeutic interventions with older adults: An overview. *Journal of Clinical Psychology, 55* (8), 927-934.

Knight, B.G. & McCallum, T.J. (1998). Adapting psychotherapeutic practice for older clients: Implications of the contextual, cohort-based, maturity, specific-challenge model. *Professional Psychology: Research and Practice, 29* (1), 15-22.

Knight, B.G. & Satre, D.D. (1999). Cognitive behavioral psychotherapy with older adults. *Clinical Psychology: Science and Practice, 62*(2), 188-203.

Koder, D.A., Brodaty, H., & Anstey, K.J. (1996). Cognitive therapy for depression in the elderly. *International Journal of Geriatric Psychiatry, 11*(2), 97-107.

Koenig, H.G., George, L.K., & Peterson, B.L. (1998). Religiosity and remission of depression in medically ill older patients. *The American Journal of Psychiatry, 155,* 536-542.

Kroenke, K. (1997). Discovering depression in medical patients: Reasonable expectations. *Annals of Internal Medicine, 126,* 463-465.

Laidlaw, K. (2001). Empirical review of cognitive therapy for late life depression: Does research evidence suggest adaptations are necessary for cognitive therapy with older adults? *Clinical Psychology and Psychotherapy, 8,* 1-14.

Lebowitz, B.D., Pearson, J.L., Schneider, L.S., Reynolds, C.F., III, Alexopoulos, G.S., Bruce, M.L. et al. (1997). Diagnosis and treatment of depression in late life: Consensus statement update. *Journal of the American Medical Association, 278*(14), 1186-1190.

Lenze, E. J., Rogers, J.C., Martire, L.M., Mulsant, B.H., Rollman, B.L., Dew, M.A. et al. (2001). Association of late-life depression and anxiety with physical disability: A review of the literature and prospectus for future research. *American Journal of Geriatric Psychiatry, 9*(2), 113-135.

Leung, S.N. & Orrell, M.W. (1993). A brief cognitive behavioural therapy group for the elderly: Who benefits? *International Journal of Geriatric Psychiatry, 8*(7), 593-598.

Lyketsos, C.G. & Olin, J. (2002). Depression in Alzheimer's disease: Overview and treatment. *Biological Psychiatry, 52,* 243-252.

MacKinlay, E. (2002). Mental health and spirituality in later life: Pastoral approaches. *Journal of Religious Gerontology, 13,* 129-147.

Mays, W. (2005, June). Resolution on mental health and substance abuse services and interventions. *Second Annual Indiana Mental Health and Aging Conference,* Indianapolis, IN.

McInnis-Dittrich, K. (2002). *Social work with elders: A biopsychosocial approach to assessment and intervention.* Boston: Allyn & Bacon.

McIntosh, J.L., Santos, J.F., Hubbard, R.W., & Overholser, J.C. (1994). *Elder suicide: Research, theory, and treatment.* Washington, DC: American Psychological Association.

McWha, J.L., Pachana, N.A., & Alpass, F. (2003). Exploring the therapeutic environment for older women with late-life depression: An examination of the benefits of an activity group for older people suffering from depression. *Australian Occupational Therapy, 50,* 158-169.

Mohlman, J. (2004). Psychosocial treatment of late-life generalized anxiety disorder: Current status and future directions. *Clinical Psychology Review, 24*(2), 149-169.

Mosher-Ashley, P.M. & Barrett, P.W. (1997). *Life worth living: Practical strategies for reducing depression in older adults.* Baltimore, MD: Health Professions Press.

Mossey, J.M., Knott, K.A., Higgins, M., & Talerico, K. (1996). Effectiveness of a psychosocial intervention, interpersonal counselling, for subdysthymic depression in medically ill elderly. *Journal of Gerontology: Biological Sciences, Medical Sciences, 51,* 172-178.

Nadal, M. (2000). *Program design to ameliorate learned helplessness and depression in the elderly with arthritis.* UMI Dissertation Services, ProQuest Information and Learning, Ann Arbor, MI. 2000.

National Institute of Mental Health (2006). *Older adults: Depression and suicide facts.* Retrieved 3/20/06 from http://www.nimh.nih.gov/publicat/elderlydepsuicide.cfm

Nordus, I.H. & Pallesen, S. (2003). Psychological treatment of late life anxiety: An empirical review. *Journal of Consulting and Clinical Psychology, 71,* 643-651.

Oxman, T.E., Dietrich, A.J., & Schulberg, H.C. (2003). The Depression Care Manager and Mental Health Specialist as collaborators within primary care. *American Journal of Geriatric Psychiatry, 11*(5), 507-516.

Paluska, S.A., & Schwenk, T.L. (2000). Physical activity and mental health: Current concepts. *Sports Medicine, 29,* 167-180.

Pinquart, M. & Sorenson, S. (2001). How effective are psychotherapeutic and other psychosocial interventions with older adults? A meta-analysis. *Journal of Mental Health & Aging, 7,* 207-243.

Raicu, R.G. & Workman, R.H., Jr. (2000). Management of psychotic and depressive features in patients with vascular dementia. *Topics in Stroke Rehabilitation, 7*(3), 11-19.

Roose, S.P., Sackeim H.A., Krishnan, K.R., Pollock, B.G., Alexopoulos, G., Lavretsky, H. et al. (2004). Antidepressant pharmacotherapy in the treatment of depression in the very old: A randomized, placebo-controlled trial. *American Journal of Psychiatry, 161,* 2050-2059.

Rose, C., Wallace, L., Dickson, R., Ayres, J., Lehman, R., Searle, Y. et al. (2002). The most effective psychologically-based treatments to reduce anxiety and panic in patients with chronic obstructive pulmonary disease (COPD): A systematic review. *Patient Education & Counseling, 47,* 311-318.

Sadavoy, M. & LeClair, J.K. (1997). Treatment of anxiety disorders in late life. *Canadian Journal of Psychiatry, 42,* 28S-34S.

Scogin, F. & McElreath, L. (1994). Efficacy of psychosocial treatments for geriatric depression: A quantitative review. *Journal of Consulting and Clinical Psychology, 62,* 69-74.

Scogin, F., Shackelford, J., Rohen, N., Stump, J., Floyd, M.,, McKendree-Smith, N. et al. (2001). Residual geriatric depression symptoms: A place for psychotherapy. *Journal of Clinical Geropsychology, 7,* 271-283.

Scogin, F., Welsh, D., Hanson, A., Stump, J., & Coates, A. (2005). Evidence-based psychotherapies for depression in older adults. *Clinical Psychology: Science & Practice, 12,* 222-237.

Sheikh, J.I. & Cassidy, E.L. (2000). Treatment of anxiety disorders in the elderly: Issues and strategies. *Journal of Anxiety Disorders, 14*(2), 173.

Simon, G.E., Von Koroff, M., Piccinelli, M., Fullerton, C., & Ormel, J. (1999). An international study of the relations between somatic symptoms and depression. *New England Journal of Medicine, 341,* 1329-1335.

Singh, N.A., Stavrinos, T.M., Scarbek, Y., Galambos, G., Liber, C., & Fiatarone Singh, M.A. (2005). A randomized controlled trial of high versus low intensity weight training versus general practitioner care for clinical depression in older adults. *Journal of Gerontology: Biological Sciences, Medical Sciences, 60,* 768-776.

Sirey, J.A., Bruce, M.L., & Alexopoulos, G.S. (2005). The Treatment Initiation Program: An intervention to improve depression outcomes in older adults. *American Journal of Psychiatry, 162,* 184-186.

Stanley, M.A., Beck, J.G., & Glassco, J.D. (1996). Treatment of generalized anxiety in older adults: A preliminary comparison of cognitive-behavioral and supportive approaches. *Behavior Therapy, 27*(4), 565-581.

Stanley, M.A. & Novy, D.M. (2000). Cognitive-behavior therapy for generalized anxiety in late life: An evaluative overview. *Journal of Anxiety Disorders, 14*(2), 191-207.

Steffens, D.C. (2004). Depression in the elderly: A timely update. *Primary Psychiatry, 11,* 30.

Stein, M.B. & Barrett-Connor, E. (2002). Quality of life in older adults receiving medications for anxiety, depression, or insomnia: Findings from a community-based study. *American Journal of Geriatric Psychiatry, 10,* 568-574.

Thomas, W. (1996). *Life worth living: How someone you love can still enjoy life in a nursing home–The Eden Alternative in action.* Acton, MA: VanderWyk & Burnham.

Thompson, L., Coon, D.W., Gallagher-Thompson, D., Sommer, B.R., & Koin, D. (2001). Comparison of desipramine and cognitive-behavioral therapy in the treatment of elderly outpatients with mild-to-moderate depression. *American Journal of Geriatric Psychiatry, 9*(3), 225-240.

Tsang, H.W.H., Cheung, L., & Lak, D.C.C. (2002). Qigong as a psychosocial intervention for depressed elderly with chronic physical illnesses. *International Journal of Geriatric Psychiatry, 17*(12), 1146-1154.

Uncapher, H. (2000). Physicians less likely to offer depression therapy to older suicidal patients than to younger ones. *Geriatrics, 55*(4). 82.

Uncapher, H. & Areán, P.A. (2000). Physicians are less willing to treat suicidal ideation in older patients. *Journal of the American Geriatrics Society, 48,* 188-192.

U.S. Department of Health and Human Services (1999). *Mental health: A report of the surgeon general–Executive summary.* Rockville, MD: US DHHS.

Walker, D.A. & Clarke, M. (2001). Cognitive-behavioral psychotherapy: A comparison between younger and older adults in two inner city mental health teams. *Aging and Mental Health, 5*(2), 197-199.

Wampold, B., Minami, T., Baskin, T., & Callen Tierney, S. (2002). A meta-(re)analysis of the effects of cognitive therapy versus 'other therapies for depression.' *Journal of Affective Disorders, 68,* 159-165.

Wang, J.J. (2005). The effects of reminiscence on depressive symptoms and mood status of older institutionalized adults in Taiwan. *International Journal of Geriatric Psychiatry, 20*(1), 57-62.

Wernert, J. (2005, June). Challenges of the aging brain. *Second Annual Indiana Mental Health and Aging Conference,* Indianapolis, IN.

Wetherell, J.L. (1998). Treatment of anxiety in older adults. *Psychotherapy, 35,* 444-458.

White, H., McConnell, E., Clipp, E., Branch, L.G., Sloane, R., Pieper, C. et al. (2002). A randomized controlled trial of the psychosocial impact of providing internet training and access to older adults. *Aging & Mental Health, 6,* 213-221.

Yang, J.A. & Jackson, C.L. (1998). Overcoming obstacles in providing mental health treatment to older adults: Getting in the door. *Psychotherapy, 35*(4), 498-505.

Zesiewicz, T.A., Gold, M., Chari, G., & Hauser, R.A. (1999). Current issues in depression in Parkinson's disease. *American Journal of Geriatric Psychiatry, 7*(2), 110-118.

Chapter 8

Alzheimer's Disease and Related Dementias

Sara Sanders, PhD
Carmen Morano, PhD

Hearing the words "dementia" or "Alzheimer's disease" (AD) is a dreaded event for older adults and their support systems. These words carry a life sentence of progressive loss in cognitive functioning and an increasing dependence on others. Unlike some other chronic, age-related health conditions, there is no cure for dementia. Thus, the sense of hopelessness that is felt by these individuals and their familial care-givers may seem insurmountable.

Recognition of memory loss as a disease process rather than a normal part of aging occurred at the beginning of the 20th century. In 1907, German psychiatrist Alois Alzheimer identified the symptoms of dementia, specifically AD, in a young woman named Augusta D. Dr. Alzheimer found that certain composites developed in the brains of individuals who suffered from symptoms of progressive memory loss, but were not seen in the other psychiatric patients he treated. It is now understood that these composites are amyloid plaques and neuro-fibulary tangles, the hallmarks of a diagnosis of AD (Mace & Rabins, 2001).

Although professionals in the medical community recognized that memory loss was not a normal part of aging, during the next 75 years many older adults continued to believe the contrary and expect significant memory loss to occur during the aging process. Until the early 1980s, it was uncommon for individuals to receive a formal diagnosis of dementia or AD. Instead, the condition was generally referred to as "senility," "hardening of the arteries," or just "old age." Due in part to the increased attention to aging demographics in the United States and a significant increase in research funding by the National Institutes of Health, a greater interest in AD and its personal and societal implications developed. Scientific advances have examined the role of genetics in AD, specifically in early onset dementia, and the potential for effective treatments to slow the progression of the disease, delaying its onset and ultimately finding a cure (Epple, 2002). Regardless of these strides, there still remains a great need for education of health-care providers and the public about AD and related dementias, and specifically about developing psychosocial interventions for those diagnosed.

Much of the focus on dementia has been given to the impact of this condition on familial caregivers. While caregivers experience a range of emotional, psychological, and physical effects during their "caregiving career," the individuals with the diagnosis also experience a range of emotional and psychological reactions as they slowly lose their memory and grasp on present reality. Additionally, individuals with dementia often develop a range of behavioral changes that occur as a result of the changes in their cognitive status. Thus, it is necessary for a variety of treatments, specifically psychosocial treatments, to be implemented throughout the disease course to assist in addressing the emotional, psychological, and behavioral changes that occur as a result of the dementia. These treatments will help ensure the best quality of life for diagnosed individuals until their death (Kasl-Godley & Gatz, 2000).

For the most part, the interventions highlighted in the literature have focused on the pharmacological treatments that address the problematic behaviors exhibited by the person with dementia and on strategies that address the mental health issues experienced by caregivers (Desai & Grossberg, 2001). Slowly, a body of literature is developing that examines non-pharmacological, psychosocial interventions for individuals with the diagnosis of dementia. The purpose of this article is to examine the psychosocial interventions specifically designed for individuals diagnosed with a non-reversible form of dementia, such as AD. As suggested by Bates, Boote, and Beverly (2004), "psychosocial approaches to dementia care form an important part of modern-day non-pharmacological treatment" (p. 645). Despite the obvious importance of non-pharmacological treatment strategies, the depth of scientific rigor in the study of psychosocial interventions varies tremendously (Bartels, Haley, & Dums, 2002). The specificity of the intervention, the sampling strategy, and the measurement of key outcomes are just some of the limitations of the studies in this area (Bates et al., 2004). The interventions described in this review represent some of the important strategies that address a wide range of behaviors and moods manifested by individuals with dementia.

DEMOGRAPHICS/PREVALENCE OF PROBLEM

As of 2005, 4.5 million individuals in the United States were diagnosed with dementia. This number is expected to increase to a range of 11.3 to 16 million by 2050 (Alzheimer's Association, 2005; Herbert, Scherr, Bienia, Bennett, & Evans, 2003). Dementia is one of the largest groups of chronic illnesses impacting older adults. While AD remains the most common form of dementia, other forms include Lewy Body disease, Multi-infarct dementia, frontal-lobe dementia, and Parkinson's related dementia. In fact, there are over 70 different types of dementia, with AD accounting for over 50% of all cases (Alzheimer's Association, 2005). While each form of dementia causes memory loss, the disease progression, the impact on the individual, and the types of prescribed treatment may vary. While many of the behaviors resulting from the different types of dementia are similar to those of AD, the onset of behavioral changes may vary. For example, persons diagnosed with AD have been found to exhibit a more gradual decline in cognitive functioning, while a person with a multi-infarct dementia will experience more rapid or unpredictable changes (Alzheimer's Association, 2004). The duration of AD lasts between three and 20 years. Approximately, 70% of all individuals with AD are cared for at home for the entire course of the disease; however, 50-70% of all residents in long-term care facilities have some form of dementia (Alzheimer's Association, 2005; Ganzer & England, 1994).

Even though AD is assumed to have no gender, race, or socioeconomic boundaries, there are several demographic characteristics that place people at a greater risk for developing the disease (Alzheimer's Association, 2002). Age is one of the primary risk factors for Alzheimer's disease. It is estimated that one out of 10 individuals over the age of 65 and as many as one out of two over the age of 85 will develop AD (Alzheimer's Association, 2004; Brown & Kleist, 1999; Evans, Fundenstein, Albert et al., 1989). Since AD is associated with older age and women still live longer than men, more women receive a diagnosis. Race has also been examined as an important factor in the onset of Alzheimer's disease. According to the Alzheimer's Association (2002), the overall prevalence of Alzheimer's disease among African Americans is 14-100% higher than it is among other racial groups.

NATURE OF THE PROBLEM

The progression of AD is gradual and unrelenting. As the disease progresses from the early to middle to late/end stages, individuals gradually lose their short-term memory, ability to perform activities of daily living (ADLs) and instrumental activities of daily living (IADLs), their ability to recognize time, people, and places, and to reason and judge environments. During the end stages, individuals with AD typically die in a state of being non-verbal, non-ambulatory, and unresponsive to cues from their environment (Hurley & Volicer, 2002). Throughout the progression of the disease, it is common for individuals to experience a variety of personality, mood, and behavioral transformations that can be distressing for familial caregivers. Personality changes, such as having laughter or tears at inappropriate times, a loss of initiative, and a change in interest or participation in activities, are some of the hallmarks of AD that can continue throughout the disease course. Mood changes include depression and/or mania, anxiety, psychosis, and withdrawal from routine activities. For some individuals, the mood changes occur upon the onset of the memory loss or in response to the memory loss. For others, however, the mood changes occur as the memory loss and confusion become more pronounced. The behavioral changes are often more difficult than the mood changes for family members because these mark the intensity of the disease process and the degree of impairment that has occurred. Some of the most common and frustrating behavioral changes include agitation, wandering, sleep disturbances, changes in communication patterns, lack of sexual inhibitions, and sundowning, which is characterized by late afternoon confusion due to changes in lighting, tiredness, stress, or lack of activities. The behavioral changes associated with Alzheimer's disease are often the trigger event for families to initiate services through formal support networks, including respite, adult day care, and long-term care (Alzheimer's Association, 2004). The mood and behavioral changes that accompany AD and related dementia are the centerpiece of most pharmacological and psychosocial interventions.

CONSEQUENCES OF ALZHEIMER'S DISEASE

The overall impact of AD on the individual, family, and society is staggering. Unfortunately, the costs will only increase as more individuals age and receive the diagnosis. Far beyond the financial costs, affected individuals experience multiple intra- and interpersonal losses throughout the course of the disease (Rentz, Krikorian, & Keys, 2005). Changes in status, identity, roles, activities, and responsibilities within the family are some of the most significant losses. Other losses include the loss of independence, recognition of one's environment, and orientation to present, past and future time. These losses become more pronounced as the disease progresses.

As a result of the behavioral manifestations which occur in 90% of all individuals with dementia (Grossberg & Desai, 2003), caregivers experience a range of physical and mental health conditions, including burden and depression, as well as changes in socialization patterns and overall social contact (Rodriguez, Leo, Girtler, Vitali, Grossi, & Nobili, 2003). Numerous researchers have defined the caregiving experience as an unrelenting process of grief and loss that is seldom recognized by others (Meuser & Marwit, 2001; Sanders & Corley, 2002; Sanders,

Morano, & Corley, 2002; Walker & Pomeroy, 1996). The focus on the caregivers is understandable; however, it has unfortunately resulted in the research and clinical communities devoting limited attention towards exploring psychosocial interventions for the person with AD.

In addition to the emotional costs that impact the individual with AD and the caregiver, there are financial costs that affect the individual, family, and society overall. Estimates suggest that families spend approximately $12,500 to $30,000 per year in out-of-pocket medical and nursing costs for affected individuals (Delagarza, 2003; Rice et al., 1993). Beyond the familial costs, the economic impact of dementia reaches into larger societal structures. Much of the current costs of AD are felt by U.S. businesses in expenses for caregivers and affected individuals. Koppel (2002) indicated that the total cost of AD to U.S. businesses is approximately $61 billion, with much of these costs related to caregiver issues, including absenteeism, temporary leave from work, and employee assistance programs ($36.5 billion), as well as healthcare expenditures ($24.6 billion). The Alzheimer's Association has cited that the total costs of AD are over $100 billion. However, Koppel argued that this number may be low. In addition to the costs of AD to businesses, the government pays over $50 billion in health-related expenses.

EMPIRICAL RESEARCH

The majority of the intervention literature specific to individuals with AD has focused on medication and medical trials (see Cummings, 2004, for review) in an attempt to determine strategies to slow or stop the progression of the disease. The ultimate goal of researchers, geriatric health professionals, and families is to find a cure for AD. As stated in much of the public awareness literature distributed by the National Alzheimer's Association, a "world without Alzheimer's disease" is the hope and dream although this vision has yet to be achieved. Even though pharmacological advances have been significant, not all individuals with AD benefit from these treatments. Thus, the demand for psychosocial interventions is great. This review of empirical literature details only the research on psychosocial interventions that utilized samples of individuals with AD or a related form of dementia. Four inclusion criteria were used to select studies on psychosocial interventions that utilized samples of individuals with AD or a related dementia. First, the study had to address interventions specific to individuals with AD or a related dementia, not their formal or informal caregivers. Second, the interventions tested had to address the problematic behavioral changes or the mood state of individuals as a result of AD or a related dementia. Third, the intervention could not be testing a pharmacological treatment strategy at the same time that it was testing a psychosocial approach (e.g., medical clinical trials could not be included as part of psychosocial intervention). Finally, the articles had to be published after 1985, as the movement towards evidence-based psychosocial interventions started to occur in the late 1980s with increased interest taking place in the 1990s.

The following databases were used in an extensive search for psychosocial intervention literature: Psychinfo, Medline, Cinahl, Social Work Abstracts, and Ageline. Given the inclusion criteria outlined above, a total of 14 studies were reviewed that tested psychosocial interventions for individuals with dementia and met the criteria outlined above (Table 1). Many of the psychosocial interventions, such as validation therapy, cognitive behavioral therapy, psychotherapy, and life review/reminiscence models have been administered in both individual and group formats; however, research has used more group models. The following review will examine psychosocial interventions that can be administered in both formats.

Psychotherapy groups are one mode of addressing changes in the mood of individuals with AD. Cheston, Jones, and Gilliard (2003) examined the effectiveness of community-based psychotherapy groups for improving the mood of individuals with Alzheimer's disease or another form of dementia. The intervention consisted of 10 group sessions, with each lasting approximately 75 minutes. The size of the groups ranged from six to 10 participants. The sessions focused on the impact of the memory loss on the person and his/her relationships. Individuals were interviewed approximately five to 10 weeks prior to the group, one week before the group started, one week after the group was terminated, and at 10 weeks post-group. Among the 19 people who participated in all phases of the research process and completed the clinical groups, levels of depression increased prior to the start of the group, but decreased during the intervention and remained consistent at the 10 week post-test assessment. Anxiety decreased during the intervention period but increased slightly during the post-test period.

Similar to psychotherapy groups, wellness groups have also been utilized to improve the overall mental health of individuals with AD.

TABLE 1. Review of Interventions for Individuals with Alzheimer's Disease or a Related Dementia

Author/date	Population	N	Intervention	Outcome
Cahn-Weiner, Malloy, Rebok, & Ott (2003)	Community-based	24	Memory Training	MT–improved recall and recognition
Camberg et al. (1999)	Long-term care residents	54	Simulated Presence Therapy	SP–-reduced behavioral manifestations and improved well-being
Cheston, Jones, & Gilliard (2003)	Community-based, adult day care	42	Group Psychotherapy	GP–improved depression and anxiety
Goldwasser, Auerbach, & Harkins (1987)	Long-term care residents	27	Reminiscence Therapy vs. Support group vs. No treatment	RT–effective in reducing depression in long-term care residents
Head, Portnoy, & Woods (1990)	Community-based settings and long-term care residents	10	Reminiscence Group	RT–increased communication in community and long-term care settings
Kipling, Bailey, & Charlesworth (1999)	Day hospital	3	Cognitive Behavioral Therapy	CBT–improved ability to relax; greater social participation; improved memory and awareness
Kovach et al. (2004)	Long-term care residents	78	Balancing Arousal Controls Excess	BACE–decreased level of agitation
Lantz, Buchalter, & McBee (1997)	Long-term care residents	14	Wellness Group	WG–decreased agitation
Morton & Bleathman (1991)	Long-term care residents	5	Validation Therapy vs. Reminiscence Therapy	Effectiveness varied by individual; no significant findings
Orten, Allen, & Cook (1989)	Long-term care residents	56	Reminiscence Therapy vs. No treatment	No conclusive findings on effectiveness of RT
Spector et al. (2003)	Long-term care residents and adult day care	210	Cognitive Stimulated Therapy	CST–improved cognitive ability and quality of life
Tabourne (1995)	Long-term care residents	32	Life Review	LR–improved social interaction, disorientation, and life review
Toseland et al. (1997)	Long-term care residents	88	Validation Therapy vs. Social Contact vs. Usual Care	VT–less verbal and physical aggression; SC and UC–more effective at reducing the use of physical restraints and psychotropic medications
Woods & Ashley (1995)	Long-term care residents	27, 9	Simulated Presence Therapy	SPT–effective in reducing social isolation and decreasing agitation and aggression

Lantz, Buchalter, and McBee (1997) provided a group therapy intervention (Wellness Group) to enhance the self-esteem and self and body awareness of individuals with dementia in a nursing facility. The intervention consisted of one-hour sessions, and ran for 10 weeks. The therapy sessions included discussion and relaxation exercises such as breathing techniques, muscle relaxation, guided imagery, and tactile stimulation. Eight individuals were assigned to the treatment groups and six individuals were in the no treatment condition, which consisted of routine facility treatment programs. Group composition was based on the cognitive status and severity of dementia of the resident. No post-test data were collected. The results indicated that the group therapy program was effective in reducing agitation in residents, as compared to the no treatment group. Interviews with nurses revealed that knowledge about self and body awareness was deemed beneficial. The authors found that the concept of a Wellness Group benefited the entire facility by using techniques that "focus on resident strengths and individual coping skills, and allow[ing] direct care staff to become partners in the therapeutic effort" (p. 555).

Life review treatment has been found to be a viable strategy in addressing the overall mental health and outlook of individuals with AD or a related dementia. Tabourne (1995) researched how the self-esteem of nursing home residents with AD or a severe cognitive dysfunction could be improved through a life review group. Tabourne was particularly interested in whether the self-esteem of past participants of a life review group could be improved by serving as an assistant to new participants in a similar life review group format. The effects of the life review program on disorientation, social interaction, and facilitating the life review process were also measured. Thirty-two residents were assigned to either the intervention condition, a life review program, or the control condition, which consisted of recreation activities without the prompting for reminiscence. The interventions lasted for 12 weeks and met two times each week. The life review program addressed life events from birth to death. Eight of the residents served as "veteran participants." The veteran participants, as well as the new participants, were randomly assigned to each treatment group within the participating facilities. The areas of discussion were presented through props or activities associated with elements and stages of life. The results from the study demonstrated that those individuals who participated in the life review group had decreased disorientation, greater recognition of time, person, place, and interest in activities, greater social interaction, and higher levels of self-worth, acceptance of past and present. However, participation in the life review group did not impact the participants' overall appraisal of self-esteem. The veteran facilitators showed improved communication ability and changes in self-esteem, although it was unclear if this finding was a result of their facilitator role or participation in the group process a second time.

Like life review, reminiscence groups have also been used to improve the well-being of individuals with AD or a related dementia. Studies of reminiscence groups started to develop in the late 1980s. In 1987, Goldwasser, Auerbach, and Harkins examined the effectiveness of a nursing home-based reminiscence group on depression and overall memory status, including cognitive and behavioral functioning, for individuals with memory loss. Thirty individuals with moderate levels of dementia were randomly assigned to three treatment conditions: a reminiscence group that met for 30 minutes twice weekly for five weeks, a support group that met for 30 minutes twice weekly for five weeks, and a no treatment condition. Three individuals dropped out of the study, so the total number of participants was 27. The researchers found that the reminiscence group produced statistically significant changes in lowering the level of depression of residents in the reminiscence group compared to residents who were in the support group or no treatment condition. There were no changes in overall cognitive or behavioral functioning of individuals between the three group conditions.

Orten, Allen, and Cook (1989) also conducted a study on the effectiveness of reminiscence groups on social behavior in older adults with dementia residing in nursing homes. A total of 56 moderately demented residents in two different nursing facilities were randomly assigned to an experimental (reminiscence group) or control (no treatment) condition. Reminiscence therapy was provided weekly for 16 sessions lasting approximately 45 minutes each session. The control condition consisted of the routine activities of daily living provided by the facilities, but no special treatment. It was noted that individuals who receive routine treatment "generally do not participate in creative program activities" (Orten, Allen, & Cook, 1989, p. 77). No clear results were found in this study. The researcher concluded that it was impossible to provide "unqualified support for this procedure [reminiscence group]" (p. 85). It is suggested that the skills of the facilitator of the group may dictate the success of the intervention.

In another study on reminiscence, Head, Portnoy, and Woods (1990) examined the effectiveness of reminiscence groups as compared to routine group activities in improving the interaction between staff and individuals with AD or a related dementia in both community and facility settings. Ten individuals, all having moderate to severe cognitive impairment, participated in the groups. People were chosen for the groups if they had "clear evidence of cognitive impairment" (p. 296). The groups met for one hour, once a week for six weeks. Results indicated that in the community-based setting, the participants spoke more to the staff during the reminiscence group, whereas during the alternative group there were no significant differences in the amount of contact that took place between the participant, the staff, and other group members. In the institutional setting, all interaction occurred between the staff and the participant in both the reminiscence and regular activity group. Head and colleagues found that in the institutional setting, residents contributed more during the reminiscence sessions than the usual activity sessions.

The premises of cognitive behavioral therapy have been examined with individuals with AD and other progressive dementia. For instance, Kipling, Bailey, and Charlesworth (1999) utilized a cognitive behavioral therapy intervention with three men with probable mild to moderate dementia. It was hypothesized that the cognitive behavioral group would improve affect and behavioral manifestations, as well as the individuals' knowledge about their memory impairment. The intervention consisted of seven weekly, one hour group cognitive behavioral therapy sessions that also included a psycho-educational component and some form of task completion. Pre-test and post-test measures were taken; however, the time of data collection was not reported. Following the intervention, all participants had a greater ability to relax, and two participants had improved mood. All three men reported improved use of their memory and greater awareness of their cognitive limitations. Finally, the results showed that the men experienced increased participation in social activities, including shopping and interacting with others.

Validation therapy is a well-recognized strategy for addressing the problematic behaviors associated with AD. Toseland et al. (1997) compared the effectiveness of three group-based interventions: validation therapy, social contact, and a usual care (control). The sample consisted of 66 individuals with moderate dementia in four long-term care facilities. Data on psychosocial functioning, agitation, positive behaviors, and the use of psychotropic medications were collected at baseline (two weeks prior to the intervention), three months, and one year. Each group met for a 30-minute session, four times each week for 52 weeks. Toseland et al. concluded that even though validation therapy was effective in addressing depression and aggressive behavior, it was not as effective as the social contact groups or usual care groups in diminishing the use of restraints and psychotropic medications. Additionally, validation therapy was not as effective as the social contact or usual care groups in diminishing physically aggressive behavior.

Validation therapy was also studied by Morton and Bleathman (1991). These researchers were interested in the effectiveness of a weekly validation therapy group for improving the mood, behavior, and levels of communication in four individuals with dementia, who were studied as separate case studies. One individual did not complete the study due to an unexpected death. Ten weeks of baseline data were collected, followed by 20 weeks of data during the validation therapy group, and finally 10 weeks of reminiscence therapy. Validation therapy was effective in improving the social interactions of two individuals; however, one participant's interaction increased following reminiscence therapy and one individual had decreased interaction in both therapy settings.

One of the struggles experienced in dementia care is balancing overstimulation with sensory deprivation. The Balancing Arousal Controls Excesses (BACE) program (Kovach et al., 2004) was evaluated for its effectiveness in reducing agitation in a randomized control study with 78 residents with dementia in long-term care facilities. Thirty-six were assigned to the BACE intervention and 42 were in a control group. The BACE intervention organizes the schedule of activities in an effort to achieve a "balance between the time a person spends in high-arousal and low-arousal state" (Kovach et al., 2004; p. 800). In two prior studies, the researchers had established that more than 1.5 hours of high or low arousal without change contributed to agitation of the residents (Kovach & Schlidt, 2001; Kovach & Wells, 2002). This study first measured the amount of agitation and arousal of the resident every 15 minutes during a one-day period to identify those residents who spent greater than 2.5 hours in an aroused state without change (Phase 1). Once these residents were identified, the researchers worked with the staff to develop a balanced arousal plan, so residents spent no more than 1.5 hours in either high or low arousal activities (Phase 2). Once developed, this plan was implemented during Phase 3 which always occurred within seven days of the initial measurement period of Phase 1. The researchers reported that participants who had more than 2.5 hours of arousal *in-balance* during Phase 1 had a significant decrease in agitation with the more balanced arousal time during Phase 3.

Similar to the BACE program, cognitive stimulation is another treatment approach that has been used with individuals with AD or a related dementia to assist with behavioral manifestations. Spector et al. (2003) examined the effectiveness of cognitive stimulation therapy for individuals with dementia in addressing issues of quality of life, communication, problematic behaviors, depression, and functioning. Ninety-seven individuals were in the intervention group, while 70 were in the control condition. The comparison condition consisted of a regular activity program at a long-term care facility or adult day care center. The intervention, cognitive stimulation, consisted of 14 sessions that occurred biweekly for seven weeks. Each session lasted approximately 45 minutes. The intervention format utilized a variety of topics, such as money, games, or famous people, as well as multi-sensory stimulation to assist in improving the quality of life, communication ability, behavior, depression, and overall functioning of respondents. Results suggested that cognitive stimulation was beneficial in improving memory, as measured by the Mini Mental Status Examination, and overall quality of life of the respondents. Communication ability also showed improvement. The intervention did not positively impact the behavior of the participants.

Another intervention for individuals with progressive dementia consists of strategies to enhance memories not yet affected by the disease process. Cahn-Weiner, Malloy, Rebok, and Ott (2003) researched the effectiveness of memory training for 34 individuals with probably Alzheimer's disease. The sample was randomly assigned to two treatment conditions, a memory training group and a control group, both lasting six weeks. Assessments occurred six-weeks prior to the intervention, immediately after the intervention, and eight weeks post-intervention. The assessments measured the participants' recall, reasoning, recognition, and naming ability, as well as their overall cognitive status and daily functioning. After completing the six-week memory training program, patients in the treatment group demonstrated no significant change in neurological test performance or memory functioning as compared to the control group. Additionally, the reported ADL performance did not differ between the treatment and control group. The researchers concluded that overall memory functioning remained relatively stable across the four months of the study for both the treatment and control group.

Simulated presence therapy (SPT) is another strategy used to address the behavioral manifestations in individuals with AD or a related dementia. SPT consists of creating a sense of comfort for the person with AD by replicating an experience with one's primary caregiver in some auditory way, such as a tape recorded phone conversation or listening to the caregiver reminisce (Woods & Ashley, 1995). The goal of SPT is to alter the environment of the individual with AD so that the feeling of people and experiences that bring the most comfort are present. When SPT is administered appropriately, it is hoped that the frequency of behavioral manifestations will diminish. Woods and Ashley conducted a two-part study to examine the effectiveness of SPT for individuals with dementia. In the first part of the study, they were interested in determining the types of individuals with dementia who would benefit most from SPT. Twenty-seven individuals with some form of moderate to moderately severe cognitive impairment who resided at four different nursing facilities participated. Each individual received SPT when they experienced a problematic behavior for one month. Each simulated presence tape lasted approximately 15 minutes. Woods and Ashley found that SPT was most effective in residents who were socially isolated, followed by agitated and aggressive.

In the second part of the study by Woods and Ashley (1995), pre-test/post-test data were collected on nine residents with moderate Alzheimer's disease or a related dementia. Each resident received SPT two times each day for a period of two months to assist with problematic behaviors. It was determined that problematic behaviors improved 91% of the time with simulated presence therapy. Aggression improved 91%, agitation improved 96%, and social isolated improved 86% of the time.

In a later study, Camberg et al. (1999) also studied the impact of SPT on agitation and social withdrawal among nursing home residents with AD. Fifty-four individuals participated in SPT, consisting of memories being replayed to the individual with dementia through a telephone or audiotapes. Three treatments were studied: simulated presence, a placebo which consisted of audiotapes of people reading articles from a newspaper, and a usual care group. The treatments were administered for a period of 17 days over a course of four weeks. The intervention was withdrawn 10 days following the treatment period. Direct observation was used to collect data on the residents' well-being. Camberg et al. (1999) found that SPT was more effective than the other treatments in reducing agitation and improving withdrawn behavior. They concluded that SPT was effective in enhancing the well-being of individuals with dementia and decreasing the manifestations of problematic behaviors.

TREATMENT SUMMARY

As a whole, studies of the effectiveness of interventions for individuals with dementia have had mixed results. The impact of these interventions was determined not only by the type of treatment employed (e.g., reminiscence, validation), but also by other variables, such as intervention administration protocol and characteristics of the person with dementia. While some of the interventions examined seemed to be effective in addressing the mood and behavioral manifestations of the individuals with dementia, the results for all of the studies must be interpreted cautiously. Some possible complicating factors include small sample sizes, lack of randomization to groups, and the lack of clarity about study participants' disease stage.

Across all studies reviewed, the most common outcome variables were depression, anxiety, self-esteem and self-awareness, agitation and behavioral manifestations, and socialization and communication with others. For the majority of studies, it was found that the psychosocial intervention of interest was effective in positively impacting the specified outcome. As a result of the particular intervention, depression, anxiety, and agitation decreased (Camberg et al., 1999; Cheston, Jones, & Gilliard, 2003; Goldwasser, Auerbach, & Harkins, 1987; Lantz, Buchalter, & McBee, 1997; Toseland, 1997; Woods & Ashly, 1995) and social interactions, awareness, and recognition increased (Head, Portnoy, & Woods, 1990; Kipling, Bailey, & Charlesworth, 1999; Morton & Bleathman, 1991; Spector et al., 2003; Tabourne, 1995). As seen in the review of literature, the majority of psychosocial interventions that are being employed for individuals with dementia are being administered in a group format, typically with people in the middle or moderate stages of the disease process. The use of individually-based psychosocial interventions still seems to be in the infancy stage, thus suggesting the need for further intervention development and empirical testing. However, based upon the effectiveness of the interventions reviewed, it suggests that these, too, may be effective for dementia care in an individual format.

CONCLUSION

Despite the growth in the use of psychosocial approaches in dementia care, several steps need to occur to assist in evaluating the overall effectiveness of these forms of treatment. Most importantly, more research is needed on psychosocial interventions for individuals with dementia.

This research should entail the use of larger sample sizes, clearer intervention strategies, interventions in both individual and group formats, and interventions for both community and facility-based individuals with dementia. Opie and colleagues (1999) stated that

> Non-pharmacological strategies . . . are promoted as safe, humane, and at least as effective as medications, but the evidence for this view is sometimes lacking. This deficiency should be rectified, however, to ensure that treatment strategies are firmly based on the evidence acquired through rigorously conducted scientific trials. (p. 790)

This was further echoed by Bates, Boote, and Beverly (2004) who argued that there is "a paucity of well-designed studies focusing on the effectiveness of psychosocial interventions" for individuals with mild, but also all, stages of dementia (p. 653). Beck (2001) also touched upon this issue, but further emphasized the need to address the overall methodology of the research on psychosocial interventions. Issues related to sampling strategies and theoretically grounded outcome measures are just two of the methodological limitations found in many of the studies of psychosocial interventions. Additionally, the lack of a randomized sampling strategy draws into question the overall validity of the intervention and the results that are produced. While randomization is not always feasible, it is important to consider other strategies for increasing the rigor of psychosocial intervention studies, such as having larger sample sizes, increasing the homogeneity of the sample, and using well-established outcome measures.

Similarly, many of the psychosocial approaches that are widely used in practice, such as validation therapy and early-stage support groups for individuals with dementia, need more empirical testing. The literature on these methods provides essential knowledge about how the particular treatment should be implemented, but not on their overall effectiveness. Kasl-Godley and Gatz (2000), in a review of the literature on psychosocial interventions for individuals with dementia, repeatedly argued that many psychosocial approaches including psycho-dynamic therapies, life review/reminiscence, support groups, and cognitive/behavioral approaches have not been well-researched, specifically with individuals with some of the specific types of dementia. Thus, practitioners who choose to employ these intervention strategies are judging the effectiveness of the approach based upon research that has been conducted on unrelated or dissimilar populations or on their clinical experience, not actual empirical testing.

Third, the research on psychosocial interventions for individuals with dementia needs to expand the sampling strategies to include respondents who are living in the community, as well as in long-term care communities. In the studies reviewed, the majority of samples were based on individuals living in long-term care facilities. Thus, little is known about the effectiveness of psychosocial interventions for community-based individuals with dementia. This is particularly important given that many persons of color, such as African American and Hispanics, are more apt to provide care in the community for the entire duration of the disease instead of utilizing a long-term care facility. Additionally, since the vast majority of care for persons with dementia is provided in the community, the need for research in community-based settings is much overdue.

Moreover, the sampling strategy should be expanded to include individuals with dementia from diverse racial and ethnic backgrounds. With statistics suggesting that the number of African Americans over the age of 65 is expected to grow to over 7 million by 2030 and the incidence of AD is higher among African Americans (Alzheimer's Association, 2002), it is critical that researchers examine the types of psychosocial interventions that work most effectively with this population. Additionally, with the continual emphasis on culturally competent social work practice, one needs to understand how the effectiveness of interventions may vary based on the culture or ethnicity of individuals. Just as research with caregivers from more diverse backgrounds is expanding (Dilworth-Anderson, Williams, & Gibson, 2002; Morano, 2003), research including more diverse persons with dementia must also expand.

There is also a need to expand the literature on interventions for individuals at the late and end stage of Alzheimer's disease or a related dementia. Some empirical attention has been given to the early stage of the disease, however, the majority of the focus has been placed on the middle stages, which are typically the most difficult due to the radical personality and behavioral changes that occur. Little is known about the appropriate types of treatment that should be provided at the end stages of this disease. Knowledge of these types of psychosocial interventions would be beneficial for a variety of health providers, including hospital staff, long-term care professionals, and hospice providers.

Finally, greater attention needs to be given to measuring the desired outcomes of the intervention. Given the challenges with self-report measures for individuals with dementia, much of the evidence on the effectiveness of the intervention is based on observational data. Consequently, the findings of any study will in part depend on the perception of the observer (i.e., family member, formal or institutional care providers, or the researcher), how the observation is measured, the purpose of the study, and a host of other variables. Thus, what is considered to be a measurement of success by one set of researchers may not be considered success by others. As this base of literature grows, the publishing of observation protocols for measuring the effectiveness of interventions for individuals with dementia is necessary. Clearly articulated protocols for the design and evaluation of any evidence-based inter-vention are important for understanding what worked under what conditions. Thus, it will also provide future researchers with a foundation on which to build.

The full impact of AD and related dementia is resonating throughout society. The economic costs of this disease impact families, health-care systems, businesses, and social structures. The emotional, psychological, and physical burdens of this disease impact the person with dementia, his/her family, as well as the formal support networks that provide assistance. Historically, those individuals impacted by AD and related dementias have felt helpless in their struggle to deal with behavioral, emotional, and cognitive changes. Now, with more advanced medical knowledge, pharmacological treatments, and psychosocial interventions, the unaddressed behavioral and mental health aspects can be better treated, thereby improving the overall well-being of all involved.

TREATMENT RESOURCE APPENDIX

www.vfvalidation.org

This web site provides information about Validation Therapy, a method for communicating with very old people. In addition to articles and books, the best introduction to Validation Therapy is through a *Workshop* or *Course*, many of which are given by Naomi Feil, developer of the Validation Method.

Links are provided to several practice and resource manuals including:

- *The Validation Breakthrough: Simple Techniques for Communicating with People with "Alzheimer's-Type Dementia,"* 2nd edi-

tion, 2002, 352 Pages. By Naomi Feil, revised by Vicki deKlerk-Rubin, this is the standard reference on Validation.
- *The Validation Training Program: Training Manual for the Instruction of Validation*, By Evelyn Sutton and Naomi Feil
- *V/F Validation: The Feil Method*
  This book tells how to help disoriented old-old people. It teaches those who care for and about disoriented old-old how to: recognize the signs of disorientation, the physical, emotional and social factors leading to confusion, and how to help confused old-old in each stage. By Naomi Feil and Vicki deKlerk-Rubin

In addition, this web site contains a bibliography of articles on the impact of Validation Therapy that have been published in the professional literature.

www.alz.org

The Alzheimer's Association, the world leader in Alzheimer research and support, is the first and largest voluntary health organization dedicated to finding prevention methods, treatments and an eventual cure for Alzheimer's. This web site contains links to the latest information about the diagnosis and treatment of Alzheimer's disease. This web site provides several Resource manuals that offer practical suggestions for clinicians and family care providers. These include:

- *Communication: The Best Way to Interact with a Person with Dementia.* This practical publication provides information about some of the communication changes that accompany dementia. In addition, ways to enhance communication are provided including individuals who have sight and hearing disabilities.
  http://www.alz.org/Resources/factsheets/Communications10_5.pdf
- *Dementia Care Practice Recommendations for Assisted Living Residences and Nursing Homes.* This 32-page booklet provides detailed information about best practice strategies for people with dementia in residential facilities. The content includes working on issues of pain management, wandering, food and nutrition, falls, social engagement, and restraint free care.
  http://www.alz.org/Downloads/DementiaCarePractice Recommendations.pdf
- *Helping Children and Teens Understand Alzheimer's Disease.* This booklet focuses on younger family members' reaction to and

experience with older loved ones who have dementia. Included in the contents are typical reactions of children and teens, strategies to help them discuss their experience, and typical questions that people this age might ask. This publication includes numerous pictures of older adults and children/teens interacting. A good resource for families, as well as practitioners, who are working with families where there are children.
http://www.alz.org/Resources/FactSheets/Brochure_ChildrenTeens.pdf

• *Late Stage Care: Providing Care and Comfort During the Late Stage of Alzheimer's Disease.* This publication targets the final stage of dementia, and particular dimensions of care that are critical. Included is the importance of providing comfort and support to the person with dementia, including skin, hygiene, and nutritional care. Also included is information about types of interaction that are helpful during this stage and the importance of supporting the caregiver.
http://www.alz.org/Resources/factsheets/LateStage10_05.pdf

• *Staying Strong: Stress Relief for the African American Caregiver.* This publication provides information and resources specifically for African Americans who are in caregiving roles. Included is a stress checklist that provides care providers with a way to determine the impact of this role within their life.
http://www.alz.org/Resources/Diversity/downloads/AfAmCaregiver.pdf

• *Tools for Early Identification, Assessment and Treatment for People with Alzheimer's Disease and Dementia.* This 40-page booklet contains a wealth of information for practitioners and service providers! Several assessment protocols are included to assess functioning of the person with dementia, as well as the stressful impact on care providers. Tools for care managers are included which can assist with structuring interventions and care planning with individuals and families.
http://www.alz.org/Resources/FactSheets/CCN-AD03.pdf

http://www.atra-tr.org/atra.htm

The American Therapeutic Recreation Association (ATRA) is the largest national membership organization representing the interests and needs of recreational therapists. Recreational therapists are health-care providers using recreational therapy interventions for improved functioning of individuals with illness or disabling conditions. For additional information regarding the American Therapeutic Recreation

Association, contact us at our national office: ATRA, 1414 Prince Street, Suite 204, Alexandria, VA 22314, (703) 683-9420.

www.activitytherapy.com

This web site provides in-service and training for innovative Therapeutic Recreation and Social Service Programs for long term-care residents. The association of activity therapists is committed to helping your staff provide quality programs to fit the needs of all residents' interests and functioning levels.

www.healthandage.com

Health and Age is a web site that provides a variety of information and news on issues related to aging, as well as specifically to Alzheimer's disease. The site provides links to a number of other sites that also provide information about managing persons with Alzheimer's disease.

Books:

36 Hour Day. M. Mace & P. Rabins (1981). Johns Hopkins University Press.
Creative Aging: Awakening Human Potential in the Second Half of Life. Gene Cohen (2000). Avon Books.
The Positive Interactions Programs of Activities for People with Alzheimer's Disease. S. Nissenboim & C. Vroman (2003). Health Professionals Press.

REFERENCES

Alzheimer's Association (2002). *African Americans and Alzheimer's disease: The silent epidemic*. Alzheimer's Association, Chicago, IL.

Alzheimer's Association (2004). *Just the facts: Disease overview*. Chicago, IL.

Alzheimer's Association (2005). *Statistics*. Chicago, IL.

Bates, J., Boote, J. & Beverly, C. (2004). Psychosocial interventions for people with a milder dementing illness: A systematic review. *Journal of Advanced Nursing, 45*, 644-658.

Brown, T. & Kleist, D.M. (1999). Alzheimer's disease and the family: Current research. *The Family Journal: Counseling and Therapy for Couples and Families, 7*, 54-57.

Camberg, L, Woods, P., Ooi, W.L, Hurley, A., Volicer, L., Ashley, J., Odenheimer, G., & McIntyre, K. (1999). Evaluation of simulated presence: A personalized approach to enhance well-being in persons with Alzheimer's disease. *Journal of the Geriatric Society, 47*, 446-452.

Cheston, R., Jones, K., & Gilliard, J. (2003). Group psychotherapy and people with dementia. *Aging and Mental Health, 7,* 452-461.

Cohn-Weiner, D.A., Malloy, P.F., Rebok, G.W., & Ott, B.R. (2003). Results of a randomized placebo-controlled study of memory training for mildly impaired Alzheimer's disease patients. *Applied Neuropsychology, 10,* 215-223.

Cummings, J. (2004). Alzheimer's disease. *The New England Journal of Medicine, 351,* 56-67.

Delagarza, V.W. (2003). Pharmacologic treatment of Alzheimer's disease: An update. *American Family Physician, 68,* 1365-1372.

Dilworth-Anderson, P., Williams, I.C., & Gibson, B.E. (2002). Issues of race, ethnicity, and culture in caregiving research: A 20 year review (1980-2000). *The Gerontologist. 42*(2), 237-272.

Epple, D.M. (2002). Senile dementia of the Alzheimer's type. *Clinical Social Work Journal. 30,* 95-110.

Evans, D.A., Funkenstein, H.H., Albert, M.S. et al. (1989). Prevalence of Alzheimer's disease in a community population of older persons. *Journal of the American Medical Association, 262,* 2551-2556.

Ganzer, C. & England, S.E. (1994). Alzheimer's care and service utilization: Generating practice concepts from empirical findings and narratives. *Health and Social Work, 19,* 174-181.

Goldwasser, A.N., Auerbach, S.M., & Harkins, S.W. (1987). Cognitive, affective, and behavioral effects of reminiscence group therapy on demented elderly. *International Journal of Aging and Human Development, 25,* 209-222.

Grossberg, G. & Desai, A.K. (2003). Management of Alzheimer's disease. *Journal of Gerontology: Medical Science, 58A,* 331-353.

Head, D.M., Portnoy, S., & Woods, R.T. (1990). The impact of reminiscence groups in two different settings. *International Journal of Geriatric Psychiatry, 5,* 295-302.

Herbert, L.E., Scherr, R.A., Biernia, J.L., Bennett, D.A., & Evans, D.A. (2003). Alzheimer's disease in the U.S. population: Prevalence estimates using the 2000 census. *Archives of Neurology, 60,* 1119-1122.

Hurley, A.C. & Volicer, L. (2002). Alzheimer's disease: "It's okay mama if you want to go, it's okay." *Journal of the American Medical Association, 288,* 2324-2331.

Kasl-Godley, J. & Gatz, M. (2000). Psychosocial interventions for individuals with dementia: An integration of theory, therapy, and a clinical understanding of dementia. *Clinical Psychology Review, 20,* 755-782.

Kipling, T., Bailey, M., & Charlesworth, G. (1999). The feasibility of a cognitive behavioral therapy group for men with mild/moderate cognitive impairment. *Behavioral and Cognitive Psychotherapy, 27,* 189-193.

Koppel, R. (2002). *Alzheimer's disease: The costs to U.S. businesses in 2002.* National Alzheimer's Association, Chicago, IL.

Kovach, C.R. & Schlidt, A.M. (2001). The activity-agitation interface of people with dementia in long-term care. *Journal of Alzheimer's Disease, 16,* 169-175.

Kovach, C.R. & Wells, T. (2002). Pacing of activity as a predictor of agitation for people with dementia in acute care. *Journal of Gerontological Nursing, 28,* 28-35.

Kovach, C.R., Taneli, Y., Arch, M., Dohearty, P., Schlidt, A.M., Cashin, S., & Silva-Smith, A.L. (2004). Effect of the BACE Intervention on agitation of people with dementia. *The Gerontologist, 44*, 797-806.

Lantz, M.S., Buchalter, E.N., & McBee, L. (1997). The wellness group: A novel intervention for coping with disruptive behavior in elderly nursing home residents. *The Gerontologist, 37*, 551-556.

Lott, L. & Klein, D.T. (2003). Psychotherapeutic interventions. In *Agitation in patients with dementia: A practical guide to diagnosis and management*. Hay, D.P., Klein, D.T., Hay, L.K., Grossberg, G.T., & Kennedy, J.S. (eds.), American Psychiatric Publishing: Washington, DC.

Mace, N. & Rabins, P. (2001). *36 hour day*. Warner Books: New York, NY.

Marwit, S.J. & Meuser, T.M. (2002). Development & initial validation of an inventory to measure grief in caregivers of persons with Alzheimer's disease. *The Gerontologist, 42*(6), 51-65.

Meuser, T.M., & Marwit, S.J. (2001). A comprehensive, stage-sensitive model of grief in dementia caregiving. *The Gerontologist, 41*(5), 658-670.

Morano, C. (2003). The role of appraisal and expressive support in mediating strain and gain in Hispanic Alzheimer's disease caregivers. *The Journal of Ethnic & Cultural Diversity in Social Work, 12*, 2, 1-18.

Morton, I. & Bleathman, C. (1991). The effectiveness of validation therapy in dementia: A pilot study. *International Journal of Geriatric Psychiatry, 6*, 327-330.

Opie, J., Rosewarne, & O'Connor, D.W. (1999). The efficacy of psychosocial approaches to behavior disorders in dementia: A systematic literature review. *Australian and New Zealand Journal of Psychiatry, 33*, 789-799.

Orten, J.D., Allen, M., & Cook, J. (1989). Reminiscence groups with confused nursing center residents: An experimental study. *Social Work in Health Care, 14*, 73-86.

Rentz, C., Krikorian, R., & Keys, M. (2005). Grief and mourning from the perspective of the person with a dementing illness: Beginning the dialogue. *Omega, 50*, 165-179.

Rice, D.D. et al. (1993). The economic burden of Alzheimer's disease. *Health Affairs, 12*, 164-176.

Rodriguez, G., De Leo, C., Girtler, N., Vitali, P., Grossi, E., & Nobili, F. (2003). Psychological and social aspects in management of Alzheimer's patients: An inquiry among caregivers. *Neurological Science, 24*, 329-335.

Sanders, S. & Corley, C.S. (2003). Are they grieving? A qualitative analysis examining grief in caregivers of individuals with Alzheimer's disease. *Social Work in Health Care, 37*, 35-53.

Sanders, S., Morano, C., & Corley, C.S. (2002). The expression of loss and grief among male caregivers of individuals with Alzheimer's disease. *Journal of Gerontological Social Work, 39*, 3-18.

Spector, A., Thorgrimsen, L., Woods, B., Royan, L., Davies, S., Butterworth, M., & Orrell, M. (2003). Efficacy of an evidence-based cognitive stimulation therapy program for people with dementia. *British Journal of Psychiatry, 183*, 248-254.

Tabourne, C. (1995). The effects of a life review program on disorientation, social interaction, and self-esteem of nursing home residents. *International Journal of Aging and Human Development, 41*, 251-266.

Toseland, R.W., Diehl, M., Freeman, K., Manzanares, T., Naleppa, M., & McCallion, P. (1997). The impact of validation group therapy on nursing home residents with dementia. *The Journal of Applied Gerontology, 16*, 31-50.

Walker, R.J. & Pomeroy, E.C. (1996). Depression or grief? The experience of care-givers of people with dementia. *Health and Social Work, 96*, 247-254.

Woods, P. & Ashley, J. (1995). Simulated presence therapy: Using selected memories to manage problematic behaviors in Alzheimer's disease patients. *Geriatric Nursing, 16*, 9-14.

Chapter 9

Substance Abuse

Sherry M. Cummings, PhD
Brian Bride, PhD
Kimberly McClure Cassie, MSSW, MA
Ann Rawlins-Shaw, MSW

The inexorable growth of the older population that began in the last century will further increase in the coming decades with the retirement of the "baby boom" generation. As an increasing number of persons live until later years, the number of older persons struggling with substance abuse problems will also expand. Currently, it is estimated that between 1.5% and 6% of older persons experience substance abuse disorders (Fingerhood, 2000; Mirand & Welte, 1996). This number is likely to grow as the next generation of older adults, raised in the 1950s and 1960s, reaches later life. This cohort of older adults, more comfortable with alcohol and drug use and significantly larger than any previous cohort, is apt to consist of an expanded group of individuals with a history of substance use and dependence (Oslin & Blow, 2000). Older adults' increased vulnerability to the deleterious effects of alcohol presents a serious problem which is, therefore, likely to grow (Johnson, 2000). As a result, the number of older adults with a need for substance abuse treatment is expected to rise from 1.7 million in 2000 to approximately 4.4 million by 2020 (Gfroerer, Penne, Pemberton, & Folsom, 2003).

Older adults have a decreased biological ability to process alcohol and other such substances, are susceptible to psychiatric illnesses co-morbid with substance abuse such as dementia and depression, and are prone to increased morbidity and suicide when substance abuse is present (Fingerhood, 2000; Ganzini & Atkinson, 1996; Liberto, Olsin, & Ruskin, 1996). Although substance abuse represents a major public health problem and presents increased risks to older adults, to date little attention has focused on older adults with substance abuse problems or on the potential efficacy of interventions to address the needs of this population (Atkinson, 1990; Schonfeld, Rohrer, Zima, & Spiegel, 1993). As the population continues to age, social work practitioners and researchers will increasingly confront the needs of older adults with substance abuse disorders. The ability of the social work profession to respond to these needs is dependent upon the development of strategies effective for use with the older population and upon social work professionals' knowledge of such strategies.

DEMOGRAPHICS/PREVALENCE OF SUBSTANCE ABUSE DISORDERS AMONG OLDER ADULTS

The most commonly abused substance by older adults is alcohol (Crome & Crome, 2005; Guida, Unterback, Tavolacci, & Provet, 2004; King, Van Hasselt, Segal, & Hersen, 1994). The prevalence of alcohol use disorders in older adults has been generally accepted to be less prevalent than in younger groups (Johnson, 2000). The Epidemiologic Catchment Area (ECA) Study found the prevalence rates of alcohol abuse and dependence to be 1.9% and 3.1% for older men and 0.4% and 0.46% for older women, respectively (Helzer, Burnam, & McEvoy, 1991). Other studies of community-dwelling older adults aged 50 and over have found similar rates, ranging from 2 to 4%, of alcohol dependence (Black, Rabins, & McGuire, 1998; Kandel, Chen, Warner, Kessler, & Grant, 1997).

Prevalence rates of alcohol use disorders increase when studies of at-risk community samples or clinical populations in health care or psychiatric settings are considered, however. In a study of community dwelling older adults who were considered to be at-risk for psychopathology, Jinks and Raschko (1990) found that 9.6% of persons over the age of 60 met the DSM-IV (APA, 1994) criteria for alcohol abuse. Callahan and Tierney (1995) reported 10.6% of nearly 4000 primary care patients over the age of 60 had alcohol problems, based on a self-report of any drinking in the last year and a score of 2 or higher on the CAGE questionnaire. Joseph, Ganzini, and Atkinson (1995) investigated the prevalence of alcohol problems in a sample of nursing home residents aged 51 and older and found that 10% met the criteria for either alcohol abuse or dependence. Another study of nursing home residents found that 18% of the sample met the criteria for alcohol abuse (Oslin, Streim, Parmelee, Boyce, & Katz, 1997). Although Oslin et al. (1997) failed to report the age range of persons in their sample, they did report a mean age of 73.96 (SD = 10.87). Further, Holroyd and Duryee (1997) found a prevalence rate of 8.6% for alcohol dependence in a sample of outpatient, geriatric psychiatry patients over the age of 60.

In addition to alcohol, older adults have also been found to be users and abusers of illicit drugs, such as cocaine, heroin, PCP, and barbiturates (Guida et al., 2004; Mittleman, Mintzer, Maclure, Tofler, Sherwood, & Muller, 1999; Schlaerth, Splawn, Ong, & Smith, 2004). In 1992, Compton, Grant, Colliver, Glantz and Stinson (2004) found the prevalence of marijuana use among individuals aged 45-64 to be 0.6%, but a decade later the prevalence rate had increased to 1.6%. Schlaerth and colleagues (2004) examined the patterns of illegal drug use among adults aged 50 and over who presented for treatment at an inner city emergency room serving a large Latino and African-American population in Los Angeles. In 2001, the researchers found that about 0.3% of older adults presenting at the emergency department were users of illegal drugs. Almost 70% of the illegal drug users identified were male. Almost 77% were between the ages of 50 and 65, 16% between the ages of 65 and 75, and 8% were over the age of 75. The most commonly abused illegal substance was cocaine which was used by 63% of the illegal drug users, followed by opiates (16%), marijuana (14%), barbiturates (7%) and PCP (4%). Many were users of more than one illegal substance. Schlaerth and colleagues (2004) concluded that the type of drugs used by older adults tends to mirror those found in the larger population.

A major limitation of the epidemiological literature is that few studies have examined gender and ethnic differences in the prevalence of substance abuse and dependence. In the few studies that investigate gender differences in alcohol abuse, a consistent finding is that women have lower levels of consumption, are less likely to meet the criteria for alcohol abuse or dependence, and are more likely to abstain altogether (Chermack, Blow, Hill, & Mudd, 1996; Stevenson, 2005). A study of alcohol consumption, rather than incidence of abuse or dependence, among residents of San Diego County aged 65 and older, found that whites were more likely to use alcohol than African-American or Mexican-American respondents (Molgaard, Nakamura, Stanford, Peddecord, & Morton, 1990). The ECA Study (Helzer et al., 1991) found differences in the one-month incidence of alcohol abuse and dependence between African-Americans (0.82% among males, 0.34% among females) and Caucasian-Americans (1.74% among males, .42% among females). These results suggest that among the older population, African-American women are at the lowest risk of alcohol use disorders, while Caucasian men are at the highest risk. When religion measures were added to a study by Krause (2003), race differences in the odds of drinking were no longer statically significant. In the only study to look at alcohol consumption among Native Americans over the age of 60, Barker and Kramer (1996) conclude that older, urban Native Americans do not differ from other older people with respect to the consumption of alcohol.

Another significant limitation of the epidemiological and research literature related to older substance abusers is lack of definitional clarity (Fingerhood, 2000). Varying definitions of substance abuse are common. When conducting research on alcohol abuse among older adults, for example, a DSM-III/IV diagnoses of alcohol abuse/dependence may be used (Blow, Walton, Chermack, Mudd, & Brower, 2000) while others define abuse as DWI arrests (Fitzgerald & Mulford, 1992). Still others use standardized measurement tools to screen for problem drinking (Joseph, Rasmussen, Ganzini, Atkinson, 1997) or illicit drugs use such as marijuana, cocaine, opiates, or barbiturates among older adults (Guida et al., 2004; King et al., 1994; Schlaerth et al., 2004; Colliver, Compton, Gfroerer, & Condon, 2006). In some cases the use of the term "substance" can be confusing, leading the reader to wonder which specific substance is being discussed. Considerable variation is also present in drug and alcohol-related studies concerning the definition of "older persons." The age of persons considered older in drug and alcohol abuse literature ranges from 45 years and over to 75 years and above. Epidemiological and research studies concerning drug and alcohol abuse among older persons have varyingly defined "older" as 45 years and over (Kashner et al., 1992), 50 years and above (Black et al., 1998; Gfroerer, Penne, Pemberton, & Folsom, 2003; Schlaerth et al., 2004), 51 years and over (Joseph et al., 1995), 55 years and older (Blow, Walton, Chermack, Mudd, & Brower, 2000; Satre, Mertens, Areán, & Weisner, 2003; Satre, Mertens, Areán, & Weisner, 2004), over 60 years (Holroyd & Duryee, 1997; Jinks & Raschko, 1990), and ages 65 and above (Gordon, Conigliaro, Maisto, McNeil, Kraemer, & Kelley, 2003).

THEMES/NATURE OF SUBSTANCE ABUSE AMONG OLDER ADULTS

According to the age of onset of problematic drinking, older individuals with alcohol use disorders may be classified as either *early onset* or *late onset* (Fingerhood, 2000). Individuals with early-onset alcoholism have a long-standing history of drinking, but have avoided some of the usual complications associated with alcohol abuse and reached late life (Adams & Waskel, 1993; Atkinson, Tolson, & Turner, 1990; Fingerhood, 2000). For individuals with late-onset alcoholism, problematic drinking developed later in life. The role of stressors in aging, such as the loss of a spouse, health, or status is often put forth as an antecedent to drinking for late-onset alcohol abuse (Brown & Lichtenberg, 1997-8; Fingerhood, 2000). Although it is widely reported that approximately two-thirds of older adults with alcohol use disorder fall into the early-onset category (Brown & Lichtenberg, 1997-98; Fingerhood, 2000), some researchers have found the distribution of early-onset and late-onset to be much less lopsided, with 53% (Adams & Waskel, 1993) of study samples classified as early-onset. Although no firm consensus exists concerning factors leading to late-onset problem drinking, some research suggests that contributing factors include: an earlier pattern of heavy drinking, greater acceptance of one's drinking by close associates, reliance on avoidance-type coping mechanisms, and a history of responding to stress with increased alcohol consumption (Schutte, Brennan, & Moos, 1998).

Similarly, Guida and colleagues (2002) classify substance abusers as *late-in-life users* or *life-long users.* In their survey of 68 clients receiving treatment at a residential treatment center for older adults with substance abuse and mental health problems in New York City, Guida and colleagues found that about one-third of those surveyed were *late-in-life* users who began using substances after the age of 45. These individual typically started using substances following a traumatic event. The drug of choice for these individuals tended to be cocaine or crack cocaine. *Life-long users* tended to use alcohol or heroin. The precipitating cause of substance use among *life-long users* was not discussed.

Some evidence exists that older problem drinkers also suffer from poor emotional health. Many studies link depression and alcohol use in later life. Older adults who are heavy drinkers, for instance, have more depressive symptoms and lower levels of life satisfaction (Colsher & Wallace, 1990). Older problem drinkers also reported taking more medication for anxiety and depression than did non-alcohol abusers. Alcoholism and suicide are also linked in later life. However, current studies have not yet examined the primary-secondary distinction in older depressed alcoholics. So, although the association between alcohol abuse and depression is firmly established, it is not known whether depression causes alcoholism or alcoholism leads to depression in older adults (Atkinson, 1999).

Less is known about the factors associated with illegal drug use among older adults. Rosen (2004) examined the factors related to drug abuse at a methadone clinic in a small midwestern city. Rosen's study was limited to 143 African-American and Caucasian clients over the age of 50 being served by the methadone clinic. Eighty-five percent of those surveyed were between the ages of 50 and 60, 55% were African-American and 70% were male. Exposure to illegal drugs in one's neighborhood and social network was associated with increased drug use. Females in particular were three times more likely to have an adult in their household who was in need of drug treatment. No statistically significant relationship was found between drug use and financial problems, unstable living environments, race or gender.

CONSEQUENCES OF SUBSTANCE ABUSE AMONG OLDER PERSONS

Drug and alcohol abuse poses special risks for increased morbidity and mortality among older adults due to substance-specific disorders and to heightened occurrence of related diseases and disability (King et al., 1994). Adults in later years are especially sensitive to the effects of alcohol use due to a decrease in lean body mass and body water leading to higher blood alcohol concentrations. Higher alcohol concentration coupled with aging body systems result in more severe complications which occur at lower levels of alcohol intake than in younger persons (Fingerhood, 2000; Olsin & Blow, 2000). The older alcohol abuser is at a higher risk for pancreatitis, cirrhosis, hepatitis, stroke, several types of cancer, lack of vitamin absorption leading to malnutrition and chronic diarrhea, coronary artery disease, cardiomyopathy, atrial fibrillation, and high blood pressure than is the general older population (Fingerhood, 2000). Cirrhosis of the liver is one of the major risks associated with alcohol abuse. Up to 30% of alcohol abusers eventually develop cirrhosis which is among the eight leading causes of death for persons 65 years of age and over (Bortz & O'Brien, 1997; Blazer, 1995). Diseases of other organ systems are also caused or exacerbated by alcohol excess. Hepatitis, for example, occurs in 10-35% of older alcoholics (Fingerhood, 2000). Alcohol abuse is additionally associated with heart damage and can result in alcohol-induced cardiomyopathies. It is estimated that 20-30% of all cardiomyopathies are related to alcohol abuse (Regan, 1990).

Older alcohol abusers are also at risk for developing a variety of other serious medical conditions. One study of older alcoholic inpatients revealed that COPD, found in 4.6% of the general older population, was present in 30.6% of the older alcoholics studied. Peptic ulcers were also more frequent in the older alcoholics (15.3%) than in the older population at large (3.4%) (Hurt, Finlayson, Morse, & Davis, 1988). Men who consume two or more alcoholic drinks a day may be at a higher risk for ischemic stroke (Mukamal, Conigrave, Stampfer, Camargo, Ascherio, Mittleman, Rimm, Kawachi, & Willett, 2005). Heavy alcohol use is also associated with increased risk of common cancers including cancer of the liver, esophagus, larynx, colon, breast, and prostate. Additionally, older alcoholic cancer patients have lower survival rates than do older non-abusers (Fingerhood, 2000). Studies have also found a greater risk for all-cause mortality with increased alcohol use among older adults (Reid, Boutros, O'Connor, Cadariu, & Cancato, 2002). Abuse of substances other than alcohol has primarily been linked to cardiovascular disease. Based on their examination of older adults who presented to an emergency room for treatment, Schlaerth and colleagues (2004) found that the prevalence of cardiovascular disease among illegal drug abusers was 60% compared to 10% among nonusers. Similar findings linking cocaine use to cardiovascular disease has also been reported by Mittleman and colleagues (1999).

Heavy alcohol use is associated with several disorders that exacerbate functional impairment and hamper an individual's ability to perform basic activities of daily living. Peripheral neuropathy, for example, occurs in up to 45% of chronic alcohol patients due to vitamin deficiency and results in burning and numbness in the extremities. Chronic alcohol use also increases an individual's risk of falls due to the adverse effect on gait and balance. One study found older moderate to heavy drinkers had a 25% greater risk of falls than did abstainers and light drinkers (Mukamal, Mittleman, Longstreth, Newman, Fried, & Siscovick, 2004). Additionally, alcohol has a direct negative effect on bones and causes bone loss and osteoporosis, leading to increased risk of vertebral compression fractures in older women. Heavy alcohol use also accelerates and increases the loss of muscle mass that occurs in later life, further extending the risk of falls. Researchers estimate that 50% of chronic alcohol abusers have alcoholic muscle disease resulting in loss of up to 20% of the skeletal musculature (Preedy, Salisbury, & Peters, 1994). All these conditions, which damage bone, muscle and nerves, negatively impact functional ability and can severely impede mobility.

Older heavy users of alcohol are also at increased risk for psychiatric disorders including dementia and depression. One study found that men with a history of heavy drinking for five years or more had a five times greater risk for developing psychiatric disorders than had individuals with no history of heavy drinking (Saunders, Copeland, Dewey, Davidson, McWilliam, Sharma, & Sullivan, 1991). Geriatric alcohol abusers have higher rates of depression than non-drinking cohorts in the same age group (Reinhardt & Fulop, 1996). The co-morbidity of alcoholic abuse and depression in older adults is important due to the issue of suicide. People who are alcohol abusers are highly represented in the population of persons who complete suicide (Light & Lebowitz, 1991). In a research study of persons 65 and older, who were assessed after attempting suicide, Draper (1994) found that 32% had alcohol or substance abuse issues. Cognitive disability is also frequently co-morbid with alcohol use and moderate alcohol use has been linked with substantially higher risk of dementia among older adults (Reid, Boutros, O'Connor, Cadariu, & Cancato, 2002). Alcohol-induced cognitive impairment ranges from mild cognitive difficulties to more severe dementia in long-term alcoholics. Researchers estimate that 1 to 25% of the dementia cases in community-dwelling older adults are alcohol-related (Bortz & O'Brien, 1997).

Substance abuse among older adults poses negative consequences not only for individuals but also for society as a whole in terms of the heightened use of medical resources and a related increase in medical costs. Older people, age 45 and up, account for 50% of the alcohol-related costs for physician and hospital care (Kashner, Rodell, Ogden, Guggenheim, & Karson, 1992). In one study, 23% of all admissions to a Veteran's Administration hospital for patients 55 and over were due to an alcohol-related problem (Moos, Mertens, & Brennan, 1993). Studies have also found that the presence of secondary alcohol-related disorders increases charges and length of stay for older persons admitted to the hospital through emergency departments (Shadi & Szabenyi, 2005). The actual prevalence of hospitalizations and the cost of medical care due to drug and alcohol-related problems among older adults are potentially much higher than reported since drug and alcohol abuse and dependence in this population often remain undiagnosed and untreated. The consequences of substance abuse among older adults present serious challenges both for older individuals and for society as a whole. As the number of older adults with drug and alcohol abuse problems continues to grow, effective strategies for treating this vulnerable population become increasingly critical.

REVIEW OF EMPIRICAL STUDIES

The literature review of empirical studies examining alcohol and drug abuse treatments for older adults was conducted according to specific parameters. The review was limited to studies concerning the outcomes of interventions for older persons with alcohol and other substance abuse/dependence disorders. Only those studies that specifically examined outcomes for older adults were included; those studies that contained older subjects but did not specifically analyze results for this age group were excluded. No specific definition of "older adult" was established for this literature review. Rather, those studies of alcohol and drug treatment outcomes that identified study subjects as "old" or "older" were included.

The following databases were surveyed for this literature review: NIAAA alcohol and Alcohol Problems Science Database (ETOH), Psycinfo, Sociofile, Pubmed, and Ageline. Articles listed in these databases and with publication dates from 1980 to the present were examined. The vast majority of articles found concerning interventions for older substance abusers were descriptive in nature and discussed either the nature of specific programs for older adults or recommended approaches for the treatment of older substance abusers. In all, eight articles were found detailing the results of interventions for older alcohol abusers and two articles addressing the same research study were found that examined outcomes in substance and alcohol abuse treatment programs (Table 1).

A study conducted by Gordon, Conigliaro, Maisto, McNeil, Kraemer, and Kelley (2003) sought to determine if Motivational Enhancement (ME) and Brief Advice (BA) decreased the amount of alcohol consumption among the older (65 years +) population. Older patients were screened in primary care offices and were randomly assigned to three groups: ME (n = 18), BA (n = 12) and Standard Care (n = 12). The ME intervention focused on feedback, consequences of drinking and goal setting. The initial session for ME was 45-60 minutes, with two 10-15 minute sessions conducted at the second and sixth week. The BA was one 10-15 minute session that focused on feedback from a drinking assessment questionnaire dealing with the social and health implications of drinking and on advice about how to stop or reduce alcoholic consumption. Results indicated that there was a statistically significant decrease in alcohol consumption measures in ME and BA as compared to Standard Care. However, no difference in effectiveness was found between BE and ME. The authors concluded that Motivational Enhancement and Brief Advice are equally effective in reducing alcohol consumption among older patients.

The Gerontology Alcohol Project (GAP) described by Dupree, Broskowski, and Schonfeld (1984) utilized four cognitive-behavioral treatment modules specifically designed for older alcohol abusers. The modules were designed to teach clients the components of behavior chains, methods for dealing with personal and general antecedents associated with drinking, and the consequences of alcohol abuse. Dupree and colleagues collected follow-up data on 24 graduates of the program, finding a high success rate in maintaining drinking goals, significant reduction in average daily alcohol consumption, and significant improvement in community adjustment.

Carstensen, Rychtarik, and Prue (1985) conducted a long-term follow-up of persons, aged 60 and over, who completed treatment in the Alcohol Dependence Treatment Program (ADTP) of the Jackson VA Medical Center. The ADTP is a mixed-age, 28-day inpatient treatment program that provides individual counseling, alcohol education, and training in self-management and problem-solving skills, in addition to vocational assistance, marital therapy and medical attention when needed. The study's authors contacted 16 persons who had completed the ADTP between two and four years prior, finding that half were successfully abstaining from alcohol and an additional 12% significantly reduced their alcohol consumption.

A retrospective, non-randomized study conducted by Kofoed et al. (1987) compared a sample of 24 older alcoholics treated in traditional mixed-age outpatient groups with a sample of 25 older alcoholics treated in older adult peer groups. The traditional groups, which usually contained one to two older adults in each group of six to 10 people, emphasized expression of feelings and resulted in frequent peer and staff confrontation. The age-specific groups emphasized socialization and support, progressed at a slower pace, and contained less confrontation than the traditional groups. Results indicated that older patients treated in the age-specific groups had better attendance rates and completed one year of treatment at a rate four times higher than older patients in the mixed-age groups.

Kashner et al. (1992) randomly assigned 137 male alcoholic patients who were aged 45 and older to either an age-specific treatment program, or a traditional, mixed-age treatment program. Patients in both treatment groups received between two and seven days of inpatient detoxification, three to four weeks of inpatient treatment, and one year of outpatient aftercare. Both groups received individual counseling, and attended a variety of group sessions. The traditional program was oriented to problem-solving, vocational development, and life change, and staff used a more confrontational approach. The older adult-specific program was focused on developing patient self-esteem and peer relationships, employed reminiscence therapy, and used a more supportive and respectful approach. The results of the study indicated that patients receiving older adult-specific treatment were more than twice as likely to report abstinence at one year following treatment. Further, response was best for those patients over 60 years of age.

Rice, Longabaugh, Beattie, and Noel (1993) randomly assigned 229 clients undergoing outpatient alcoholism treatment to one of three 20-session treatment conditions: extended cognitive behavioral treatment (CB), relationship enhancement (RE), and vocational enhancement (VE). CB consisted of a functional analysis of the antecedents to drinking and the short- and long-range consequences of drinking. Further, CB entailed helping the client modify the association between drinking antecedents and consequences through cognitive behavioral restructuring and precluded the participation of significant others. RE focused on the client's relationship with his/her significant others and included sessions devoted to "partner's therapy" and multiple family group therapy, but also included six sessions of functional analysis. The VE treatment condition included a four-session occupational component directed at assisting the client to enhance his/her occupational role performance, in addition to six functional analysis sessions, four partner sessions, and two "family nights." The researchers were interested in two outcomes: percentage of days abstinent and percentage of heavy drinking days. Results revealed that persons aged 50 years and older did best in the extended cognitive behavioral treatment and did poorest when assigned to vocational enhancement.

Schonfeld and colleagues (2000) describe an age-specific, outpatient program for older veterans with substance abuse problems. The Geriatric Evaluation Team: Substance Misuse/Abuse Recognition and Treatment (GET SMART) Program is structured around 16 weekly group sessions using cognitive-behavioral and self-management approaches. As described by the researchers, group sessions are initially comprised of an analysis of substance use behavior to determine high-risk situations for substance use, followed by a series of modules to teach skills for coping with social pressure, isolation, uncomfortable feelings (i.e., depression, loneliness, anxiety, tension, anger, and frustration), cues for substance use, urges, and slips or relapses. Among 49 patients who were contacted after completing the GET SMART program, 55% remained abstinent six months following completion of the program while an additional 27% were abstinent at the time of follow-up, although they had experienced at least one "slip" since completing the program. Further, those who completed treatment were significantly more likely to be abstinent than those who did not complete the program.

Blow and colleagues (2000) employed a prospective, longitudinal design to investigate treatment outcomes of 90 patients over the age of 55 who participated in an older adult-specific inpatient alcoholism treatment program. This older adult-specific program included both inpatient and outpatient services, was designed to accommodate the varying medical needs of patients, and utilized a softer, less direct form of confrontation. In addition, the program included cognitive-behavioral, interpersonal, and supportive approaches, and placed a strong emphasis on the development of a therapeutic alliance with treatment staff. Results revealed that approximately half of those treated in this older adult-specific treatment program reported abstinence during the six-month follow-up period, as well as improvements in other outcomes such as general health and pain. In addition, the majority of relapses occurred in social situations in which others, usually family members, were using alcohol.

Satre, Mertens, Areán and Weisner (2003 & 2004) compared the treatment outcomes for over 1,200 participants in a Northern California HMO day hospitalization program and outpatient treatment program. The study assessed three age groups: young adults (18-39); middle adults (40-54); and older adults (55 and over). Sixty-two percent of the sample was randomly assigned into one of two treatment programs: an outpatient treatment program and a day hospitalization program. The remainder of the sample refused randomization and instead self-selected into one of the programs. Both treatment modalities were designed to meet for eight weeks with a goal of total abstinence among participants. Both treatment modalities also employed a variety of techniques including group therapy, education, relapse prevention, family-oriented treatment and individual counseling as needed. During the first three weeks, the day hospitalization group met daily for six hours and during weeks four through eight participants met four times a week for an hour and a half. The outpatient treatment group met for an hour and a half three times a week during the study. While both programs were designed to treat participants for eight weeks, those in the outpatient treatment program participated in treatment for an average of 8.5 weeks and those in the day hospitalization program participated for an average of 10.5 weeks. A statistically significant difference was found between the

TABLE 1

Author(s)	Site	Population	Gender/Race	N	Treatment	Outcome
Blow, Walton, Chermack, Mudd & Brower (2000)	IP	55 years + Diagnosis of alcohol abuse/ dependence	58.9% male 88.8% Cauc., 7.5% AA, 2.5% Hispanic	90	Older adult-specific CBT, interpersonal & supportive; treatment duration unspecified	Drinking frequency General health, Emotional distress (six months after discharge)
Carstensen, Rychtarik & Prue (1985)	VA IP	60 years + Alcohol admission Criteria not specified	100% male Ethnicity unreported	16	Non older adult-specific 28 day in-patient; education, problem-solving, self-management	Abstinence/substantial modification of drinking (two to four years after discharge)
Dupree, Broskowski, & Schonfeld (1984)	OP	55 years + Late-onset alcohol abusers	54.2% male Ethnicity unreported	48	Older adult-specific program 79 sessions-Behavioral, problem-solving, educational, risk management	Abstinence Responsible/limited drinking Community adjustment (at 12 months)
Gordon et al. (2003)	OP	Hazardous Alcohol-drinking 65+	87% male 69% white	45	Motivational Enhancement Therapy, Brief advice and Standard Care	Decrease in alcohol consumption and increase in days abstinent for ME and BA
Kashner, Rodell, Ogden, Guggenheim & Karson (1992)	VA IP	45 years + Discharged from detoxification at the VA Medical Center	100% male	137	Older adult-specific program vs. traditional program and mixed-age program; 3-4 weeks of treatment	Abstinence (six and 12 months after discharge)

Author(s)	Site	Population	Gender/Race	N	Treatment	Outcome
Kofoed, Tolson, Atkinson, Toth, & Turner (1987)	VA	54 years +	95.9% male	49	Older adult-specific "Socio-therapeutic" weekly group meetings vs. mixed-age weekly groups for 1 year	Treatment duration Treatment completion
	OP	Older alcoholics				
Rice, Longabaugh, Beattie & Noel (1993)	OP	50 years +	69% male	42	Non older adult-specific	Alcohol use (at 3 to 6 months)
		Diagnosis of alcohol abuse/ dependence	Ethnicity unreported		18 sessions—CBT vs. Relationship enhancement vs. Relationship/ enhancement	
Satre, Mertens, Areán & Weisner (2003 & 2004)	CA	18-81 years: Older adults were 55+	Of those aged 55+, 93% Caucasian, 76% male	89 (aged 55+)	8 week treatment via out-patient treatment vs. day hospitalization	Drug and alcohol abstinence (at 6 months and 5 years)
		HMO Dependency Recovery Program				
Schonfeld et al. (2000)	VA	55 years +	98.2%	110	Older adult-specific program 22 session—CBT, psycho-education, self-management	Abstinence (at six months)
	OP	Older persons with alcohol problems	Ethnicity unreported			

length of treatment for older adults and other age groups. Older adults were more likely to stay in treatment longer than those in other age groups. Aftercare involved weekly meetings for 10 months, but only 26% of the sample participated in aftercare. At six months post-intervention, 55% of older adults reported abstinence during the preceding 30 days. Participation in the day hospitalization program was a more significant predictor of abstinence than participation in the outpatient program for all participants. At five years post-interventions, older adults were more likely to report abstinence during the preceding 30 days and during the preceding year than younger adults.

TREATMENT SUMMARY

The few empirical studies that have examined outcomes associated with the treatment of older substance abusers do reveal positive outcomes. Among the alcohol abuse intervention studies, five examined the benefits of age-specific programs, two compared the results of age-specific programs with those of mixed age treatments, and one study explored the impact of a mixed-age intervention on older participants. The majority of older adult-specific programs employed CBT techniques. Researchers found that such interventions resulted in decreased alcohol consumption (Dupree, Broskowski, & Schonfeld, 1984), and increased abstinence (Blow et al., 2000; Rice, Longabaugh, Beattie, & Noel, 1993; Schonfeld et al., 2000) among the older adult participants. Other benefits reported for older adult-specific CBT-based programs include improvement in general health (Blow et al., 2002) and community adjustment (Dupree et al., 1984). The most recent age-specific study (Gordon et al., 2003) examined the impact of two brief therapies—motivational intervention and brief advice—on older problem drinkers. In recent years substance abuse researchers have focused increased attention on brief therapies, especially motivational interviewing, and have reported decreased rates of alcohol consumption and alcohol-related problem behaviors among adolescents and young to middle-aged participants. The study by Gordon and colleagues indicates that MI, and other brief treatments, can also reduce alcohol consumption among older adults. The one study that examined the efficacy of a substance abuse intervention (Satre, Mertens, Areán & Weisner, 2003 & 2004) employed a variety of therapeutic approaches including individual, group and family counseling.

The two studies that compared age-specific with mixed age alcohol abuse interventions used a combination of treatments for their older adult programs, including individual, group and reminiscence therapies that emphasized support and socialization. The older adult programs revealed better outcomes in terms of abstinence (Kashner et al., 1992; Kofoed et al., 1987) and treatment completion (Kofoed et al., 1987) than did the mixed age programs. In spite of this, it must be noted that older adults are able to derive benefits from participation in mixed age treatment programs. Carstensen, Rychtarik, and Prue (1985) examined the impact of a mixed age intervention that employed individual counseling, alcohol education, and problem-solving on older problem drinkers and reported improvement in terms of increased abstinence for half of those who participated.

It is important to note a couple of things about the research conducted by Satre and colleagues (2003 & 2004). To begin, the researchers indicated that older adults in this study were seeking treatment for both alcohol and drug dependence. It is unclear how many older adults in this sample were seeking treatment specifically for drug dependence, what types of substances were being abused, and how the treatment outcomes varied based on the type of substance used. Secondly, only 17 older females were included in this study and third, the researchers did not specify which treatment modality was more effective among older adults. They found the day treatment program to be more successful without consideration of age, but it is possible this may not have been the case when older adults were considered in isolation. Given these limitations, practitioners should be cautious before applying these techniques with older adults.

In sum, older adults with alcohol abuse disorders appear to do best when treated with a cognitive-behavioral approach (Rice, Longabaugh, Beattie, & Noel, 1993) and have better treatment compliance and outcome when treated in an older adult-specific program (Kashner et al., 1992; Kofoed et al., 1987). Further, evidence suggests that older substance abuse patients have better outcomes when treated in a more supportive, less confrontational treatment environment (Kashner et al., 1992).

CONCLUSION

In recent years, substance abuse treatment has begun to move away from generic treatment approaches that fail to identify and adjust for subgroup differences, to programs tailored to meet the needs of specific treatment to sub-populations. In past decades older adults have been underrepresented in standard substance abuse treatment programs and outcome studies. However, as evidenced by the above review, there have been some efforts to address the particular needs of older alcohol abusers in "age-specific" treatment programs. Such treatments are generally group approaches in which older individuals come together in either a discrete program designed for older alcohol abusers that is entirely age-specific, or in age-specific groups within a treatment program that treats substance abusers of all ages (CSAT, 1998). A primary assumption of an age-specific approach is that treatment is most effective when the issues dealt with are congruent with the life stage of the client (CSAT, 1998). Older substance abusers often face different issues than their younger counterparts, including loss, isolation, serious physical health problems, and other aging-related experiences (Blow et al., 2000; Schonfeld & Dupree, 1995). Social isolation, depression, and health problems may be more central to the substance use of older persons (Lemke & Moos, 2002). Therefore, age-specific programs are designed to address the challenges associated with older adulthood such as bereavement, grief, loss, loneliness, boredom, isolation, and developmental issues and how they impact substance use (Blow et al., 2000). Lastly, older adult-specific programs often embrace a supportive, non-confrontational approach in the belief that confrontation may dissuade aging substance abusers from entering into or remaining in treatment.

As can be seen from the outcome studies reviewed, cognitive-behavioral approaches are often employed in the treatment of substance abusing older adults. Such interventions are typically based on Marlatt and Gordon's (1985) relapse prevention model, identified by the National Institute on Drug Abuse (1999) as an efficacious, scientifically-based treatment approach for substance use disorders. The relapse prevention model views addictive behaviors as over-learned habits that can be analyzed and modified. As such, cognitive behavioral treatment typically consists of a functional analysis of the antecedents to substance use and the short- and long-range consequences of substance use. Treatment is designed to modify the client's association between substance use antecedents and consequences through cognitive behavioral restructuring (Rice, Longabaugh, Beattie, & Noel, 1993). Treatment programs utilizing the cognitive-behavioral approach usually employ approaches to teach clients the skills necessary to avoid relapse, such as cognitive restructuring, thought-stopping, problem-solving, self-monitoring, and self-reinforcement techniques (Schonfeld & Dupree, 2002).

With the unprecedented growth in the older population comes an increased need to address the problems older substance abusers face. The next generation to enter the ranks of older adults is the "baby boomer" generation, a group that is not only much larger than any other previous cohort but also one with much more exposure to and comfort with the use of alcohol and other substances. Studies concerning the impact of substance use on older persons indicate the deleterious effect that substance abuse has on aging systems, in terms of increased illnesses and functional impairment. As the numbers of older adults increase, social workers will increasingly encounter older clients with alcohol or drug-related disorders. In order to meet this challenge, it is critical that social workers have a deeper understanding of the nature of substance abuse in the older population and knowledge of effective treatment strategies to address this issue.

The literature review conducted for this article reveals only a handful of studies examining the efficacy of treatment programs for older substance abusers. While these studies offer important data suggesting the beneficial response of older persons to alcohol and drug treatment programs, additional research is needed to confirm and extend the findings of these studies. Further study is needed to explore differences in mixed-age and age-specific treatment outcomes. If, as many of those working in the substance abuse field believe and as studies cited above indicate, age-specific programs do produce superior results in terms of treatment compliance and outcomes, then additional research is needed to confirm these findings. It should be noted, however, that the particular treatment modalities included in the age-specific programs cited above vary significantly as do the treatment durations. Beyond the study of the overall efficacy of age-specific programs, further research is needed to examine which particular components are essential to the success of these programs.

The majority of studies described above focus on alcohol treatment outcomes for older males and only two report the ethnic composition of their subject pool. Additional research is needed on risk factors and treatments for substance abuse among older women and minorities. Women constitute 55% of the population 65 to 74 years of age and 71% of those over age 85, the fastest growing sub-population of older adults in the U.S. (Hooyman & Kiyak, 2005). The growth of older ethnic minorities is outpacing that of older Caucasians. While ethnic minorities currently represent 15.7% of persons age 65 years and over, they will comprise 33% of the older population by 2050 (NIH, 2000). Thus, in the coming years there will be increasing numbers of older women and minorities. Given the reality that older women and minorities have more disability, lower incomes and are more likely to live alone than older white males (Hooyman & Kiyak, 2005), their risk factors for substance abuse and the elements critical to their recovery may differ from those of older white males. As evident from the research studies cited above, much substance treatment research takes place at VA hospitals. In order to attract and retain older women and minorities in substance treatment programs, alternate sites and approaches for such programs may be necessary.

Another issue that must be addressed in older adult substance treatment research is that of definitional clarity. Persons defined as "older" in the above studies ranged in age from 45 years and over to 60 and above while actual participants ranged in age from 45 years to 91 years. It must be recognized that several different generations are represented within these age groups. Each of these generations grew up in different historical periods with varying norms and cultures. Their attitudes toward drinking and drug use and toward treatment may, therefore, vary considerably. In addition, persons from these different age groups are faced with divergent life challenges. While those in their 40s and 50s may be struggling with vocational and child-rearing issues, those in their 70s and above encounter increased illness, disability, and loss. Therefore, issues impacting substance use behaviors and the ability to maintain sobriety may vary tremendously. Adopting a standard definition of "older" such as 55 years and above, which was used as the definition in the majority of the studies cited above, is critical. Although 65 years is used by many governmental agencies such as Social Security and Medicare, gerontological researchers concerned with populations suffering from chronic mental health conditions often do use a slightly younger age, such as 55 years, due to the high levels of co-morbid physical, psychosocial, and medical problems experienced by persons with psychiatric disability at this age (Moak, 1996).

As can be seen from the studies noted in this review of the literature, definitions of substance abuse also vary significantly. While some researchers employ a DSM diagnosis of substance abuse or dependence (Blow et al., 2000; Rice et al., 1993), others do not specify the criteria used. In alcohol abuse research, light alcohol use is deemed acceptable by some while others define any alcohol use as abuse. Bingeing and heavy drinking are often used as these lead to an increase in physical problems (Liberto et al., 1996). While definitional confusion concerning what constitutes alcohol abuse or problematic drinking exists regardless of the age group, more uncertainty exists when dealing with the older population. In addition, due to aging physiology alcohol abuse may not present in the same way for older as for younger persons. For example, DSM criteria for substance dependence includes the development of marked tolerance, substances taken longer or in larger amounts than intended, and social, occupational or recreational activities given up. Because physical changes make older persons susceptible to higher blood alcohol concentration, marked tolerance or the consumption of larger quantities may not be present. In addition, a decrease in social, occupational, or recreational activities is not uncommon among older adults who may be experiencing medical problems, chronic conditions, or functional impairment (Brown & Lichtenberg, 1997-98).

Another issue requiring definitional clarity is the type of substance abuse that is being treated. While alcohol is thought to be the most common substance to be abused by older adults, other substances are also of concern. Colliver, Compton, Gfroerer and Condon (2006) project that in 2050 over 3.5 million adults will be illicit drug abusers, including about 3.3 million marijuana users and about 2.7 million users of prescription psychotherapeutics without medical directions. Despite these projections, research on treatment for substance abuse among older adults rarely examines interventions for any substance other than alcohol. In the rare event that substances other than alcohol are examined, it appears that researchers and practitioners are likely to submit abusers of various substances to the same interventions provided to those abusing alcohol. Researchers and practitioners alike must overcome the compassionate stereotypes that suggest that older adults do not abuse illicit substances and drugs such as heroin, cocaine, and marijuana. Substance abuse among older adults is a real problem worthy of consideration and rigorous, scholarly research is needed in order to provide practitioners with guidance as to which intervention strategies are the most effective among older adults abusing a variety of substances.

Researchers indicate that a substantial minority of older adults suffer from late onset substance abuse and suggest that the emergence of such behavior in later life is associated with loss and is amenable to treatment. While practice wisdom may indicate that late onset substance abuse is more remedial to treatment than early onset, little outcome research has been conducted to test this hypothesis. If the development of late onset substance abuse disorders is strongly influenced by challenges commonly experienced in later life such as loss of loved ones, status, and health, then prevention as well as treatment strategies are essential. For older adults who are unable to employ previously used coping strategies when facing serious life challenges, the use of alcohol or other substances may constitute an accessible, albeit, maladaptive coping mechanism. Research concerning both the risk and protective factors for the development of late substance abuse is needed. Preventive interventions that educate older adults about consequences of substance abuse and promote the use of adaptive coping strategies should be developed and tested as should early intervention programs that can effectively assist late onset abusers before serious medical, physical, or social consequences ensue.

In sum, in order to address the needs of older adults with substance abuse disorders, considerable research is needed concerning the nature of substance abuse among this population and the impact of specific treatment strategies on older adults. Such research must consider the needs and experiences of specific sub-populations of older adults such as women, minorities, and those with late onset disorders. As the population of the United States continues to age, social workers will increasingly encounter older adults with substance abuse issues. Given the serious damage that alcohol and drug abuse creates for older individuals and the high social cost in terms of medical expenses, the need for continued and expanded research in this arena is critical.

REFERENCES

Adams, S.L., & Waskel, S.A. (1993). Late onset alcoholism: Stress or structure. *The Journal of Psychology, 127*, 329-335.

Atkinson, R. (1999). Depression, alcoholism and ageing: A brief review. *International Journal of Geriatric Psychiatry, 14*, 905-910.

Atkinson, R.M. (1995). Treatment programs for aging alcoholics. In T. Beresford & E. Gomberg (Eds.), *Alcohol and aging* (pp. 186-210). New York: Oxford University Press.

Atkinson, R.M. (1990). Aging and alcohol use disorders: Diagnostic issues in the elderly. *International Psychogeriatrics, 2*, 55-72.

Atkinson, R.M., Tolson, R.L., & Turner, J.A. (1990). Late versus early onset problem drinking in older men. *Alcoholism: Clinical and Experimental Research, 14*, 574-579.

Barker, J.C., & Kramer, B.J. (1996). Alcohol consumption among older urban American Indians. *Journal of Studies on Alcohol, 57*, 119-124.

Black, B.S., Rabins, P.V., & McGuire, M.H. (1998). Alcohol use disorder is a risk factor for mortality among older public housing residents. *International Psychogeriatrics, 10*, 309-327.

Blazer, D. (1995). Alcohol and drug problems. In E.W. Busse & D.G. Blazer (Eds.), *Textbook of geriatric psychiatry* (pp. 341-356). Washington, DC: American Psychiatric Press.

Blow, F.C., Walton, M.A., Chermack, S.T., Mudd, S.A., & Brower, K.J. (2000). Older adult treatment outcome following elder-specific inpatient alcoholism treatment. *Journal of Substance Abuse Treatment, 19*, 67-75.

Booth, B.M., Blow, F.C., Cook, C.A., & Bunn, J.Y. (1992). Age and ethnicity among hospitalized alcoholics: A nationwide study. *Alcoholism: Clinical and Experimental Research, 16,* 1029-1034.

Bortz, J.J. & O'Brien, K.P. (1997). Psychotherapy with older adults: Theoretical issues, empirical findings, and clinical applications. In P.D. Nussbaum (Ed.), *Handbook of neuropsychology and aging. Critical issues in neuropsychology* (pp. 431-451). New York: Plenum Press.

Brown, K.S., & Lichtenberg, P.A. (1997-98). Substance abuse and geriatric rehabilitation. *Advances in Medical Psychotherapy, 9,* 181-191.

Callahan, C.M., & Tierney, W.M. (1995). Health services use and mortality among older primary care patients with alcoholism. *Journal of the American Geriatrics Society, 43,* 1378-1383.

Carstensen, L.L., Rychtarik, R.G., & Prue, D.M. (1985). Behavioral treatment of the geriatric alcohol abuser: A long term follow-up study. *Addictive Behaviors, 10,* 307-311.

Center for Substance Abuse Treatment (1998). *Substance abuse among older adults* (DHHS Publication No. SMA 98-3179). Rockville, MD: Substance Abuse and Mental Health Services Administration.

Chermack, S.T., Blow, F.C., Hill, E.M., & Mudd, S.A. (1996). Relationship between alcohol symptoms and consumption among older drinkers. *Alcoholism: Clinical and Experimental Research, 20,* 1153-1158.

Colliver, J.D., Compton, W.M., Gfroerer, J.C. & Condon, T. (2006). Projecting drug use among aging baby boomers in 2020. *Annals of Epidemiology, 16*(4), 257-265.

Colsher, P.L. & Wallace, R.B. (1990). Elderly men with histories of heavy drinking: Correlates and consequences. *Journal of Studies in Alcohol, 51,* 528-535.

Compton, W.M., Grant, B.F., Colliver, J.D., Glantz, M.D., & Stinson, F.S. (2004). Prevalence of marijuana use disorders in the United States 1991-1992 and 2001-2002. *Journal of the American Medical Association, 291,* 2114-2121.

Crome, I., & Crome, P. (2005). "At your age, what does it matter?"–myths and realities about older people who use substances. *Drugs: Education, Prevention & Policy, 12*(5), 343-347.

Draper, B. (1994). Suicidal behavior in the elderly. *International Journal of Geriatric Psychiatry, 9,* 655-6661.

Dupree, L.W., Broskowski, H., & Schonfeld, L. (1984). The Gerontology Alcohol Project: A behavioral treatment program for elderly alcohol abusers. *The Gerontologist, 24,* 510-516.

Fingerhood, M. (2000). Substance abuse in older people. *Journal of the American Geriatrics Society, 48,* 985-995.

Fitzgerald, J.L. & Mulford, H.A. (1992). Eldler vs. younger problem drinker "treatment" and recovery experiences. *British Journal of Addiction, 87,* 1281-1291.

Ganzini, L., & Atkinson, R.M. (1996). Substance abuse. In J. Sadavoy, L.W. Lazarus, L.F. Jarvik, & G.T. Grossberg (Eds.), *Comprehensive review of geriatric psychiatry–II* (2nd ed.). (pp. 659-692). Washington, DC, US: American Psychiatric Association.

Gfroerer, J., Penne, M., Pemberton, M., & Folsom, R. (2002). Substance abuse treatment need among older adults in 2020: The impact of the aging baby-boom cohort. *Drug and Alcohol Dependence, 69,* 127-135.

Gordon, A.J., Conigliaro, J., Maisto, A.A., McNeil, M., Kraemer, K.L., & Kelley, M. E. (2003). Comparisons of consumption effects of brief interventions for hazardous drinking elderly. *Substance Use & Misuse, 38*, 1017-1035.

Guida, F., Unterbach, A., Tavolacci, J., & Provet, P. (2004). Residential substance abuse treatment for older adults: An enhanced therapeutic community model. *Journal of Gerontological Social Work, 44*(1/2), 95-109.

Helzer, J.E., Burnam, A., & McEvoy, L.T. (1991). Alcohol abuse and dependence. In L.N. Robins & D.A. Regier (Eds.), *Psychiatric disorders in America: The Epidemiologic Catchment Area Study* (pp. 81-115). New York: MacMillan.

Holroyd, S., & Duryee, J.J. (1997). Substance use disorders in a geriatric psychiatry outpatient clinic: Prevalence and epidemiologic characteristics. *The Journal of Nervous and Mental Disease, 185*, 627-632.

Hooyman, N., & Kiyak, H.A. (2005). *Social gerontology* (7th Edition). Boston: Allyn & Bacon.

Hurt, R.D., Finlayson, R.E., Morse, R.M., & Davis, L.J. (1988). Alcoholism in elderly persons: Medical aspects and prognosis of 216 inpatients. *Mayo Clinic Proceedings, 63*, 753-760.

Jinks, M.J., & Raschko, R.R. (1990). A profile of alcohol and prescription drug abuse in a high-risk community-based elderly population. *Annals of Pharmocotherapy, 24*, 971-975.

Johnson, I. (2000). Alcohol problems in old age: A review of recent epidemiological research. *International Journal of Geriatric Psychiatry, 15*, 575-581.

Joseph, C.L., Rasmussen, J., Ganzini, L., & Atkinson, R.M. (1997). Outcome of nursing home care for residents with alcohol use disorders. *International Journal of Geriatric Psychiatry, 12*:767-772.

Joseph, C.L., Ganzini, L., & Atkinson, R. (1995). Screening for alcohol use disorders in the nursing home. *Journal of the American Geriatrics Society, 43*, 368-373.

Kandel, D., Chen, K., Warner, L.A., Kessler, R.C., & Grant, B. (1997). Prevalence and demographic correlates of symptoms of last year dependence on alcohol, nicotine, marijuana and cocaine in the U.S. population. *Drug & Alcohol Dependence, 44*, 11-29.

Kashner, M., Rodell, D.E., Ogden, S.R., Guggenheim, F.G., & Karson, C.N. (1992). Outcomes and costs of two VA inpatient treatment programs for older alcoholic patients. *Hospital and Community Psychiatry, 43*, 985-989.

King, C.J., Van Hasselt, V.B., Segal, D.L., & Hersen, M. (1994). Diagnosis and assessment of substance abuse in older adults: Current strategies and issues. *Addictive Behaviors, 19*(1), 41-55.

Kofoed, L.L., Tolson, R.L., Atkinson, R.M., Toth, R.L., & Turner, J.A. (1987). Treatment compliance of older alcoholics: An elder-specific approach is superior to "mainstreaming." *Journal of Studies on Alcohol, 48*, 47-51.

Krause, N. (2003). Race, religion, and abstinence from alcohol in late life. *Journal of Aging and Health, 15*(3), 508-533.

Lemke, S., & Moos, R.H. (2002). Prognosis of older patients in mixed-age alcoholism treatment programs. *Journal of Substance Abuse Treatment, 22*, 33-43.

Liberto, J.G., Oslin, D.W., & Ruskin, P.E. (1996). Alcoholism in the older population. In L.L. Carstensen & B.A. Edelstein (Eds.) *The practical handbook of clinical gerontology* (pp. 324-348). Thousand Oaks, CA: Sage Publications, Inc.

Light, E., & Lebowitz, B.D. (1991). *The elderly with chronic mental illness*. New York: Springer Publishing Company.

Marlatt, G.A., & Gordon, J.R. (Eds.) (1985). *Relapse prevention: Maintenance strategies in the treatment of addictive behaviors*. New York: Guilford Press.

Mirand A.I., & Welte, J.W. (1996). Alcohol consumption among the elderly in the general population, Erie County, New York. *American Journal of Public Health, 86*, 978-984.

Mittleman, M.A., Mintzer, D., Maclure, M., Tofler, G.H., Sherwood, J.B. & Muller, J. E. (1999). Triggering of myocardial infarct by cocaine. *Circulation, 99*(21), 2737-2741.

Moak, G.S. (1996). When the chronically mentally ill patient grows old. In S.M. Soreff (Ed.), *Handbook for the treatment of the chronically mentally ill* (pp. 279-293). Seattle: Hogrefe & Huber.

Molgaard, C.A., Nakamura, C.M., Stanford, E.P., Peddecord, K.M., & Morton, D.J. (1990). Prevalence of alcohol consumption among older persons. *Journal of Community Health, 15*, 239-251.

Moos, R.H., Mertens, J.R., & Brennan, P.L. (1993). Patterns of diagnosis and treatment among late middle-aged and older substance abuse patients. *Journal of Studies on Alcohol, 54*, 479-487.

Mukamal, K.J., Conigrave, K.M., Stampfer, M.J., Camargo, C.A., Ascherio, A., Mittleman, M.A., Rimm, E.B., Kawachi, I., & Willett, W.C. (2005). Alcohol and risk for ischemic stroke in men: The role of drinking patterns and usual beverage. *Ann Intern Medicine 143*(1), 11-19.

Mukamal, K.J., Mittleman, M.A., Longstreth, W.T., Newman, A.B., Fried. L.R., & Siscovick, D.S. (2004). Self-reported alcohol consumption and falls in older adults: Cross sectional and longitudinal analyses of the Cardiovascular Health Study. *Journal of the American Geriatrics Society, 52,* 1174-1179.

National Institute on Drug Abuse (1999). *Principles of drug addiction treatment: A research-based guide* (NIH Publication No. 99-4180). Washington, DC: Author.

National Institute of Health (2000). *Women of color health data book*. Washington, DC: Office of Research on Women's Health.

Oslin, D.W., & Blow, F.C. (2000). Substance use disorders in late life. In I. Katz & D. Oslin (Eds.), *Annual review of gerontology and geriatrics: Focus on psychopharmacologic interventions in late life (vol. 19)* (pp. 213-224). New York: Springer Publishing Co.

Oslin, D.W., Streim, J.E., Parmelee, P., Boyce, A.A., & Katz, I.R. (1997). Alcohol abuse: A source of reversible functional disability among residents. *International Journal of Geriatric Psychiatry, 12*, 825-832.

Preedy, V.R., Salisbury, J.R., & Peters, T.J. (1994). Alcoholic muscle disease: Features and mechanisms. *Journal of Pathology, 173*, 309-315.

Regan, T.J. (1990). Alcohol and the cardiovascular system. *Journal of the American Medical Association, 264*, 377-381.

Reid, M.C., Boutros, N.N., O'Connor, P.G., Cadariu, A., & Concato, J. (2002). The health related effects of alcohol use in older persons: A systemic review. *Substance Abuse, 23*, 149-164.

Reinhardt, J., & Fulop, G. (1996). Geriatric alcoholism: Identification and elder-specific treatment programs. In J. Lonsdale, Series Ed., *The Hatherleigh guides series: Vol. 8. The Hatherleigh guide to treating substance abuse, Part 2* (pp. 197-224). New York: Hatherleigh Press.

Rice, C., Longabaugh, R., Beattie, M., & Noel, N. (1993). Age group differences in response to treatment for problematic alcohol use. *Addiction, 88,* 1369-1375.

Rosen, D. (2004). Factors associated with illegal drug use among older methadone client. *The Gerontologist, 44*(4), 543-547.

Stevenson, J.S. (2005). Alcohol use, misuse, abuse, and dependence in later adulthood. *Annual Review of Nursing Research, 23,* 245-280.

Satre, D.D., Mertens, J., Areán, P.A., & Weisner, C. (2003). Contrasting outcomes of older versus middle-aged and younger adult chemical dependency patients in a managed care program. *Journal of Studies on Alcohol, 64,* 520-530.

Satre, D.D., Mertens, J., Arean, P.A., & Weisner, C. (2004). Five-year alcohol and drug treatment outcomes of older adults versus middle-aged and younger adults in a managed care program. *Addiction, 99,* 1286-1297.

Saunders, P.A., Copeland, J.R., Dewey, M.E., Davidson, I.A., McWilliam, C., Sharma, V., & Sullivan, C. (1991). Heavy drinking as a risk factor for depression and dementia in elderly men: Findings from the Liverpool longitudinal community study. *British Journal of Psychiatry, 159,* 213-216.

Schlaerth, K.R., Splawn, R.G., Ong, J., & Smith, S.D. (2004). Change in the pattern of illegal drug use in an inner city population over 50: An observational study. *Journal of Addictive Diseases, 23*(2), 95-107.

Schonfeld, L., & Dupree, L.W. (2002). Age-specific cognitive-behavioral and self-management treatment approaches. In A.M. Gurnack, R. Atkinson, & N.J. Osgood (Eds.), *Treating alcohol and drug abuse in the elderly.* New York: Springer Publishing Company.

Schonfeld, L., & Dupree, L.W. (1995). Treatment approaches for older problem drinkers. *International Journal of the Addictions, 30,* 1819-1842.

Schonfeld, L., Dupree, L.W., Dickson-Fuhrman, E., Royer, C.M., McDermott, C.H., Rosansky, J.S., Taylor, S., & Jarvik, L.F. (2000). Cognitive-behavioral treatment of older veterans with substance abuse problems. *Journal of Geriatric Psychiatry and Neurology, 13,* 124-128.

Schonfeld, L., Rohrer, G.E., Zima, M., & Spiegel, T. (1993). Alcohol abuse and medication misuse in older adults as estimated by service providers. *Journal of Gerontological Social Work, 21,* 113-125.

Schutte, K., Brennan, P., & Moos, R. (1998). Predicting the development of late-life late-onset drinking problems: A 7 year prospective study. *Alcoholism: Clinical Exp. Research, 22,* 1349-1358.

Shadi, S.S. & Szabenyi, S.E. (2005). Resource use of elderly emergency department patients with alcohol-related diagnoses. *Journal of Substance Abuse Treatment, 29,* 313-319.

RESOURCE GUIDE–SUBSTANCE ABUSE
AND OLDER ADULTS

*www.camh.net/Care_Treatment/Resources_for_Professionals/Older_Adults/responding_*
older_adults.pdf.
Free booklet "Alcohol Problems: Responding to Older Adults with Substance Use, Mental Health and Gambling Challenges" is available through the Centre for Addiction and Mental Health. The booklet contains information on the effects of alcohol on older adults, signs of alcohol problems, and how to talk to an older adult who has an alcohol problem.

http://www.findtreatment.samhsa.gov/
Site sponsored by the Substance Abuse and Mental Health Services Administration enables the user to locate the closest alcohol or drug abuse program based upon zip code. Program contact information is given along with information concerning types of services provided, special programs offered, and forms of payment accepted.

http://www.springerpub.com
Alcohol Problems in Older Adults Prevention and Management by Kristen Barry, PhD; David Oslin, MD; Frederic Blow, PhD–book available from Springer Publishing Company. This book provides practical materials to detect, prevent, and intervene with older adults who are at-risk and problem drinkers. This book is designed as a hands-on text for use in a range of primary and mental health-care settings.

http://pathwayscourses.samhsa.gov/aaac/aaac_intro_pg1.htm
Free on-line courses–*Prevention Pathways Any Age, It Does Matter: Substance Abuse and Older Adults*–focuses on risk factors, screening tools, prevention and treatment, legal issues, and ethical concerns. *CEU's available from NASW*
Alcohol, Medication and Older Adults for Those Who Care About or Care for an Older Adult–discusses the problems of alcohol and medication misuse in older adults, signs and symptoms, and how to talk to older adults, as well as prevention, intervention, and treatment.

http://ncadistore.samhsa.gov/catalog/productDetails.aspx?ProductID = 16523
Get Connected! Toolkit (Linking Older Adults with Medication, Alcohol, and Mental Health Resources) developed by the U.S. Department of Health and Human Services is designed for service providers who wish to engage in health promotion, prevention, screening and referrals for older adults related to the misuse of alcohol and medications. The kit includes a coordinator's guide and program support materials such as education curricula, fact sheets, handouts, forms, and resources.

http://www.niaaa.nih.gov/
Powerpoint presentation entitled "Older Adults and Alcohol Problems" that offers a wealth of information including prevalence, issues unique to older adults, co-morbid conditions, screening and detection, and prevention and treatment. Once at the NIAAA homepage, type in older adults in the search box to access the link for the presentation.

EVIDENCE-BASED INTERVENTIONS FOR SOCIAL FUNCTIONING

The previous two sections of this book addressed health, mental health, and cognitive issues of later adulthood. In this section, issues and responsibilities within social relationships and the performance of roles as they occur for special populations of older adults and caregivers are discussed. Four chapters comprise this final section and highlight changes in social functioning for particular groups of individuals–older persons with developmental disabilities and their care providers, individuals at the end of life, familial care providers of older adults, and grandparents who are raising grandchildren.

Two of the chapters, which deal with older parents of those with developmental disabilities and with grandparent care providers, highlight "off time" caregiving experiences. Both types of care providers may be in mid to late life themselves, and have the simultaneous responsibility of managing their own later life experiences and taking care of younger generations. This intersection can create a particular risk situation in the care provider's health and functioning which, in turn, can precipitate a family-level crisis. Outcome studies on interventions to enhance caregiver efficacy are included in this section as well as treatments to improve future care planning and the well-being of those who are in care receiving roles.

Another group, familial caregivers, typically represents spouses and adult children in caregiving roles. These care providers benefit from psychosocial interventions that enhance their ability to manage the tasks and stresses of care provision. In addition to helping the caregiver, some of the research indicates that such interventions can also have a positive impact on the behavior and functioning of the older care recipient.

A final chapter looks at end of life issues and care. At the point of a terminal diagnosis, several psychosocial issues are present such as enhancing the quality of life that remains for the patient and supporting those people who will continue to survive after the loved one is gone. In addition, multiple decisions often must be made as a loved one nears the end of life. Various interventions have been studied that assist family members with this complex and very personal decision-making process.

In all of these chapters, social support and psychoeducational groups have been found to be effective in helping with transitions in functioning. Group interventions provide a forum for caregivers and the bereaved to be with others who are having similar experiences, which offers validation and enhanced coping. Case management and interdisciplinary team approaches are also found within these chapters, as families often require access to resources and services as a result of their caregiving situations.

These chapters span a variety of practice contexts, similar to the other chapters within this volume. Practitioners in health care see terminal patients within hospitals, clinics and hospice settings. In addition, they may encounter care providers, as a health-related crisis may be the reason that a grandparent, older parent, or family caregiver seeks support or requires resources. However, social workers in community-based settings also will encounter these situations within their practice. A wonderful example is the school social worker who works with a grandparent within the school setting. This situation highlights the importance of all social work students to have some understanding of aging and effective practice with the older population.

Chapter 10

Individuals with Developmental Disabilities and Their Caregivers

Philip McCallion, PhD
Tara Nickle, MSW

In his consideration of persons with developmental disabilities, Janicki (1994) defines successful aging as "an individual retaining his or her capacities to function as independently as possible into old age and promoting the belief that persons who age successfully are able to remain out of institutions, maintain their autonomy and competence in all activities of daily living, and continue to engage in productive endeavors of their own choosing" (p. 146). Problem behaviors, onset or poor management of mental health concerns and inadequate planning for their aging years are the biggest barriers to such successful aging for persons with developmental disabilities. However, psychosocial interventions have the potential to alleviate these barriers and promote positive aging for older persons with developmental disabilities. The evidence for the effectiveness of such interventions will be examined within this article.

DEMOGRAPHICS AND PREVALENCE

A critical first issue is to define the population of interest. Public Law 98-527, the Developmental Disabilities and Bill of Rights Act, defines a developmental disability (DD) as a severe, chronic disability of a person which: (1) is attributable to a mental or physical impairment or some combination of those mental and physical impairments; (2) is manifest before age 22; (3) is likely to continue indefinitely; (4) results in substantial functional limitations in three or more areas of major life activity; and (5) reflects the need for a combination and sequence of special, interdisciplinary or generic care, treatment or other services which are of lifelong or extended duration and are individually planned and coordinated (McCallion & Kolomer, 2003). This definition was designed to expand the scope of populations with life-long cognitive impairments towards whom services have traditionally been targeted. People with mental retardation remain the largest group of persons with DD, while persons with Down syndrome constitute an important subgroup (Janicki & Dalton, 2001). The historic focus on persons with cognitive impairments has also resulted in greater attention to the labels used to describe such individuals. "Persons with mental retardation" has been the most common term; however, in the UK, "persons with learning disability" has been used largely interchangeably with this term. Currently in Europe, there are successful efforts to change both terms to persons with intellectual disabilities (ID). Both publicly funded formal services and intervention research for persons with developmental disabilities (DD) continue to be largely concentrated on persons with mental retardation/ID.

It is also important to note that adults with DD are experiencing increased longevity. As a result, concerns have been raised that agencies and professional staff are ill-prepared to address the increased needs of an older population with lifelong disabilities (Braddock, 1999; Seltzer & Krauss, 1994). The caregiving life of families of persons with DD now spans multiple decades and is increasingly a feature of advanced age for parents and grandparents, and of old age for siblings (McCallion & Kolomer, 2003). Many individuals with DD (almost 700,000 as of 2000) are already in households where the caregiver is older; with increasing years, they will continue to be cared for by these older caregivers. In addition, those currently being cared for by family members in their 40s and 50s (approximately two million in 2000) will have caregivers that will be in their 60s and 70s by 2020 (Braddock et al., 2001; Fujiura, 1998). Therefore, the growth in the number of older persons with DD has implications for both those with DD themselves and for their aging caregiver. For example, recognition of the critical issue of long-term planning for people with DD and interventions for families may be as important for the welfare of the person with DD as those interventions which are solely targeted at the person with DD (McCallion & Kolomer, 2003).

In terms of U.S. population estimates, it is acknowledged there are no mechanisms for complete counts of people with DD. Current estimates suggest that at least 140,000 persons with DD are over the age of 65 (Janicki et al., 2005). Life expectancy for persons with DD is estimated to have increased from an average 18.5 years in 1930, to 59.1 years in 1970, to an estimated 66.2 years in 1993 (Braddock, 1999). Based upon analyses of New York State data generalized to the U.S., Janicki and colleagues project continued growth to match life expectancy of the general population (Janicki, Dalton, Henderson, & Davidson, 1999). Compared to current estimates, the projected number of persons with DD in the 65 years plus age group is expected to double by 2020 (Janicki & Dalton, 2000). Similar growth is expected in the UK, other European countries and Australia (Hogg, Lucchino, Wang, & Janicki, 2001).

These estimates assume that aging is experienced by persons with DD at traditional age cut-offs and in ways similar to the general population. Instead, there is evidence for premature aging for persons with Down syndrome, and concerns that relatively small insults to functioning attributable to aging may have greater and earlier impact upon independence for persons with DD. Alzheimer's Disease is often cited as an example of a condition that occurs earlier and has a greater impact upon some persons with DD. In fact, dementia-related research has become an extensive line of research within the DD literature. Alzheimer's disease and other dementias (ADD) are a risk of increasing age for everyone (Brookmeyer, Gray, & Kawas, 1998) and an increasingly aging population of persons with DD is exposed to similar risks. In the United States, there may be as many as 9,000 older adults with DD possibly affected by ADD, and this number will grow threefold within the next 20 years (Janicki et al., 2005). Among persons with DD, adults with Down syndrome are generally at higher risk of ADD (Holland, Karlinsky, & Berg, 1993). For adults with Down syndrome ADD onset is earlier (age of risk begins at 35 years), the course tends to be compressed, the duration short, and the decline precipitous (Janicki et al., 1999). Concerns have been noted that existing disabilities often mask symptoms of dementia and make assessment difficult for persons with DD, and that an absence of treatment alternatives discourages diagnosis and active treatment (Janicki et al., 2005). Similar concerns have been raised about the identification and treatment of other physical and mental health issues (Janicki et al., 2002). Indeed, there are anecdotal reports that the growing focus upon dementia in aging persons with DD is leading to a "rush to diagnosis" of dementia (McCallion & Janicki, 2002) without sufficient attention to other possible and treatable causes of the symptoms noted.

NATURE AND CONSEQUENCES OF PROBLEM

The prevalence of mental disorders is reported to be significantly higher among persons with DD than in the general adult population, with estimates ranging from 33% to 70% (Griswold & Goldstein, 1999). Some experts argue that mental health concerns prevalent earlier in life decline with age. For example, a recently completed systematic study of the health needs of persons with DD aged 40 and over, living in group homes in two catchment areas of New York State, found that psychiatric and behavioral disorders tended to decline in frequency with increasing age while cardiovascular diseases and sensory impairments increased with age (Janicki et al., 2002). However, this picture is confused by coexisting problems such as language disorders, impaired mobility, and hearing or visual impairments that may worsen with advancing age. In addition, it is likely that older age will be accompanied by health changes and conditions for which the person with DD is unprepared. The lack of preparation may have psychosocial consequences, which may be addressed or prevented through intervention.

Grief and loss concerns among persons with DD are particularly difficult for service providers (McCallion & McCarron, 2004). The commonly held view was that persons with DD did not understand and were unable to express grief at the deaths of friends and loved ones. More recently, there has been recognition that people with DD do experience grief and loss, yet express these emotions differently and in different time frames. Prior to this understanding, there had been an incorrect tendency for others to view grief expression in persons with DD as out of time sequence or as representing some other form of mental health concern. With a better understanding of the experience of grief, there is now recognition that interventions are possible and appropriate (McCallion & McCarron, 2004).

A more unique aging-related concern of persons with DD is futures planning. Heller and Factor (1991) found that almost 75% of family care providers of persons with DD (aged 30 years and older) did not make future living arrangements for their family member. Often, too, there was a reluctance to speak of future living arrangements with the individual's siblings. The expectations of other family members assuming care responsibilities were often implied rather than formally documented (Bigby, 1996). Yet, some evidence exists that persons with DD for whom future planning was implemented had better outcomes in terms of quality of life than did those for whom such planning did not occur (Heller et al., 2000).

In sum, there are a variety of issues that many aging individuals with DD have to face as they age. These include retirement, changing social roles, vulnerability to mental illness onset, and loss of physical/sensory abilities (Lynch, 2004). In addition, issues of maintaining independence, dealing with age-specific mental health concerns, preparing for major life transitions, planning for greater independence from caregivers, and dealing with end of life concerns become prominent for persons with DD in later years (McCallion & Kolomer, 2003).

EMPIRICAL LITERATURE

To review the empirical literature on the older population with disabilities, electronic searches were carried out in several databases. The following databases were examined: EBSCO, Ingenta, Ageline, Psych Info, using population terms (intellectual disability, developmental disability, mental retardation, and Down syndrome) in combination with intervention terms (psychosocial, therapeutic, intervention), with and without the word aging. Inclusion criteria were articles published in the last 10 years that were either specifically targeted at, or were relevant to, aging persons. Because of premature aging issues, the definition of aging is more complex in the DD literature than for other populations. As suggested by the World Health Organization (Janicki, 2000), age 50 and above was used as a criterion for aging. As well as individual studies, 10 review articles on psychosocial and behavioral interventions were identified through this process and their reference lists were manually reviewed to further identify studies of interest.

Over 50 articles were identified addressing a variety of interventions being used by clinicians with adults with DD; however, less information was available on their use with older adults with DD. A further concern was that most reported studies continue to target people with ID, meaning there was even less literature on persons with other types of DD. A total of ten intervention studies targeted at older persons with DD were ultimately identified.

This search process also yielded articles that offered an opportunity to consider the overall literature on interventions for adults with ID, and other DD. This literature provides a useful context for understanding treatment evidence for older persons with DD. For example, in a survey of clinical psychologists in ID service settings concerning the types of interventions employed, Nagel and Leiper (1999) found that respondents used cognitive-behavioral (35%), humanistic/person centered (31%) and psychodynamic (17%) methods. These findings suggest that clinical staff in ID services frame their work within formalized approaches, but such reports are not sufficient to establish that there is widespread reliance on evidence-based interventions in this field. Indeed, a recent review article by Hatton (2002) concluded that there was little support to suggest intentional use of evidence-based interventions (psychosocial or otherwise) for persons with ID and mental health problems. Instead, clinicians were found to draw from a small number of case studies where descriptions of behavioral interventions appear to suggest effectiveness, and from case series/uncontrolled trials where cognitive-behavioral or psychodynamic therapy have appeared to have some success with depression, anxiety, psychosis, anger, or offending behaviors. Nevertheless, some consensus reports have been constructed concerning various interventions with older adults who have disabilities.

Consensus Reports

An expert consensus panel reported on by Prout and Nowak-Drabik (2003) examined 92 studies of psychotherapy with persons with ID over a 30-year period. Studies that included adults with DD comprised 62% of the research examined; unfortunately, adulthood was not divided further to identify those studies that included older adults. In order to select studies, the researchers used the following criteria: the research had face-to-face application of techniques; techniques were drawn from established psychological principles; the therapist was qualified by training and experience to understand the techniques; the intention of therapy was to assist individuals in modifying their feelings, values, attitudes, and behaviors; psychotherapy did not include interventions primarily conducted by paraprofessionals; and psychotherapy did include interventions of counseling and training that met the other criteria. Each study was evaluated by three expert raters with backgrounds in psychology and research methodology. One consensus rating focused on the study *outcome* which was defined as the amount of change exhibited by participants after exposure to an intervention. The outcome rating scale was from 1 (no significant change) to 5 (marked change on all outcomes identified within the study). A second dimension, *effectiveness,* was the degree of benefit for the study participants. This second dimension was a clinical indicator about the extent or relevance of change for study participants. Effectiveness ratings were scored as 1 (minimal) to 5 (marked effectiveness). Consensus was defined as at least two raters assigning the same rating score. The outcome and effectiveness consensus ratings showed an 87% agreement rate.

The intervention studies with adults had higher outcome ratings (3.14) than either research involving children (2.91) or adolescents (3.09). The adult score indicates that the studies achieved significant change on more than two thirds of the outcome measures within the research. Ratings on the effectiveness dimension were highest for research with children (2.90), followed by adults (2.74) and adolescents (2.55). These scores indicate that for all populations, achieved outcomes had significant benefits. In conclusion, the researchers recommended that psychotherapy be considered as a viable form of intervention for people with DD. However, the authors also found serious concerns with this literature such as findings from case studies/single system designs, a lack of adequate controls, poorly or vaguely described client/intervention characteristics, an absence of treatment manuals/protocols, vague or omitted outcome data, and ill-suited or investigator developed outcome measures. They recommended that intervention research with this population include greater degrees of methodological rigor.

In an attempt to narrow the intervention modalities to various treatment types, Beail (2003) provides expert commentary on cognitive-behavioral therapy (CBT) and psychodynamic psychotherapy research in adults with DD. CBT studies were classified as either enhancing problem-solving or increasing anger management. Problem-solving studies (n = 2) focused on assertiveness and skills training groups. One study concluded that skills training had positive outcomes for participants as compared to controls, but a second study reported no differences between treatment and control groups. For anger management (n = 5), CBT protocols produced modest positive gains with men of borderline intelligence who had criminal histories. Research with other populations did not report significant impacts for adults with DD, however.

Psychodynamic interventions (n = 5) also provided limited data about effectiveness. Problem conditions that were treated using psychodynamic modalities included decreasing dysfunctional behaviors and psychological distress. In one study, a psychodynamic treatment group comprised of persons with maladaptive or criminal behavior resulted in fewer behavioral problems after six months. In a second study, adults experiencing health conditions had fewer psychological symptoms after participating in a group intervention. Overall, Beail concluded that few CBT or psychodynamic studies were undertaken with methodological rigor, and outcomes were inconclusive about the impact of these interventions for people with DD.

Despite these reservations, three classes of non-pharmacological interventions have been recommended to address psychiatric concerns and problem behaviors of persons with ID and other DD in a consensus guideline developed by Rush and Francis (2000). An expert panel was asked to rate seven psychosocial interventions for children, adolescents and adults. In addition, other characteristics were also considered in rating the effectiveness of approaches including the level of retardation, psychiatric diagnoses and behavioral issues. Three interventions were the most highly recommended for all clients with DD: applied behavior analysis, managing the environment, and client/family education. *Applied behavior analysis* encompasses behavioral analysis techniques intended to build more appropriate or functional skills and to reduce problem behaviors. *Managing the environment* approaches are designed to reduce problem behaviors by rearranging the physical and/or social conditions that appear to provoke such behaviors. *Client/family education* programs are designed to help persons with DD and/or families understand more about the behavioral and psychiatric problems that may accompany DD and how they may be managed. Regardless of age, the consensus guideline recommends these approaches for a variety of DSM-IV disorders experienced by persons with DD, including major depressive disorder, PTSD, OCD, bipolar disorder, schizophrenia and other psychotic disorders, GAD, conduct disorder, substance abuse or dependence, and adjustment disorder. Supportive counseling and psychotherapy were not as highly recommended as a treatment approach for persons with ID and other DD.

Individual Studies

Several individual research studies have provided evidence for psychosocial intervention effectiveness specifically with older adults with DD. In some studies, older adults with ID were participants but family members were the primary targets. In the literature on psychosocial interventions specifically for older persons with ID and other forms of DD, 10 intervention studies have been identified (see Table 1). Seven studies are focused upon futures planning interventions (Bigby, Ozanne, & Gordon, 2002; Botsford & Rule, 2004; Heller, Miller, Hsieh, & Sterns, 2000; Heller, Factor, Sterns, & Sutton, 1996; Mahon & Goatcher, 1999; Reilly & Conliffe, 2002; Smith, Majeski, & McClenny, 1996) with the remaining three studies focused on coping with aging-related change (Hammel, Lai, & Heller, 2002; Kessel, Merrick, Kedem, Borovsky, & Carmeli, 2002; Lynggaard & Alexander, 2004). All studies have strong educational components, and the futures

TABLE 1. Interventions for Older Adults with DD and Their Caregivers

Authors/Date	Population	N	Intervention	Outcome
Bigby, Ozanne, & Gordon (2002)	Older parents caring at home for an adult offspring with ID	55	Case management	Carers had better experience with futures planning, more access to services, and greater emotional support.
Botsford & Rule (2004)	Older parents caring at home for an adult offspring with ID	28	Group intervention, six two hour sessions weekly	Intervention group showed significantly greater increases in knowledge and awareness of planning resources, competence and confidence to plan, and advancement in the planning process.
Hammel, Lai, & Heller (2002)	Adults with DD age 35 and older seeking to transition from institutional to community-based settings	109	Targeted, later life assistive technology and environmental intervention (AT-EI)	More than 70% of participants had higher functioning with AT after intervention as compared to control.
Heller, Factor, Sterns, & Sutton (1996)	Adults with DD age 50 and over or 35 and over with Down syndrome; staff members; family	70 Adults with DD; 48 Staff members; 14 Family members	Person-centered training program of 17 two hour weekly sessions with adults with DD; one six hour training for staff and family members	Intervention group gained significantly more knowledge of skills/concepts, and more leisure participation (for those living at home). --- Intervention group decreased in life satisfaction, the comparison group increased.
Heller, Miller, Hsieh, & Sterns (2000)	Adults with DD age 50 and over or 35 and over with Down syndrome, staff and family	60 Adults with DD; 51 Staff members; 14 Family members	Person-centered training program of 17 two hour weekly sessions with adults with DD; one six hour training for staff and family members	Intervention group gained significantly more knowledge of skills/concepts in the curriculum and made more choices over time. --- 87% of participants met or partially met goals they set in training.

Authors/Date	Population	N	Intervention	Outcome
Kessel, Merrick, Kedem, Borovsky, & Carmeli (2002)	Older adults with ID in residential care experiencing loss of physical abilities affecting living, independence, or QOL	9	Group intervention on functional disabilities, ten sessions	Positive changes in attitude and improved self-esteem, and less extreme behavioral reactions.
Lynggaard & Alexander (2004)	Persons with ID living in residential home with people with ID diagnosed with dementia	4	Group intervention aimed at understanding dementia with six weekly one hour sessions	Participants showed more knowledge, support/empathy.
Mahon & Goatcher (1999)	Older adults with DD in need of retirement planning	20	Individualized later-life planning intervention	Intervention group showed significantly greater increases in leisure and life satisfaction.
Reilly & Conliffe (2002)	Families and other carers of adults with ID	31	Futures planning	Participants reported a reduction in anxiety and stress surrounding planning issues.
Smith, Majeski, & McClenny (1996)	Parents aged 50 and over of adult offspring with DD	30	Group intervention for permanency planning; six 1.5 hour sessions weekly	Participants residing with adult offspring found information on permanency planning and support services most helpful.

planning interventions are more often targeted at family members, with the person with ID as an indirect beneficiary.

Future Planning Interventions. In terms of building evidence-based practice, only one study within the group of seven futures planning studies used an experimental design (Botsford & Rule, 2004). In this study, data were collected from mothers, who ranged in age from 49 to 82 years, and were assigned to either a treatment or control group. Caregivers who participated in the intervention group (n = 14) attended six, two-hour sessions to increase permanency planning for their adult children with DD. The group sessions focused on psycho-education, problem-solving, and supportive interactions. The first two and last sessions consisted primarily of parents' discussions and interactions. Sessions 3-

5 involved speakers on residential, financial, and legal resources followed by group discussion. A control group (n = 14) was also included. Analysis of post-intervention data indicated that intervention group participants had significantly greater knowledge and awareness of planning resources, competence and confidence in future planning for their son or daughter, and advances in their own planning process than did the control group.

The remainder of studies used quasi-experimental, or pre- and post-intervention designs to determine intervention effectiveness. Smith et al. (1996) also employed a group intervention for older parents. Four groups were run in the Baltimore and Washington, DC area, with two for those parents whose child lived at home and two where the child lived outside the family residence. A total of 30 parents were involved in the intervention, and their average age was 65.3 years. Each group attended six sessions of 1.5 hours duration each week. Various topics related to permanency planning were included in the session such as family support services, living options, legal and financial issues, relaxation techniques, permanency planning and emergency planning. A pre- and post-data collection strategy was employed focusing on how helpful the participants found the groups to be with respect to eight potential futures planning outcomes. Results indicated that participants who resided with their offspring found content on the permanency planning and support service sessions as most helpful. Interestingly, however, the non-residential parents rated the group sessions most helpful overall.

An Australian case management program for older parents was also evaluated (Bigby et al., 2002). Older parents who were caring for adult children with DD in the home were included in the intervention. A total of 55 caregivers were involved, with an age range of 50 to 91 years. The sons and daughters in care ranged in age from 18 to 54 years of age. The case management program provided caregiver support, assistance with future planning, and skill development for the person with DD. At post-intervention, the highest gains for the care providers were in the areas of future planning, getting access to support services, and receiving emotional support.

An Irish study included 31 families in a futures planning intervention (Reilly & Conliffe, 2002). Families were involved in topics such as later life planning processes, residential planning, social planning, health care, asset management, and family supports. In a post-test only design, participants reported a reduction in anxiety and stress in future planning issues. In addition, families engaged in greater discussion about future planning issues.

Heller, Factor, Sterns and Sutton (1996) implemented a person-centered training program for adults with DD who were 50 and over, or 35 and older with Down syndrome. Seventy adults with mild to moderate intellectual disability participated, with their ages ranging from 35 to 87 years. Their outcomes were compared to a group receiving usual treatment. Participants attended 15, two-hour sessions. Residential support staff (n = 48) and participants' family members (n = 14) attended one six-hour training session. In addition, participants, staff and family members participated jointly in one, three-hour planning session. Data were collected at pre- and six months post-test. At post-test, the participants had gained significantly more knowledge of skills and concepts for planning than had adults with DD who had not gone through the training. Those participants who lived at home also reported greater leisure participation. Interestingly, however, the intervention group decreased in life satisfaction and the usual care comparison group had increased scores.

Heller et al. (2000) replicated this intervention with older adults who participated in vocational day programs in Ohio and Illinois. The same selection criteria were applied and resulted in a sample of 60 individuals who ranged in age from 35 to 84 years. Small group trainings consisting of five to seven individuals were provided in weekly two-hour sessions. The intervention lasted for 17 weeks, and also involved program staff and family members. Data were collected pre-intervention and at six months post-intervention. The results indicated that the treatment group gained significantly greater knowledge in the area of future planning, and made more choices in future care options. However, no significant difference was found for the life satisfaction scores between treatment and control groups.

A study of individualized late life planning was implemented by Mahon and Goatcher (1999) and focused on improving life and leisure satisfaction. An intervention group (n = 10) was compared to a control group (n = 10) with pre- and post-test measures. The intervention group participated in an average of 25.5 sessions that included various leisure and retirement issues, and planning processes with family and significant others. At post-test, the intervention group had higher scores on leisure and life satisfaction than had control group members.

Age-Related Changes. Other studies evaluated interventions to assist persons with DD and their families cope with age-related changes. Lynggaard and Alexander (2004) administered a psycho-educational group intervention (n = 4) for persons with DD who were living in residences with others who had dementia. Six sessions of one-hour duration were administered weekly. The topics included how memory works, problem-solving, and living with people who have dementia. Post-intervention data from residential staff were collected at three points: one week post-intervention, and one and six months post-intervention. Staff indicated that participants in the intervention demonstrated greater degrees of knowledge and support for residents with dementia than exhibited prior to the intervention.

In an Israeli study evaluating older adults with DD who were experiencing physical losses, a psycho-educational group was implemented with nine individuals who had moderate intellectual impairments (Kessel et al., 2002). The group intervention provided information to the participants (ages 39 to 56 years) on losses associated with aging and physical changes. Ten sessions were provided with topics ranging from body perception, feeling shame related to disability status, maintaining autonomy, and mourning and bereavement. In this pre-post test design, the participants reported a more positive sense of self-esteem, lower behavioral reactions, and more positive attitudes toward the aging process upon completion of the intervention.

Residential transitions, a high-risk time for adults with disabilities, was the focus of an intervention designed to assist institutionalized residents with the move to community-based settings (Hammel et al., 2002). The sample (n = 109) ranged in age from 35 to 89 years. The intervention involved both assistive technology (AT) and environmental interventions (EI) to provide modifications in the community-based residence to which the individual was transitioning. The intervention included an individualized AT-EI assessment and home visits (ranging from 1-12 per person) to complete the modifications. Compared to their initial level of functioning, over 70% of the participants had higher rates of functioning with the AT-EI modifications. In addition, the average number of AT-EI interventions was 12.8 per individual. Those individuals who were living in the community had higher functioning scores overall than individuals who resided in institutions regardless of the presence of an AT-EI intervention.

Treatment Summary

In the futures planning interventions that have been evaluated, there was strong reliance on group rather than individual approaches. The methodologies used appeared to place value upon the mutual support which families experience as part of a group, but the direct involvement of the person with DD varied. There was also an expectation that work would be completed between sessions. The future planning interventions was a modality where intervention manuals were well-developed.

Similarly, the three interventions targeting persons with DD also relied upon group approaches. In addition, they were designed to be mindful of cognitive, developmental, and speech/language deficits as well as aging associated changes. Modifications of interventions for people with disabilities included simplifying language, presenting information at a slower rate, repeating information for clarity, checking for comprehension of concepts, using concrete language, and employing nonverbal and visual communication strategies. Sessions were also of shorter duration than typical for non-disabled populations.

Overall, interventions that assist DD persons cope with age-related transitions proved to be a relatively underrepresented type of research. The few studies that were found dealt with important psychosocial issues (e.g., residential transitions, physical changes), yet samples were small and few outcomes were examined. Clearly, the aging of the DD population and their care providers will require that additional research in this area be conducted.

CONCLUSION

It is a challenge to develop an evidence base for psychosocial interventions for older adults with DD. Small sample numbers, underrepresentation of persons with non-ID developmental disabilities, difficulties in delivering interventions due to the dearth of trained staff, and the impact of co-morbid conditions as well as preexisting disabilities make it more difficult to build such an evidence base. However, the desire for people with DD to live similar lives to the general population should be no less important as persons with DD age.

The beginning body of evidence for futures planning interventions demonstrates that the accumulation of such evidence is possible but even for this intervention modality more work is needed. Similarly, the single intervention found for maintaining independence through the use of technology shows what is possible. These important first steps need to be followed up with more rigorous studies. Two additional issues must also be addressed: extending the interventions to people with DD where the disability is not ID, and ensuring that the interventions are not only extended to those with the highest levels of cognitive functioning and communication skills but also to lower functioning individuals.

The absence of studies of strictly behavioral interventions was surprising. On the one hand, an argument can be made for relying upon the broad research evidence for behavioral interventions with a variety of populations (Strumey, 2005). However, if such interventions are to be widely used and recommended, rigorous consideration and replication of behavioral interventions with older persons with DD must be a priority. Consent and service delivery issues will also always be more challenging with persons with DD than with other aging populations. Yet, there are examples, particularly in the dementia care area (see for example McCallion, McCarron & Force, 2005 and McCallion, Nickle & McCarron, 2005), of researchers forming translational research partnerships with providers so that research studies both address issues of critical interest for persons with DD and their caregivers and utilize increasingly rigorous designs. A similar approach is needed to build a base for a systematic body of studies to accumulate evidence for other types of psychosocial interventions.

A final concern is the value placed upon levels of evidence. In most considerations of evidence-based practice the greatest value is placed upon studies that include randomized control trials, particularly where findings have been replicated by more than one investigator and where a meta-analysis supports positive findings. There are relatively small numbers of persons with DD currently in the aging population, and consent, random assignment and replication are more difficult issues. Despite need, it may simply not be possible to develop the same range of intervention studies as for the general population. Not seeking to determine what is effective is not acceptable, but holding too rigorously to standards for evidence may stymie efforts to initiate studies and develop interventions for particularly vulnerable populations such as older adults with DD. Therefore, it is important to welcome efforts to build evidence for practice rather than simply point out the limitations of the evidence available. For this reason, all studies that are cited within this chapter are recognized as contributing to the evidence base.

TREATMENT RESOURCE APPENDIX

Research, Rehabilitation and Training Center on Aging with Developmental Disabilities
http://www.uic.edu/orgs/rrtcamr

This RRTC specifically focuses on older adults who have a developmental disability. The site offers the latest in research in the area of supporting healthy aging in the population, supporting care providers, and fostering disability and aging-friendly environments. There is also a link to literature and resources within the field.

Website on Intellectual Disabilities, Aging and Dementia Maintained by the University at Albany
http://www.albany.edu/aging/IDD/index.html

On this site, there are a number of resources listed as well as links to other related sites. The online magazine, *The Frontline of Learning Disabilities,* is featured and the current issue has several articles on dementia in the population with an intellectual disability. Other information on this site includes a toolkit on assisting care providers of adults with disabilities, and content on sexuality.

The ARC
www.thearc.org/

The ARC of the United States advocates for the rights and full participation of all children and adults with intellectual and developmental disabilities. Together with a network of members and affiliated chapters, this organization seeks to improve systems of supports and services; connect families; inspire communities and influence public policy. On the site, there are publications, videos, and a directory of local chapters.

National Center for the Dissemination of Disability Research
http://www.ncddr.org/

The NCDDR scope of work responds directly to the National Institute on Disability and Rehabilitation Research (NIDRR) concern for increasing the effective use of NIDRR-sponsored research results in shaping new technologies, improving service delivery, and expanding decision-making options for people with disabilities and their families. The site provides information standards for quality of care for people with disabilities, and an overview of current disability-related research.

National Down Syndrome Society
http://www.ndss.org/

The mission of the National Down Syndrome Society is to benefit people with Down syndrome and their families through national leadership in education, research and advocacy. The site contains information and resources specific to this syndrome, and provides locator services for each state.

LITERATURE AND REPORTS

Debrine, E., Caldwell, J., Factor, A., & Heller, T. (2003). *The future is now: A future planning training curriculum for families and their adult relatives with developmental disabilities.* Chicago, IL: RRTC-UIC.

Bouras, N. (2000). *Psychiatric and behavioural disorders in mental retardation.* Cambridge: Cambridge University Press.

Davidson, P.W., Prasher, V.P., & Janicki, M.P. (Eds.) (2003). *Mental health, intellectual disabilities, and the aging process.* London: Blackwell Press.

Janicki, M.P. (2000). *Ageing and intellectual disabilities: Improving longevity and promoting healthy ageing.* Ageing and Intellectual Disabilities Special Interest Research Group (SIRG) of The International Association for the Scientific Study of Intellectual Disability (IASSID). *www.IASSID.org.*

Five Reports Developed in Collaboration Between IASSID and the World Health Organization

Janicki, M.P. & Dalton, A.J. (Eds.) (1999). *Dementia, aging, and intellectual disabilities: A handbook.* Philadelphia: Brunner/Mazel.

McCallion, P. & Janicki, M.P. (2002). *Intellectual disabilities and dementia. A two cd-rom self-instructional training package.* Albany, NY: NYS Developmental Disabilities Planning Council.

Rush, J. & Francis, A. (2000). Expert consensus guidelines series: Treatment of psychiatric and behavioral problems in mental retardation. *American Journal on Mental Retardation, 105* (3), 159-228.

Thorpe, L., Davidson, P., & Janicki, M. (2001). Healthy ageing–Adults with intellectual disabilities: Biobehavioural issues. *Journal of Applied Research in Intellectual Disabilities,* 14, 218-228.

Wilkinson, H. & Janicki, M.P. (2002). The Edinburgh Principles with accompanying guidelines and recommendations. *Journal of Intellectual Disability Research,* 46 (3), 279-284.

AAMR/IASSID Dementia Documents
http://www.aamr.org/dementia_docs.shtml

TEST BATTERY for the Diagnosis of Dementia in Individuals with Intellectual Disability
http://www.aamr.org/Bookstore/Downloadables/Battery/Battery_Test.pdf

Report of the Working Group for the Establishment of Criteria for the Diagnosis of Dementia in Individuals with Intellectual Disability under the auspices of the AAMR and IASSID.

PRACTICAL GUIDELINES for the Clinical Assessment and Care Management of Alzheimer and Other Dementias Among Adults with Mental Retardation
http://www.aamr.org/Bookstore/Downloadables/Practical/practical_guidelines.pdf

Report of the AAMR-IASSID Workgroup on Practice Guidelines for Care Management of Alzheimer Disease Among Adults with Mental Retardation.

DIAGNOSIS OF DEMENTIA in Individuals with Intellectual Disability
http://www.aamr.org/Bookstore/Downloadables/Practical/dementia.pdf

Report of the AAMR-IASSID Working Group for the Establishment of Criteria for the Diagnosis of Dementia in Individuals with Intellectual Disability.

REFERENCES

Beail, N. (2003). What works for people with mental retardation? Critical commentary on cognitive-behavioral and psychodynamic psychotherapy research. *Mental Retardation, 41* (6), 468-472.

Bigby, C. (1996). Transferring responsibility: The nature and effectiveness of parental planning for the future of adults with intellectual disability who remain at home until mid-life. *Australian Society for the Study of Intellectual Disability, 21* (4), 295-312.

Bigby, C., Ozanne, E., & Gordon, M. (2002). Facilitating transition: Elements of a successful case management practice for older parents of adults with intellectual disability. *Journal of Gerontological Social Work, 37* (3/4), 25-43.

Botsford, A.L. & Rule, D. (2004). Evaluation of a group intervention to assist aging parents with permanency planning for an adult offspring with special needs. *Social Work, 49* (3), 423-431.

Braddock, D. (1999). Aging and developmental disabilities: Demographic and policy issues affecting American families. *Mental Retardation, 37,* 155-161.

Braddock, D., Emerson, E., Felce, D., & Stanliffe, R.J. (2001). Living with circumstances of children and adults with mental retardation and developmental disabilities in the United States, Canada, England and Wales. *Mental Retardation and Developmental Disabilities Research Reviews, 7* (2), 115-121.

Brookmeyer, R., Gray, S., & Kawas, C. (1998). Projections of Alzheimer's disease in the United States and the public health impact of delaying disease onset. *American Journal of Public Health, 88,* 1337-1342.

Fujiura, G.T. (1998). Demography of family households. *American Journal of Mental Retardation, 103,* 225-235.

Griswold, K.S. & Goldstein, M.Z. (1999). Issues affecting the lives of older persons with developmental disabilities. *Psychiatric Services, 50,* 315-317.

Hammel, J., Lai, J., & Heller, T. (2002). The impact of assistive technology and environmental interventions on function and living situation status with people who are ageing with developmental disabilities. *Disability and Rehabilitation, 24* (1/2/3), 93-105.

Hatton, C. (2002). Psychosocial interventions for adults with intellectual disabilities and mental health problems: A review. *Journal of Mental Health, 11* (4), 357-373.

Heller, T. & Factor, A. (1991). Permanency planning for adults with mental retardation living with family caregivers. *American Journal on Mental Retardation, 96,* 163-176.

Heller, T., Miller, A.B., Hsieh, K., & Sterns, H. (2000). Later-life planning: Promoting knowledge of options and choice-making. *Mental Retardation, 38* (5), 395-406.

Heller, T., Factor, A., Sterns, H., & Sutton, E. (1996). Impact of person-centered later life planning training program for older adults with mental retardation. *Journal of Rehabilitation,* Jan/Feb/Mar, 77-83.

Hogg, J., Lucchino, R., Wang, K., & Janicki, M.P. (2001). Healthy aging–Adults with intellectual disabilities: Ageing and social policy. *Journal of Applied Research in Intellectual Disabilities, 14* (3), 229-25.

Holland, A.J., Karlinsky, H., & Berg, J.M. (1993). Alzheimer's disease in persons with Down syndrome: Diagnostic and management considerations. In J.M. Berg, H. Karlinsky, & A.J. Holland (Eds.), *Alzheimer's disease, Down Syndrome, and their Relationship* (pp. 96-114). Oxford: Oxford University Press.

Janicki, M.P. (1994). Policies and supports for older adults with mental retardation. In M.M. Seltzer, M.W. Krauss, & M.P. Janicki (Eds.), *Life course perspectives on adulthood and old age.*Washington, DC: American Association on Mental Retardation.

Janicki, M.P. (2000). *Ageing and intellectual disabilities: Improving longevity and promoting healthy ageing.* Geneva: World Health Organization.

Janicki, M.P. & Dalton, A.J. (2000). Prevalence of dementia and impact on intellectual disability services. *Mental Retardation, 38,* 277-289.

Janicki, M.P., Dalton, A.J., Henderson, C.M., & Davidson, P.W. (1999). Mortality and morbidity among older adults with intellectual disability: Health services considerations. *Disability and Rehabilitation, 21* (5/6), 284-294.

Janicki, M.P., Dalton, A.J., McCallion, P., Baxley, D.D., & Zendell, A. (2005). Group home care for adults with intellectual disabilities and Alzheimer's disease. *Dementia, 4* (3), 361-385.

Kessel, S., Merrick, J., Kedem, A., Borovsky, L., & Carmeli, E. (2002). Use of group counseling to support aging-related losses in older adults with intellectual disabilities. *Journal of Gerontological Social Work, 38* (1/2), 241-251.

Lynch, C. (2004). Psychotherapy for persons with mental retardation. *Mental Retardation, 42* (5), 399-405.

Lynggaard, H. & Alexander, N. (2004). 'Why are my friends changing?' Explaining dementia to people with learning disabilities. *British Journal of Learning Disabilities, 32* (1), 30-34.

Mahon, M.J. & Goatcher, S. (1999). Later-life planning for older adults with mental retardation: A field experiment. *Mental Retardation, 37* (5), 371-382.

McCallion, P., & Janicki, M.P. (2002). *Intellectual disabilities and dementia.* Albany, NY: NYS Developmental Disabilities Council. A two cd-rom training package.

McCallion, P. & McCarron, M. (2004). Intellectual disabilities and dementia. In K. Doka (Ed.) *Living with grief: Alzheimer's disease* (pp. 67-84).Washington, DC: Hospice Foundation of America.

McCallion, P. Nickle, T., & McCarron, M. (2005). A comparison of reports of caregiver burden between foster family care providers and staff caregivers of persons in other settings. *Dementia, 4* (3), 401-412.

McCallion, P. & Kolomer, S.R. (2003). Aging persons with developmental disabilities and their aging caregivers. In B. Berkman & L Harootyan (Eds.), *Social work and health care in an aging world* (pp. 201-225). New York: Springer.

McCarron, M., Gill, M., McCallion, P., & Begley, C. (2005). Health co-morbidities in ageing persons with Down syndrome and Alzheimer's dementia. *JIDR, 49,* 560-566.

McCarron, M. & Lawlor, B.A. (2003). Responding to the challenges of ageing and dementia in intellectual disability in Ireland. *Ageing and Mental Health, 7* (6), 413-417.

Nagel, B. & Leiper, R. (1999). A national survey of psychotherapy with people with learning disabilities. *Clinical Psychology Forum, 129,* 14-18.

Prout, H.T. & Nowak-Drabik, K.M. (2003). Psychotherapy with persons who have mental retardation: An evaluation of effectiveness. *American Journal on Mental Retardation, 108* (2), 82-93.

Reilly, K.O. & Conliffe, C. (2002). Facilitating future planning for ageing adults with intellectual disabilities using a planning tool that incorporates quality of life domains. *Journal of Gerontological Social Work, 37* (3/4), 105-119.

Rush, J. & Francis, A. (2000). Expert consensus guidelines series: Treatment of psychiatric and behavioral problems in mental retardation. *American Journal on Mental Retardation, 105* (3), 159-228.

Seltzer, M.M. & Krauss, M.W. (1994). Aging parents with coresident adult children: The impact of lifelong caregiving. In M.M. Seltzer, M.W. Krauss, & M.P. Janicki

(Eds.) *Life course perspectives on adulthood and old age* (pp. 3-18).Washington, DC: American Association on Mental Retardation.

Smith, G.C., Majeski, R.A., & McClenny, B. (1996). Psychoeducational support groups for aging parents: Development and preliminary outcomes. *Mental Retardation, 34*, 172-181.

Sturmey, P. (2005). Against psychotherapy with people who have mental retardation. *Mental Retardation, 43* (1), 55-57.

Chapter 11

Treatment at the End of Life

Deborah P. Waldrop, MSW, PhD

End-of-life care has gained recognition as an important interdisciplinary clinical domain during the past three decades largely because scientific and medical advances have changed the nature of dying in the US. Rapid developments have both lengthened the dying process and underscored the need to develop new ways of providing care as death approaches. Advances in the treatment of life-limiting illness have typically focused on medical issues and on treating the physical symptoms that accompany the final stage of a terminal illness. However, because the lengthening life span has made more choices available at the end of life, there is also greater need for evidence-based psychosocial treatment to diminish some of the prolonged emotional, psychological, social, and spiritual distress that accompanies dying (Institute of Medicine [IOM], 1997). Physical symptoms have been treated more often than psychosocial symptoms but there is growing awareness that psychosocial care is an essential element of quality at the end of life (Georges, Onwuteaka-Phillipsen, van der Heide, van der Wal, & van der Mas, 2005; National Institutes of Health, 2005). Longer periods of psychosocial distress can include questioning, uncertainty, anxiety, fear, financial burden and anticipatory loss (Lunney, Foley, Smith, & Gelband, 2003). Both terminally ill older adults and their caregivers can be helped by interventions that address the need for information, education, preparation, communication, emotional support, and advocacy (Morrison & Meier, 2003). This paper presents a review of evidence-based psychosocial treatments at the end of life for both older adults and their caregivers.

Because the terms "end-of-life care," "palliative care" and "hospice" are often used interchangeably, their definitions are critical. *End-of-life care* refers broadly to the physical, psychological, spiritual and practical dimensions of care that is provided for people who are dying in various environments which range from the high acuity of an intensive care unit (ICU) or emergency department (ED) to less formal home settings (IOM, 1997). *Palliative care* refers to the comprehensive management of physical, psychological, social, spiritual and existential needs but it is not limited to end-of-life care and is often provided to people who experience chronic pain. Palliative medicine focuses primarily on symptom management such as preventing, relieving, reducing, or soothing the discomfort of incurable, progressive illnesses but it does not focus on a cure (Last Acts, 2002; Lipman, 2000). *Hospice* organizations provide both end-of-life and palliative care in nursing homes, hospice inpatient units and home settings for people whose illness is expected to end in death within six months. Optimal end-of-life care is highly individual and results from the integration of personal desires and values, respect for family, and social and cultural contexts. It also involves a unique and individual combination of preventive, life-prolonging, rehabilitative and palliative measures, which meet both the physical and psychosocial needs of older people who are dying and of their family members (Morrison & Meier, 2003).

End-of-life care is provided on a continuum which often begins with a terminal prognosis, continues through the active decline which accompanies the dying process and is available as bereavement care for family members after the person's death. How and where end-of-life care occurs influences the type of the psychosocial treatment that is provided. Moreover, the fragile and changeable nature of a terminal illness makes the establishment and implementation of behavioral treatments and evidence-based research challenging (Ferrell & Hastie, 2003). Evidence-based research of medical interventions for symptom management (involving some randomized clinical trials) has been more prevalent than research involving psychosocial treatment, which is currently in a much earlier phase of development.

DEMOGRAPHICS AND PREVALENCE

Death and loss are universal human experiences. However, when, where and how people die is influenced by the availability of medical treatment as well as the social and historical contexts. Death at the turn of last century typically followed an acute infectious illness, life expectancy peaked by age 65, and most people died at home. The combined influence of both medical advances and changing health-care benefits have altered the nature of dying during the 20th century in two ways: (1) the age of death continued to rise and (2) hospitals increasingly became the most common place of death (IOM, 1997). Currently, most people die in later life and the overall life expectancy in 2003 was 77.6 years of age. The estimated age-adjusted death rate in the US has been steadily declining since 1900, reaching a record low of 831.2 per 100,000 in 2003 but the age-adjusted death rate for people over age 65 is higher (Centers for Disease Control [CDC], 2002). Between ages 65-74 the rate was 2,314.7 deaths per 100,000 people; from ages of 75-84 the death rate is 5,556.9 per 100,000; and after the age of 85 the death rate increases to 14,828.3 per 100,000 people. These statistics indicate that now most people die after age 65 (National Center for Health Statistics, 2004). The majority of people continue to die in hospitals but changing health-care resources have increased the utilization of other environments for care such as home, nursing home, and hospice residences or inpatient units at the end of life (CDC, 2004).

Presently, the five overall leading causes of death in later life are heart disease, cancer, cerebrovascular disease, chronic respiratory disease and influenza (National Center for Health Statistics, 2004). Although heart disease and cancer are the leading causes of death for all older people, other leading causes of death differ by gender and race. For men, the third, fourth and fifth causes of death are chronic low respiratory disease, cerebrovascular disease, and influenza. For women, they are cerebrovascular disease, chronic low respiratory disease, and Alzheimer's disease. Overall, for all races the third and fourth causes of death are cerebrovascular disease and chronic low respiratory disease. However, for Blacks, the third, fourth and fifth leading causes of death are cerebrovascular disease, diabetes and chronic lung disease. For Native Americans and Alaskan Natives, the third, fourth and fifth leading causes of death are diabetes, cerebrovascular disease and chronic respiratory disease. Racial, cultural and economic differences influence access to and disparities in both general medical services as well as end-of-life care. Primary barriers to optimum end-of-life care include lack of insurance, differential use of primary care, patient/family mistrust, as well as provider insensitivity and an inadequate number of providers from minority groups (Krakauer, Crenner, & Fox, 2002).

How people die is highly individual and is influenced by the unique combination of several factors including diagnoses, the duration and shape of the illness trajectory, and the environment in which end-of-life care is provided. Each of these factors shape the person's dying experience (Wennberg, McAndrew Cooper, & Tolle, 2003). Three distinct trajectories of dying have been identified and described: (1) sudden death from an unexpected cause, (2) steady decline from a progressive disease with a terminal phase, and (3) an advanced illness marked by slow decline and periodic crises, but ending in a seemingly "sudden" death (IOM, 1997). Longer periods of living with a terminal illness have increased the importance of developing evidence-based treatments that can alleviate suffering (Engle, Fox-Hill, & Graney, 1998). Psychosocial issues at the end of life include caregiving needs, financial burden, transportation, the existence of anxiety and depression, and the need for social support and communication within the family as well as with providers (Morrison & Meier, 2003). Where people die is influenced by both social and disease-related factors. Older people typically die in one of four environments: (1) hospitals, (2) nursing homes, (3) inpatient hospice units or (4) home. However, there is substantial regional variation in location of death (Centers for Disease Control, 2002) that influences the availability of hospital beds and community supports for people who are seriously ill and dying. Hospital deaths can occur in emergency rooms (EDs), intensive care units (ICUs) or on acute care floors. In Portland, Oregon, for example, only 35% of adult deaths occur in hospitals compared to over 50% in New York City (Morrison & Meier, 2003). ICUs and EDs are unique clinical settings where death occurs frequently and there is a professional culture of "rescue therapy" which involves technological and invasive interventions (Rubenfeld & Curtis, 2001). Nursing home deaths can occur in skilled nursing facilities, sub-acute or regular long-term care units with no particular end-of-life attention or they may be moderated by an in-house nursing home end-of-life team or by an external hospice team that comes regularly to assist with managing symptoms and end-of-life care. Home deaths can occur with either: (1) no formal end-of-life care assistance, (2) intermittent assistance through a home health agency, or (3) with formal end-of-life care guidance through a hospice organization (including 24-hour telephone availability and regular in-home assistance).

THEMES AND NATURE OF END-OF-LIFE CARE

Evidence-based treatment in end-of-life care has previously been explored through systematic reviews that have focused on only one aspect of end-of-life such as a specific disease (cancer), the management of one symptom (pain), or on one treatment such as a specific medication (Lorenz et al., 2004). A different, more inclusive organizing framework for the systematic review of end-of-life care was presented in a recent report that was commissioned by the Association for Health Care Research and Quality, and incorporated four cross-cutting themes. This new framework is based on the assumption that there is an essential interrelationship between the disease process, existence of multiple symptoms, coexisting patient and family needs, and ongoing interactions about planning and care with health-care professionals. This framework underscores the importance of examining end-of-life care within the social context. Describing interrelated aspects of end-of-life care, the themes that were used in this review include: (1) patient experience, (2) caregiver experience, (3) advanced care planning, and (4) continuity of care (Lorenz et al., 2004). The psychosocial aspects of dying which are integrated within these four themes are communication between patient and caregiver, client satisfaction, caregiving, depression, and anxiety.

Patient experiences involve a combination of multiple physical and psychological symptoms of dying, which are often found in clusters (e.g., dyspnea, anxiety, fatigue and anorexia). One or more major chronic illnesses (e.g., diabetes, hypertension) are often superimposed on age-related changes such as decreased organ function and progressive functional decline from osteoarthritis or gait disturbances (McQuay, Moore, & Wiffen, 2004; Morrison & Meier, 2003). Non-disease-specific markers of decline include increasing frailty, functional dependence, cognitive impairment, symptom distress, and family support needs. Disease-specific markers include symptomatic congestive heart failure, chronic lung disease, dementia, or recurrent infections (Morrison & Meier, 2003). Symptoms such as pain and discomfort are indicators of distress and signal the need for intervention. During the terminal phase of an illness there are often multifaceted symptoms and new causes of suffering (Furst & Doyle, 2005). Moreover, people who are actively dying often experience multiple coexisting physical and psychosocial symptoms. Although randomized clinical trials can ascertain when one symptom-specific treatment is more effective, the presence of two or more makes the interrelationship between symptoms difficult to isolate.

Caregiver experiences involve learning to provide physical hands-on care while simultaneously anticipating death and loss; ultimately, bereavement is experienced. Family members and friends who provide care during a life-limiting illness experience an emotional process that parallels and reflects the terminally ill person's decline. Caregivers face physical, emotional, financial and social challenges that are related to the terminally ill person's deteriorated status. Caregiving continues throughout each stage of an ongoing illness and accompanies transitions between levels of care (e.g., transfer from hospital to nursing home or inpatient hospice).

Advance care planning involves anticipating issues and challenges that the patient and family will experience during the later stages of an illness and specifying how people want to be treated as they decline (IOM, 1997). Death can become a protracted and negotiated process with health-care providers and family members making difficult decisions about the use or discontinuation of life-prolonging technologies such as feeding tubes, ventilators and intravenous fluid while simultaneously dealing with psychosocial issues such as facilitating family communication and saying goodbye (Morrison & Meier, 2003). Advance care planning includes the completion of advance directives, discussion of do not resuscitate orders (DNR), and the establishment of surrogate decision-makers to uphold personal choices at the end of life. Initially, advance care planning was established primarily as a legal process but the concept has been broadened to encompass discussions about honoring individual wishes (Lorenz et al., 2004). An example of a new approach to advance care planning is the Five Wishes program, which addresses medical and legal decisions. Beyond those decision-making domains, however, the Five Wishes program also helps people put into words various things they want family members to know (Aging with Dignity, 2004).

Continuity of care is defined as "the degree to which a series of discrete health-care events is experienced as coherent, connected and consistent with the patient's medical needs and personal context" (Lorenz et al., 2004, p. 76). Continuity of care is a process that can be characterized by ongoing relationships with health-care providers so that the care is provided in an integrated, consistent or seamless fashion and health-care information follows the person when he or she transfers between settings. Most people receive care in multiple settings which can include providers' offices, hospitals, emergency rooms, their homes, and possibly nursing homes (National Consensus Project, 2004) Communication between individuals, families and health-care providers within and across these environments is a central component in continuity of care (IOM, 1997).

There has been an evolution in the way that people think about dying within the past century and now, most people would prefer to die at home rather than in a hospital or other institutional setting (Last Acts, 2002b). The growing recognition that good end-of-life care is an interrelationship between patient and caregiver experiences, advanced care planning and attention to the continuity of care between settings represents an important reconceptualization of the field. However, there remains a gap between the changing nature of end-of-life care and the way that most people die.

CONSEQUENCES

Death is a process rather than a moment in time for many older adults. As a result, there is a need for balance between the possibilities for and actualization of "a good death," defined as one with dignity (Proulx & Jacelon, 2004). Three core domains of a good death have been identified as the psychosocial/spiritual, physical and clinical aspects (Schwartz, Mazor, Rogers & Reed, 2003). In addition, Steinhauser and colleagues (2000) investigated providers', patients' and caregivers' perspectives of a "good death" and found six major themes: pain and symptom management, clear decision-making, preparation for death, completion of unfinished tasks, contributing to others and the affirmation of the whole person. Death with dignity has been described as involving physical comfort, autonomy, meaningfulness, usefulness, preparedness, and interpersonal connection (IOM, 1997). These psychosocial concepts have become central in both end-of-life care practice and research, however, it is important to note that there are no claims-based quality indicators of psychosocial care (Earle et al., 2003); thus psychosocial outcomes are not routinely being measured by health-care providers.

The quality of life during the advanced stages of disease is often poor and characterized by inadequately treated physical distress, fragmented care, poor communication between doctors, patients and families, and enormous strains on family caregiver and support systems (Morrison & Meier, 2003). People have come to fear both a technologically overtreated death as well as a lingering death. Conversely, following a terminal prognosis, some health-care professionals withdraw from active care for people who are dying and their family members. Such abandonment and untreated physical and emotional stress can be as frightening as over-treatment (IOM, 1997, p. 15). Growing awareness of the essential interrelationship between the disease process, the existence of multiple physical and psychosocial symptoms, coexisting patient and family needs, and communication with health-care professionals is shaping both the delivery of clinical end-of-life care and research aimed at improving outcomes.

A serious consequence of neglecting psychosocial end-of-life care is that older adults may approach death with fear, anxiety, and uncertainty about what is occurring. They may also have no opportunity to resolve unexpressed feelings or deal with unresolved, fragmented relationships, which can result in psychosocial distress and existential suffering. Family caregivers who have not received psychosocial care as a loved one is dying, may also feel responsible for a loved one's unmanaged symptoms, have unanswered questions or experience unresolved guilt, and be surprised by the death when it occurs. Family caregivers may miss opportunities for meaningful final communication, live with unanswered questions about the dying process, and they may ultimately attempt to adapt to a major loss while dealing with unresolved issues and unsettled memories of the death experience.

EMPIRICAL LITERATURE

This review of empirical studies examining psychosocial aspects of treatment for older adults and their caregivers who are facing an approaching death was conducted according to specific parameters. The following databases were surveyed for this literature review: Medline, Cancer Lit, Psychinfo, CINAHL, Social Work Abstracts and Ageline. Hand searches of the sources used in several systematic reviews were also conducted. Articles listed in these databases and with publication dates from 1980 to the present were examined. Two types of searches were conducted in each database. First, the keywords "psychosocial and intervention," "end-of-life or dying" and "old or older" were used. If articles met the end-of-life and psychosocial criteria they were searched for the age of participants and included if a majority of the sample was over age 65. Articles that did not specify participants' ages or did not include older adults were excluded. Overall, 52 articles matched the keyword search but only four reported findings of evidence-based research. A second search was conducted using the keywords "grief or bereavement and intervention," and "old or older." A total of 45 articles matched the search criteria but only six reported evidence-based findings. The results of both searches are described in the treatment summary and presented in Table 1.

End-of-Life Care Intervention Studies

End-of-life care intervention studies have focused in great part on the management of physical symptoms. Primarily managed with medication, symptoms such as anorexia, nausea, vomiting, and bleeding can be

TABLE 1. Evidence-Based Treatments in End-of-Life Care and Bereavement

End of Life Care Intervention Studies

Author(s)	Setting	Population	N	Treatment	Sessions	Outcome
Ratner, Norlander, & McSteen (2001)	Home	HHC patients	84	Advance Care Planning	1-3	Decision about location for end-of-life care honored by care professionals
Schrader, Horner, Eidsness, Young, Wright, & Robinson (2002)	Hospital	patients	50	Palliative Care Team	1 multi-disciplinary consult	Symptom management; satisfaction improved
Ringdal, Jordhoy, & Kaasa (2002)	Hospital	Hospital Patients Caregivers	434 p 312 cg	Palliative Medicine Unit	100 days	Satisfaction with EOL care improved
Corner et al. (2003)	Transfer from hospital to home	Cancer patients	76	Macmillan nursing[1]	28 days	Symptoms decreased, QOL improved, anxiety decreased

Bereavement Intervention Studies

Author(s)	Setting	Population	N	Treatment	Sessions	Outcome
Reich & Zautra (1989)	Community	Bereaved spouses	62	Individual control exercise	4 biweekly sessions	personal mastery mixed, engagement increased
Tudiver, Hilditch, Permaul & McKendree (1992)	Community	Bereaved spouses (men)	113	Mutual aid	9 weekly sessions	social adjustment, support, and anxiety improved
Levy, Derby & Martinkowski (1993)	Community	Bereaved spouses	159	Support group	1-2 sessions	Adaptation/psych. sx improved for tx. and control groups
Lieberman & Yalom (1992)	Community	Bereaved spouses	56	group therapy	8, 80-minute sessions	Improved role function and mental health
Caserta & Lund (1993)	Community	Bereaved spouses	258	self-help groups	4 (min)	reduced depression/ grief for those with lower competencies
Segal, Chatman, Bogaards & Becker (2001)	Community	Bereaved spouses	30	emotional disclosure intervention	4, 20-minute sessions	distress, intrusive thoughts decreased,
Caserta, Lund & Obray (2004)	Community	Bereaved spouses	84	Pathfinders project	11-week class	coping, health care daily mgt improved

1. Macmillan nursing is person-specific clinical intervention to: (1) improve physical symptoms, (2) improve emotional state, (3) provide advice and information, (4) offer support, and (5) improve perceptions of overall quality of care

controlled (Lipman, Jackson, & Tyler, 2000). Previous intervention literature has also described family caregiving interventions including mutual-aid support groups, individual counseling, and behavioral intervention strategies for caregivers (Corcoran, Fairchild-Kienlen, & Harakal Phillips, 2000). This section presents prospective research which includes evidence-based studies in the psychosocial care of patients and caregivers during the terminal phase of an illness.

Advance Care Planning was conducted by using structured social work visits to prepare families for likely scenarios near the end of life. Ratner, Norlander and McSteen (2001) followed a case series of people (N = 84) who were identified by their home health agency nurses as having a life-limiting illness and then referred for social service assessment. The group was followed for a minimum of six months with home care services other than hospice. The outcome of the intervention was to obtain and uphold patient and family preferences for place of death. The intervention established patient-family preferences for end-of-life care and 82% wanted care at home. Study outcomes indicated that 75% of the deaths occurred at home or in a hospice residence and 61% used hospice services during the study. These preferences were discussed with the patient's nurse and physician. The efficacy of the intervention is underscored by results that indicate 69% had died by the end of the study and no patient who died at home had expressed the wish to die elsewhere. Others who expressed the desire to die in home-like settings (nursing homes or home-like residential hospice settings) were able to do so. This study brings an important contextual component to evidence-based treatment research for older adults and their families by setting the study within the home context and involving both terminally ill older adults and their family members in the discussion. The results of both decision-making and interventions that occur within the family-environmental context provide insight about how to understand and meet individual needs at life's end.

Patient and caregiver experiences were the focus of an intervention study by Schrader, Horner, Eidsness, Young, Wright, and Robinson (2002). This hospital-based study employed palliative interventions that included symptom management, spiritual dialogue, psychosocial counseling, guidance on advance directives and family conferences during the course of hospitalization. The interventions were delivered to 50 patients and their caregivers by a palliative care consultant team (physician, clinical nurse specialist, social worker, chaplain and dietician). The outcome measures included pain, functional impairment, anxiety, constipation, dyspnea, family anxiety, depression, nausea, nutrition, psychosocial matters, spiritual matters, and quality of life. Data was collected to determine change between the time of admission to two days after discharge to see if symptoms had changed. The statistically significant changes were: reduced anxiety, improved quality of life indicators (perception of practical matters being addressed, greater understanding of information, and perception of less wasted time), reduced pain, better nutritional status, and less constipation. This study highlights the essential interrelationship between professionals from different disciplines who each bring different perspectives to the complex patient-family issues that are inherent in both the end-of-life experience and the provision of meaningful interventions.

Patients' symptoms and caregiver anxiety were studied by Corner, Halliday, Haviland, Douglas, Bath, Clark, Normand, Beech, Hughes, Marples, Seymour, Skilbeck and Webb (2003). Symptom management interventions were provided for people with advanced cancer (N = 76; 43 were over age 65). Provided by a clinical nurse specialist, Macmillan nursing is a person-specific clinical intervention to: (1) improve physical symptoms, (2) improve emotional state, (3) provide advice and information, (4) offer support, and (5) improve perceptions of overall quality of care. In this study, Macmillan nursing was provided to patients for 28 days. Patients' quality of life was measured at three, seven and 28 days during the intervention. Caregivers were interviewed before and after the intervention. Emotional and cognitive functioning as well as anxiety scores all improved. Patients' emotional and cognitive functioning improved and anxiety declined but physical functioning deteriorated. It is important to note that these study results were influenced by patients' rapidly declining condition. Caregivers' anxiety about the patient declined. This study underscores the importance of triangulation; by combining standard quantitative measures with narrative accounts that were collected from patients and caregivers, this intervention documented improved psychosocial functioning during the active dying process.

Caregiver satisfaction was compared between families of terminally ill patients (N = 112; Median age = 57) in a palliative medicine unit (PMU) and 68 others in a conventional care (Median age = 53) program (Ringdal, Jordhoy, & Kaasa, 2002). Intervention was provided in the PMU by a multidisciplinary team consisting of doctors and nurses. Follow-up visits were made by a community-based health-care service that consisted of nurses with specialized training. The PMU consultant team coordinated the care and was available for supervision, advice, and home visits. Visits focused on involving family members, providing information about treatment, care and prognoses, and follow-up available after the death. The control group received conventional care that was shared among hospital departments and the community according to diagnosis and medical need but without well-defined follow-up. The FAMCARE Scale was used to measure satisfaction in both groups of caregivers, one month after the person's death. Higher satisfaction was found among caregivers whose relative was treated by the PMU even after controlling for factors such as the relationship to the deceased, gender and age, duration of time in the study and place of death. Satisfaction is described as an important measure of the quality of end-of-life care and strongly linked with the availability of professionals and with the coordination of care. This study underscores the importance of satisfying patient-caregiver needs and suggests an important link between how family members' experiences with end-of-life caregiving may influence their experiences in bereavement.

Bereavement Intervention Studies

Previous intervention literature about bereavement counseling has described individual grief counseling, family counseling, or bereavement support groups (See Stroebe, Hansson, Stroebe, & Schut, 2001 and Worden, 2002 for reviews). Studies have often focused on bereaved spouses but there is growing recognition about the differences in the grief experiences for people who have had different types of losses (Jordan & Niemeyer, 2003). Few studies have focused specifically on the bereavement of older adults whose family members received end-of-life care. Most often, adult participants are included in bereavement studies and interventions, without controlling for age. This review presents findings from studies that included older adult participants.

Perceived control in bereavement was the focus of a study by Reich and Zautra (1989). Participants from one of two at-risk groups were either (1) recently disabled or (2) recently bereaved; each group was matched with non-risk controls. Participants were randomly assigned to a placebo-contact group (social contact), a no-contact control group, or a four-session/10-week intervention. The intervention involved four separate but interrelated intervention sessions that were aimed at behavioral change. The sessions were (1) Examining Personal Choices, (2) The Happiness Project, (3) The Coping Project and (4) Balancing Happiness and Coping. The interventions involved behavioral change techniques such as stimulus or reminder cards and daily log sheets that were aimed at enhancing control in daily living. Personal mastery, psychological well-being and distress, positive and negative affect, and activities of daily living were measured at third, fourth, fifth and sixth months after the intervention. Participants in the intervention demonstrated mixed effects on personal mastery, but increased engagement in desirable activities. However, the effects of the intervention began to fade by six months after the intervention. In addition, the effects were more pronounced for people in the disabled group.

Self-esteem and role strain were measured in bereaved spouses (N = 56; Median age = 57) who received either a brief group therapy intervention (N = 36) or no treatment (N = 20) (Lieberman & Yalom, 1992). The treatment group attended eight 80-minute sessions. A comparison of group participants and the untreated controls demonstrated modest improvement on role functioning mental health measures and mourning for a year following the intervention. Although there were significant changes in self-esteem and role strain for the treatment group, the absence of other differences suggest that group therapy did not have a powerful effect.

Mutual aid groups were provided as an intervention for bereaved husbands. Tudiver, Hilditch, Permaul and McKendree (1992) used a randomized controlled design that involved a community sample. Men who had lost their wives within the previous year (N = 113) were randomly assigned into treatment (N = 61; Average age = 62) or a control group (N = 52; Average age = 65). The intervention consisted of nine weekly semi-structured peer group sessions that focused on the grief process, diet, new relationships, exercise, and life-style issues. The control group was asked to wait eight months before being offered treatment. Grief resolution was measured as psychological distress (depression and anxiety), social adjustment and social support, and each variable was measured at two, eight and 14 months after entry to the study. The treatment group's mean scores were almost always higher than the control group although there was no statistical significance. Measures of social adjustment, social support, and anxiety improved for both groups but did not show statistically significant differences. Tudiver and colleagues pose three possible explanations for the lack of a treatment effect. First, because 26 participants were lost to follow-up during the course of the study, the authors suggest that men who had adapted to the loss more quickly may have dropped out of the intervention. Tudiver et al. also suggest that the course of male adaptation in bereavement may be longer than the intervention period in this study; thus, change would have become evident after the 14-month measurement. Finally, the authors suggest that an intervention that highlights grief reactions may actually hinder rather than facilitate recovery by regularly focusing participants on their losses, and therefore, preclude measures of positive change.

Support group membership for bereaved spouses was studied as an intervention to facilitate adaptation in bereavement (Levy, Derby, & Martinkowski, 1993). Bereaved spouses (N = 114 women and 45 men; mean age = 61) were recruited during the first 18 months of their bereavement. Following an initial interview, participants joined one of 15 different bereavement support groups. Treatment and control groups were determined by self-selection. Treatment (or group membership; N = 37) was defined as having attended two or more support groups. Both groups were assessed for adaptation at entry to the program and again at six, 13 and 18 months after the death. Adaptation was measured as social support, group involvement, depression, anger, anxiety, subjective stress and psychotropic medication use. Members of both the treatment and control groups demonstrated significant declines in depression, anger, anxiety, subjective stress and psychotropic medication use over the 18 months. Controlling for demographic variance, initial level of distress and perceived levels of social support, the findings indicate that neither the type of group membership nor level of group involvement was associated with significant declines in depression, anger, anxiety, subjective stress and medication use. The number of meetings attended was found to decrease levels of anger and psychotropic medication use at 18 months.

Caserta and Lund (1993) explored the relationship between a self-help group intervention for bereaved spouses (N = 295; Mean age = 67) and the participants' individual (intrapersonal) resources on their depression and grief in bereavement. Intrapersonal resources were defined as self-esteem, competencies (e.g., social and interpersonal skills, instrumental skills for daily living) and life satisfaction. Participants were assigned to either a short (8-week), long (12-week) or control group (no meetings) condition. Participants' intrapersonal resources had a greater influence on depression and grief than did the self-help group intervention. Participants with lower competencies reported reduced depression and grief with greater meeting attendance, but the opposite was true for those with high competencies. Depression eventually decreased among those with high competencies who attended the self-help group meetings for more than eight weeks. Caserta and Lund suggest that those with greater competencies were able to express and feel more depressive elements of bereavement, earlier in the process, whereas those with lower competencies benefited from meeting others and exchanging information. In addition, the authors posit that support group attendance may not be sufficiently stimulating or helpful for people with ample resources.

Structured emotional disclosure was used as an intervention to facilitate adaptation after a spouse's death. Segal, Chatman, Bogaards, and Becker (2001) studied 30 bereaved older adults (N = 23 wives; 7 husbands; age range = 51-85). Participants were asked to discuss their thoughts and feelings about the death of their spouse in four 20-minute sessions. Follow-up evaluations were conducted for one year. Findings indicated that depression, hopelessness, intrusive thoughts and avoidance decreased following the intervention. In addition, decreased negative thoughts were correlated with lower levels of depression, hopelessness, intrusive images, and avoidance. However, there were therapeutic but no significant treatment effects for depression, hopelessness or avoidance. The therapeutic effects remained one year after the death.

Bereavement interventions for improved functional abilities were the focus of a structured intervention study with 84 bereaved spouses who were age 50 and older (Caserta, Lund, & Obray, 2004). The completion of self-care activities, assumption of responsibilities that had belonged to a spouse, and social connection with the larger community were facilitated by using the Pathfinders project as an intervention. The Pathfinders demonstration project provided health and wellness information in an environment that emphasized self-care, daily living skills, and the use of community resources. Participants attended one of five 11-week class sequences. Incremental (and statistically significant) improvements were found in active coping, health care participation, household management, home safety, and nutritional self-care skills. Nearly all participants reported using some of the content and about 70% requested more information after the classes.

TREATMENT SUMMARY

In summary, evidence-based psychosocial treatment in end-of-life care has focused on outcomes which include quality of life, end-of-life preferences, satisfaction, and emotional and cognitive functioning. These interventions include situation-specific consultation, information, and education. Most evidence-based bereavement intervention programs have focused on the expression of loss and grief issues but one study included here specifically focused on bereavement interventions that can facilitate adaptation to changed daily functioning and routines (Caserta, Lund, & Obray, 2004).

Each of the four end-of-life care studies that were reviewed focused targeted interventions on the changing needs of terminally ill older adults and only one included caregivers. Two studies included interventions that were provided by multidisciplinary teams and demonstrated how this approach is beneficial for enhancing the end-of-life experience for both people who are terminally ill and their families. Two of the studies featured central nursing roles (Corner et al., 2003) and one featured the social work role in advance care planning (Ratner et al., 2001). These studies underscore the multifaceted nature of end-of-life care, and suggest that quality of life is enhanced by simultaneous attention to the physical and psychosocial issues that become central as death approaches (e.g., education, symptom resolution and planning).

The evidence-based bereavement studies that were identified focused specifically on the experiences of bereaved spouses. Six of the studies report on group interventions and one presents an individual intervention. Reported outcomes suggest that functioning during bereavement has primarily been measured as psychological and cognitive functioning. Most bereavement intervention programs have focused on the expression of loss and grief issues. Caserta and colleagues (2004) investigated bereavement interventions that can facilitate adaptation to changed daily functioning and routines (Caserta, Lund & Obray, 2004). This new direction seems particularly germane for bereaved caregivers who may have experienced altered daily routines for months to years before the death.

CONCLUSION

The results of the seven bereavement studies suggest that the field of bereavement intervention would be strengthened and enhanced by future studies that include caregivers who seek care on their own. To date, bereavement research has primarily been conducted with participants who have been recruited, rather than with people who have pursued treatment of their own accord (Schut, Stroebe, VanDen Bout, & Terheggen, 2001). Each study reported here, involved participants who were recruited for a structured, time-limited intervention; none involved participants who sought treatment independently. In addition, issues of culture, race, ethnicity and socioeconomic status influence the nature of end-of-life care and are important for inclusion as the field of psychosocial end-of-life care grows. In summary, studies discussed here focused on improving functioning and mental health during bereavement by facilitating adaptation through behavioral changes.

Most of the bereavement studies reviewed report either limited or no treatment effects. Reich and Zautra (1989) found that the effects of their intervention began to fade by six months; Lieberman and Yalom (1992) suggest that their results indicate that group therapy did not have a powerful effect; Tudiver and colleagues found no statistical significance between treatment and control groups; Levy et al. (1993) found that neither the type of group membership nor level of group involvement was associated with declines in psychosocial distress; and Caserta and Lund (1993) suggest that preexisting competencies influence the outcomes of bereavement intervention. These findings challenge the assumption that providing bereavement counseling is an effective element of end-of-life care. It is important to note that this outcome mirrors other reviews in the field of bereavement counseling (Jordan & Neimeyer, 2003; Kato & Mann, 1999). After summarizing the findings of four systematic reviews of bereavement counseling, Jordan and Neimeyer (2003) concluded that the scientific basis for accepting the efficacy of bereavement counseling is weak and suggest three possible explanations. First, formal intervention in bereavement may not be needed much of the time. Mourners may be able to work through and integrate their losses without structured assistance. Second, grief counseling as it is currently conceptualized and defined may be ineffective or delivered at the wrong times (e.g., too early or too late). Finally, there may be methodological problems in outcome studies such as the lack of control groups, or random assignment may mask the benefits of an intervention. Because the experiences of grief and bereavement are intensely individual, personal, and differ with the type of loss, these findings suggest important challenges and opportunities for investigating new and more effective means for helping individuals who need assistance after the death of a family member.

End-of-life care has developed as an integral component of comprehensive care for older adults as a direct result of the lengthening life span and changing nature of dying. Presently, longer periods of living with dying have led to increasing numbers of options for care during the dying process, as well as a sharpening focus on how evidence-based treatment can diminish symptoms of both physical and psychosocial distress. There has been increased energy and attention to developing language, shared assumptions and professional standards for providing end-of-life care. Evidence-based studies of symptom management have been most frequently conducted in oncology practice and have focused on physical (rather than psychosocial) symptom management. Additional trials with other populations, for example, people who are dying with one or more coexistent chronic conditions or with Alzheimer's Disease, will further identify and clarify effective interventions (Lorenz et al., 2004; Lipman et al., 2004). Few randomized control trials have been used in evaluating psychosocial treatment, thus suggesting the importance of focused studies that can advance new approaches which diminish psychosocial features of suffering at the end of life.

The future offers many opportunities for deepening and enhancing the limited knowledge about factors that facilitate and advance care for people who are dying and their families. Many new and promising programs and interventions are reported in the literature but have not yet been evaluated for their effectiveness. In addition, because end-of-life care occurs in a variety of settings, it is important that measures be tested across settings (Lorenz et al., 2004). The National Institutes of Health and the National Institute on Nursing Research have created initiatives that specifically ask for research in exploring the interconnection between coexisting symptoms. Because end-of-life care is, by its nature, fundamentally interdisciplinary, researchers are urged to develop new, multifaceted approaches to the problems that still remain in alleviating suffering as older people face death. Finally, growing interest in complementary and alternative treatments suggest the importance of evaluating the effectiveness of these methods for the relief of psychosocial symptoms. Clearly, recent progress in improving care for the dying on many levels predicts future success in the enhanced use of evidence-based treatment in end-of-life care for older adults.

TREATMENT RESOURCE APPENDIX

Standards of Care and Educational Materials

American Psychological Association (2004)
End of life issues and care.
http://www.apa.org/pi/eol/homepage.html

Various topics about end-of-life decisions are discussed, and the experience of both the patient and family are considered. Each topic is discussed in a narrative form which is easily read and can be shared with patients' families. In addition, the topics include references if additional content is desired.

Association of Oncology Social Work (2001)
Standards of Practice.
http://www.aosw.org/mission/standards.html

Oncology social workers provide intervention throughout all phases of the cancer continuum, from prevention, diagnosis, survivorship, through terminal care, and bereavement. Services are delivered in a wide variety of settings including specialty cancer centers, general hospitals and health systems, ambulatory centers, home health and hospice programs, community-based agencies, and private practice settings. This web site provides information on the organization, links to various publications about end-of-life issues, information about the annual conference, and a directory of members of the orgniazation.

Center to Advance Palliative Care (2004)
http://www.capc.org/

(CAPC) is dedicated to increasing the availability of quality palliative care services in hospitals and other health-care settings for people with life-threatening illnesses, their families, and caregivers. Included at this site are resources and publications that deal with various terminal illnesses and conditions. A sample of the publications that can be accessed at this site are:

- *Living and Dying Well with Cancer: Successfully Integrating Palliative Care and Cancer Care Treatment.* In the past several years, the Institute of Medicine and professional associations in oncology have put forth a new and hopeful vision for improving the comfort and quality of life for patients with advanced cancer and their families. This vision foresees a continuum of cancer care that integrates two seemingly disparate models of care–aggressive cancer treatment and palliative care–and eliminates the "terrible choice" between life-prolongation and quality of life that is currently imposed on patients and providers alike. This monograph reports on the hopeful results of demonstration projects in four leading cancer centers, each awarded grants from Promoting Excellence in End-of-Life Care, a national program of the Robert Wood Johnson Foundation.

- *Palliative Care Perspectives.* A new book on palliative care serves as an introduction to palliative care for both physicians and non-physicians. Drawing on his personal experience as a clinician and educator, the book addresses a range of topics from an overview on death and dying in the modern world to discussions of very practical issues in the practice of palliative care, including pain and symptom management, communication skills and the art of the palliative care consult.
- *Integrating Palliative Care into the Continuum of Cancer Care.* This monograph contains recommendations that address different aspects of care, and are designed to improve comfort and quality of life for patients with HIV/AIDS and their families. They are focused in the areas of physical and psychological care, clinical education, research, policy and funding. The recommendations call for reintroducing palliative care within the continuum of HIV disease-specific care and suggest basic steps toward accomplishing this goal.

End of Life Palliative Education Center (2004)
http://epec.net/EPEC/Webpages/about.cfm.

Uses conferences, training and online learning to advance professional knowledge in end-of-life and palliative care.

End of Life and Palliative Education Resource Center (2004)
http://www.eperc.mcw.edu/

The purpose of EPERC is to share educational resource material among the community of health professional educators involved in palliative care education. A wealth of information is included for both educators and practitioners. Included are sample syllabi, case studies, CD Roms, PowerPoint Presentations, modules, and other educational related items.

National Association of Social Workers (2003)
Standards for practice in palliative and end of life care.
http://www.naswdc.org/practice/bereavement/standards/standards0504New.pdf

All social workers, regardless of field of practice, work with clients who face life-limiting illness, either in themselves or a loved one. These standards are designed to enhance social workers' knowledge, values, methods and sensitivity to end-of-life care.

National Consensus Project (2004)
Clinical practice guidelines for quality palliative care.
http://www.nationalconsensusproject.org/

The guidelines describe core precepts and structures of clinical palliative care programs divided into eight dedicated sections: Structure and Processes of Care, Physical Aspects of Care, Psychological and Psychiatric Aspects of Care, Social Aspects of Care, Spiritual, Religious and Existential Aspects of Care, Cultural Aspects of Care, Care of the Imminently Dying Patient, Ethical and Legal Aspects of Care.

Clinical Practice Guidelines and Programs

Aging with dignity (2004). Five Wishes. http://www.agingwithdignity. org/5wishes.html
The Five Wishes document is designed to help people express desires for treatment in serious illness. It is a unique version of a living will and addresses medical, personal, emotional and spiritual wishes.

Fins, J.J., Peres, J.R., Schumacher, J.D., Meier, C. (2003). *On the road from theory to practice. A resource guide to promising practices in palliative care near the end of life.* http://www.lastacts.org.
This resource guide reports innovative practices and identifies barriers to excellent care. The report makes recommendations for improvements and promising practices across settings such as hospital, long-term care/home care, and hospices. The criteria for selecting promising practices were:

1. Potential for improving quality of care for seriously and/or terminally ill patients and their families
2. Potential for being adapted in different settings
3. Uniqueness
4. Degree of interest to health-care professionals working in terminal and palliative care
5. Usefulness of the tools developed.

Raveis, V. (2000). Facilitating older spouses' adjustment to widowhood: A preventive intervention program. *Social Work in Health Care, 29*(4), 13-32.

The features of a preventive mental health intervention developed to assist late middle-aged and older spouses' (aged 50-80) psychosocial adjustment to spousal death from cancer and facilitate their transition to widowhood are described. The program includes emotional support, facilitated grief work and open discussion both before and after the death. High-risk criteria are used to target spouses at risk for morbid bereavement outcomes.

Lists of Measures for Assessment

Toolkit of Instruments to Measure End of Life Care (TIME)
www.chcr.brown.edu/pcoc/bibliographies.htm

Lorenz, K., Lynn, J., Morton, S.C., Dy, S., Mularski, R., Shugarman, L., Sun, V., Wilkinson, A.M., Maglione, M., & Shekelle, P.G. End-of-life care and outcomes. http://www.ahrq.gov/clinic/epcsums/eolsum.pdf

REFERENCES

Aging with dignity (2004). Five wishes. Retrieved May 15, 2004 at: http://www.agingwithdignity.org/5wishes.html

Caserta, M.S. & Lund, D.A. (1993). Intrapersonal resources and the effectiveness of self-help groups for bereaved older adults. *The Gerontologist, 33*(5); 619-629.

Caserta, M.S., Lund, D.A., & Obray, S.J. (2004) Promoting self-care and daily living skills among older widows and widowers: Evidence from the pathfinders' demonstration project. *Omega: Journal of Death and Dying, 49(3)*, 217-236.

Centers for Disease Control (2002). Leading causes of death. Retrieved on April 15, 2005 at http://www.cdc.gov/nchs/fastats/lcod.htm

Centers for Disease Control (2004). Health care in America: Trends in utilization. Retrieved on October 31, 2005 at http://www.cdc.gov/nchs/data/misc/healthcare.pdf

Corcoran, J., Fairchild-Kienlen, S., & Harakal Phillips, J. (2000). Family treatment with caregivers of the elderly. In J. Corcoran (Ed.). *Evidence-based social work practice with families: A lifespan approach.* New York, NY: Springer.

Corner, J., Halliday, D., Haviland, J., Douglas, H.R., Bath, P.l., Clark, D., Normand, C., Beech, N., Hughes, P.l., Marples, R., Seymour, J., Skilbeck, J., & Webb, T. (2003). Exploring nursing outcomes for patients with advanced cancer following intervention by Macmillan specialist palliative care nurses. *Journal of Advanced Nursing, 41(6)*, 561-574.

Earle, C.C., Park, E.R., Lai, B., Weeks, J.C., Ayanian, J.Z., & Block, S. (2003). Identifying potential indicators of the quality of end-of-life cancer care from administrative data. *Journal of Clinical Oncology, 21(6)*, 1133-1138.

Engle, V.F., Fox-Hill, E., & Graney, M.J. (1998). The experience of living-dying in a nursing home: Self reports of black and white older adults. *Journal of the American Geriatrics Society, 46(9)*, 1091-1096.

Ferrell, B. & Hastie, B. (2003). Interventions at the end of life. In C.W. Given, B. Given, V.L. Champion, S. Kazachik, & D.N. DeVoss (Eds.). *Evidence-based cancer care and prevention.* New York: Springer.

Furst, C.J. & Doyle, D. (2005). The terminal phase. In D. Doyle, G. Hanks, & N.I. Cherny (Eds.) *Oxford textbook of palliative medicine.* New York: Oxford Press.

Georges, J.J., Onwuteaka-Philipsen, B.D., van der Heide, A., van der Wal, G., & van der Maas, P.J. (2005). Symptoms, treatment and "dying peacefully" in terminally ill cancer patients: A prospective study. *Supportive Care in Cancer,* 13(3), 160-168.

IOM (1997). *Approaching death: Improving care at the end of life.* Washington, DC: National Academy Press.

Jordan, J.R. & Niemeyer, R.A. (2003). Does grief counseling work? *Death Studies, 27,* 765-786.

Kato, P.M. & Mann, T. (1999). A synthesis of psychological interventions for the bereaved. *Clinical Psychology Review, 19,* 275-296.

Krakauer, E.L., Crenner, C., & Fox, K. (2002). Barriers to optimum end-of-life care for minority patients. *Journal of the American Geriatrics Society, 50(1),* 182-190.

Last Acts (2002a). Precepts of palliative care. Retrieved May 15, 2004 from http://www.lastacts.org.

Last Acts (2002b). Means to a Better End: A Report on Dying in America Today (2002). Retrieved September 22, 2005 at http://www.rwjf.org/files/publications/other/meansbetterend.pdf

Levy, L., Derby, J.E., & Martinkowski, K.S. (1993). Effects of membership in bereavement support groups on adaptation to conjugal bereavement. *American Journal of Community Psychology, 21(3),* 361-381.

Lieberman, M.A. & Yalom, I. (1992). Brief group psychotherapy for the spousally bereaved: A controlled study. *International Journal of Group Psychotherapy, 42(1),* 117-132.

Lipman, A.G., Jackson, K.C., & Tyler, L.S. (2004). *Evidence-based symptom control in palliative care: Systematic reviews and validated clinical practice guidelines for 15 common problems in patients with life-limiting diseases.* Binghamton, NY: The Haworth Press.

Lipman, A.G. (2004). Evidence-based palliative care. In A.G. Lipman, K.C. Jackson, & L.S. Tyler (Eds.). *Evidence-based symptom control in palliative care: Systematic reviews and validated clinical practice guidelines for 15 common problems in patients with life-limiting diseases,* pp. 1-11. Binghamton, NY: The Haworth Press.

Lorenz, K. & Lynn, J., Morton, S.C., Dy, S., Mularski, R., Shugarman, L., Sun, V., Wilkinson, A., Maglione, M., Shekelle, P.G. (2004). *End-of-life care and outcomes.* Evidence Report/Technology Assessment No. 110. AHRQ Publication No. 05-E004-2. Rockville, MD: Agency for Healthcare Research and Quality.

Lunney, J.R., Foley, K.M., Smith, T.J., & Gelband, H. (2003). *Describing death in America: What we need to know.* Washington, DC.: National Academies Press.

McQuay, H.J., Moore, A., & Wiffen, P. (2004). The principles of evidence-based medicine. In D. Doyle, G. Hanks, N. Cherny, & K. Calman (Eds.). *Oxford textbook of palliative medicine,* pp. 119-127.

Morrison, R.S. & Meier, D. (2003) Introduction. In R.S. Morrison & D. Meier (Eds). *Geriatric palliative care,* pp. xxi-xxix. New York, NY: Oxford.

National Center for Health Statistics. Health, United States 2004. Retrieved September 23, 2005 at http://www.cdc.gov/nchs/hus.htm

National Center for Health Statistics (2005). Deaths/mortality. Retrieved on April 22, 2005 at: http://www.cdc.gov/nchs/fastats/deaths.htm.

National Consensus Project (2004). Clinical practice guidelines for quality palliative care. Retrieved April 1, 2005 at http://www.nationalconsensusproject.org/

National Institutes of Health (2005). State-of-the-science conference statement: Improving end-of-life care. Retrieved on February 20, 2005 at http://consensus.nih.gov/PREVIOUSSTATEMENTS.htm#EndOfLifeCare

Proulx, K. & Jacelon, C. (2004). Dying with dignity: The good patient versus the good death. *American Journal of Hospice and Palliative Medicine, 21(2)*, 116-120.

Ratner, E., Norlander, L., & McSteen, K. (2001) Death at home following a targeted advance-care planning process at home: The kitchen table discussion. *Journal of the American Geriatrics Society, 49(6)*, 778-81.

Reich, J.W. & Zautra, A.J. (1989). A perceived control intervention for at-risk older adults. *Psychology and Aging, 4(4)*, 415-424.

Ringdal, G.I., Jordhoy, M.S., & Kaasa, S. (2002). Family satisfaction with end-of-life care for cancer patients in a cluster randomized trial. *Journal of Pain and Symptom Management, 24(1)*, 53-63.

Rubenfeld, G.D. & Curtis, R.J. (2001). End-of-life care in the intensive care unit: A research agenda. *Critical Care Medicine, 29(10)*, 2001-2006.

Schrader, S.L., Horner, A., Eidsness, L., Young, S., Wright, C., & Robinson, M. (2002). A team approach in palliative care: Enhancing outcomes. *South Dakota Journal of Medicine, 55(7)*, 269-78.

Schut, H., Stroebe, M.S., VanDen Bout, J., & Terheggen, M. (2001). The efficacy of bereavement interventions: Determining who benefits. In M.S. Stroebe, R.O. Hansson, W. Stroebe, & H. Schut (Eds.). *Handbook of bereavement research*, pp. 705-737. Washington, DC: American Psychological Association.

Schwartz, C.E., Mazor, R.K., Rogers, J.M.Y., & Reed, G. (2003). Validation of a new measure of concept of a good death. *Journal of Palliative Medicine, 6(4)*, 575-584.

Segal, D.L., Chatman, C., Bogaards, J.A., & Becker, L.A. (2001). One-year follow-up of an emotional expression intervention for bereaved older adults. *Journal of Mental Health and Aging, 7(4)*, 465-472.

Steinhauser, K.E., Clipp, E.C., McNeilly, M., Christakis, N.A., McIntyre, L.M., & Tulsky, J.A. (2000). In search of a good death: Observations of patients, families, and providers. *Annals of Internal Medicine, 132(10)*, 825-832.

Stroebe, M.S., Hansson, R. O., Stroebe, W., & Schut, H. (2001). *Handbook of bereavement research*. Washington, DC: American Psychological Association.

Tudiver, F., Hilditch, J., Permaul, J.A., & McKendree, D.J. (1992). Does mutual help facilitate newly bereaved widowers? Report of a randomized controlled trial. *Evaluation and the Health Professions, 15(2)*, 147-162.

Wennberg, J.E., McAndrew Cooper, M., & Tolle, S.W. (2003). Variability in end-of life care in the United States. In R.S. Morrison & D.E. Meier (Eds.). *Geriatric palliative care*, pp. 3-16. New York, NY: Oxford.

Werth, J.L., Gordon, J.R., & Johnson, R.R. (2002). Psychosocial issues near the end of life. *Aging & Mental Health, 6(4)*, 402-412.

Worden, W. (2002). *Grief counseling and grief therapy*. New York: Springer.

Chapter 12

Familial Caregivers of Older Adults

Kimberly McClure Cassie, MSSW, MA
Sara Sanders, PhD

HELPING THE CAREGIVER:
EVIDENCE-BASED PSYCHOSOCIAL INTERVENTIONS
FOR FAMILIAL CAREGIVERS OF OLDER ADULTS

Providing care for older adults has been a role that families have assumed for centuries. Traditionally viewed as an honor and one's duty to older relatives, caregiving has played a critical role in ensuring that the dignity and quality of life for older adults is maintained despite their health status. Over the last 30 years, the demand on familial caregivers has radically increased due to demographic transitions in society. In addition, it is important to recognize that caring for an older adult is only one of the many responsibilities faced by family caregivers. Many must also juggle the responsibility of caring for minor children and grandchildren, as well as the demands associated with employment. Social workers and other health-care providers must be knowledgeable about evidence-based psychosocial interventions in order to effectively assist family caregivers in coping with the many challenges they face throughout their caregiving careers.

Caregivers of older adults face many obstacles as they balance family, career, and caregiving demands. Caregivers are at an increased risk for burden, stress, depression, and a variety of other mental and physical health complications associated with the challenges that accompany the caregiving role (Adkins, 1999; Gallant & Connell, 1998). Geriatric professionals play a critical role in the care of caregivers. Their services, including therapy, support groups, respite, and advocacy are often the lifelines that keep older adults at home for longer periods of time where they receive the best care the caregiver can provide. It is not uncommon for caregivers to receive some form of pharmacological therapy to treat the physical and mental health changes that may occur throughout their caregiving career. However, while pharmacological forms of treatment are invaluable, medications only may not be sufficient to treat the needs of caregivers. As such, geriatric professionals also have a responsibility to intervene with caregivers through psychosocial interventions. This paper provides an overview of caregiving, a summary of evidence-based psychosocial research on interventions for family caregivers of older adults, and recommendations for future interventions.

DEMOGRAPHICS/PREVALENCE

In 2002 there were more than 36 million adults in the United States who are aged 65 and older (Administration on Aging, 2003a). By 2030, the number of individuals aged 65 and over is expected to reach 71.5 million, with the largest increase in the oldest-old, who are those aged 85 and over (Administration on Aging, 2003a). Half of those aged 85 and older need assistance with personal care (U.S. Bureau of the Census

Statistical Brief, 1995) that requires the help of some form of caregiver. While many assume that the majority of care provided to older adults occurs in long-term care facilities, the bulk of care for this population is actually provided by 22.4 million informal and unpaid family caregivers (Administration on Aging, 2003b). Estimates from the National Family Caregiver Association (2000) indicate that close to 27% of the adult population has provided care to a disabled, chronically ill, or aged relative in the past year.

While there is great diversity among familial caregivers, the average caregiver is a 46-year-old female with some college education caring for a widowed female (National Alliance for Caregiving and AARP, 2004). Yet variations in this profile exist on multiple levels including gender, race, ethnicity, age, and socioeconomic status. Current statistics suggest that 61% of all caregivers are women, while 39% are men. Most caregivers are between the ages of 35-49 years old (32%), followed by those 50-64 (30%), 18-34 (26%), and finally those over age 65 (13%). Forty-two percent of caregivers report an annual income of over $50,000 per year (National Alliance for Caregiving and AARP, 2004).

THEMES/NATURE OF THE PROBLEM

While caregiving is a valued societal resource, it does not come without costs at an economic and personal level. The overall economic cost of caregiving is staggering. In 1997, the annual cost of informal caregiving was estimated at $196 billion, compared to $32 billion spent on in-home care and $83 billion spent on nursing home care (Arno, Levine, & Memmot, 1999). By 2004, this number had grown to over $257 billion (National Alliance for Caregiving and AARP, 2004). Many of the costs of caregiving are paid directly by the primary caregiver due to a lack of financial resources or adequate health-care coverage among care recipients. MetLife (1999) reported familial caregivers spent an average of $20,000 in out-of-pocket expenses over a two to six year period on care-related expenses for their care recipients. This is particularly daunting with more than 50% of all caregivers earning less than $50,000 per year (National Alliance for Caregiving and AARP, 2004).

One of the greatest struggles for caregivers is balancing caregiving demands with employment and, in many cases, children still living at home. In 1997, the National Alliance for Caregiving and AARP reported that there were approximately 14 million employed caregivers. Research suggests almost 60% of family caregivers have been employed while simultaneously caring for an older adult (National Alliance for Caregiving and AARP, 2004). More than half of all working caregivers are employed on a full-time basis, while 12% work part-time (National Alliance for Caregiving and AARP, 2004).

U.S. businesses and corporations are also feeling the impact of caregiving. It was estimated that the cost of family caregiving to U.S. businesses ranged from $11 to $29 billion in 1997 (MetLife, 1997). Included in this estimate were costs associated with replacing lost employees, increased absenteeism, workday interruptions, and decreased productivity (MetLife, 1997). Many companies offer services through employee assistance programs to help caregivers balance their multiple demands, but the overall wear and tear on caregivers is still apparent. Many caregivers find it virtually impossible to balance the demands of a career with caregiving responsibilities. Ten to 31% of family caregivers have given up employment in order to care for an older adult (National Alliance for Caregiving and AARP, 2004). A study conducted by MetLife (1997) revealed that 11% of family caregivers took a leave of absence to care for an older adult, 7% cut their hours, moving from full-time to part-time employment, 6% left the work force completely, and 4% applied for early retirement. In another study, 40% of employed caregivers reported that caregiving affected their opportunities for advancement in their careers (MetLife, 1999). More specifically, 29% were unable to accept promotion or training opportunities and 25% were unable to accept a transfer (MetLife, 1999).

Research has found racial differences in the manner in which informal caregivers respond to balancing employment demands with caregiving responsibilities. While one may assume that employed caregivers would provide fewer hours of caregiving and use formal services at a higher rate than non-employed caregivers, the contrary has been found among African American care providers. Bullock, Crawford, and Tennstedt (2003) found that employment status was not a factor that predicted formal service use. Instead, it was suggested that employed African Americans subscribe to cultural values of family relatives providing care to the elderly. Similar findings were reported by Fredriksen-Goldsen and Farwell (2004) who found that employed minority caregivers, even though more economically disadvantaged, provided more care to elderly relatives in terms of hours and types of care than did Caucasian caregivers. Additionally, the employed minority caregivers reported less caregiver strain than did their employed Caucasian counterparts. These studies point to the uniqueness of informal caregivers and the need for culturally competent services.

CONSEQUENCES OF THE PROBLEM

While caring for an older friend or relative can have intrinsic rewards, there are also a variety of negative consequences associated with caregiving. Because of the multiple demands placed on caregivers, they are at an increased risk of physical and mental stress. Research starting in the early 1980s has indicated that informal caregivers are at a greater risk for a variety of mental health conditions, such as depression, anxiety, stress and burden, as well as a variety of physical health problems. In fact, Adkins (1999) reported that 25-85% of all caregivers suffer from depression and other aversive caregiving reactions.

There are multiple factors that contribute to the depression and burden that are experienced by caregivers. Changes in the care recipient's physical, functional and cognitive status, the nature and type of caregiving demands, as well as the nature of the relationship between the caregiver and care recipient can all impact caregiver depression and burden (Sherwood, Given, Given, & Von Eye, 2005). Other factors contributing to caregiver burden and depression include the caregiver's emotional and psychological status, coping strategies, and the availability of formal and informal support systems. The aversive reactions of caregiving are particularly important to address given their significant correlation with abuse of the care recipient (Beach et al., 2005) and increased caregiver health problems. Unfortunately, many caregivers provide care in isolation because social support is neither available nor accessible. Research has revealed that 60% of all family caregivers do not receive assistance from paid professional supportive services and 30% do not receive unpaid assistance (National Alliance for Caregiving and AARP, 2004). Given this information, it is easy to understand the overwhelming burden and stress many caregivers face. Despite the negative ramifications of informal caregiving, 55%-90% of caregivers report positive outcomes as a result of caring for an older adult (Butler, Holkup, & Buckwalter, 2001; Cohen, Gold, Shulman, & Zucchero, 1994; Farran, 1997).

Caregivers play a critical role in our society. Therefore, a primary focus of gerontological professions should be on supporting these valuable resources. The personal, social, and economic costs of caregiving will only increase with the growing number of older adults. The following literature review will examine nonpharmacological interventions to treat the mental and physical health concerns reported by caregivers.

EMPIRICAL LITERATURE

Research on the effectiveness of nonpharmacological interventions with family caregivers of older adults has been conducted by a variety of disciplines including nursing, occupational therapy, psychology and social work. To identify research studies for inclusion in this review several search terms were used including caregivers, older adults, dementia, interventions, evidence-based treatments, and meta-analysis. Only research conducted in the past 20 years was included in this review. PsychINFO, PubMed, Cinahl, Academic Search Premier and the Cochrane databases were searched. Over 5,000 articles were identified. Clinical drug trials were excluded and 97 articles remained. Meta-analyses of randomized controlled studies, as well as well-designed controlled studies with and without randomization were included in this paper. Sixteen studies met these requirements and are included in this empirical literature review. A review of empirical literature from these fields revealed four distinct types of treatment modalities that are available for practitioners working with family caregivers. Treatment modalities found in these studies include: (1) individual interventions occurring between the practitioner and a single caregiver; (2) group interventions occurring between one or more practitioners and multiple caregivers; (3) multi-modal interventions involving a variety of treatment modalities; and (4) technology-based interventions.

Individual Interventions

Individual interventions are therapeutic treatments that occur between the practitioner and a single-family caregiver or caregiver unit and can include counseling, problem-solving, skill-building, and psychoeducational interventions, among others. These practice approaches can be delivered through agency-based settings or in the caregiver's home. Several researchers have explored the effectiveness of individual interventions among family caregivers. Table 1 provides a summary of these studies.

Buckwalter and colleagues (1999) and Gerdner, Buckwalter and Reed (2002) explored the effects of the Progressively Lowered Stress Threshold (PLST) model, a psychoeducational intervention emphasizing the effect of the environment on people with dementia. Buckwalter and colleagues (1999) conducted a multi-state, longitudinal study over a four-year period in Iowa, Minnesota, Arizona and Indiana. The sample included 245 caregivers who provided four or more hours of care per day to people with dementia. Participants were randomly assigned to a treatment group and to a routine care comparison group. Those in the treatment group received an average of three to four hours of in-home interventions and regular follow-up phone calls over a six-month period of time. The intervention consisted of the creation of individualized care plans with caregiver training, written educational materials, and referrals to supportive services in the community. Researchers found that those in the treatment group were less depressed, less tired, and less tense at six months post-intervention than those in the comparison group. At 12 months post-intervention those in the treatment group continued to be less tired and less tense than those in the comparison group, however, there was not a statistically significant difference in depression between the groups.

In Gerdner and colleagues' study of PLST (2002), 237 caregivers of people with moderate to severe dementia were randomly assigned into a treatment group (n = 132) and a comparison group (n = 105). The treatment group received an in-home psychoeducational nursing intervention. The intervention included the creation of a care plan with a structured routine for the person with dementia, education regarding environmental modifications, and referrals to community-based services. Participants in the treatment group received four hours of services in their home. The comparison group received routine care with generic information during two 1-hour home visits. Findings suggest the intervention resulted in improved caregiver response to challenging behavior problems in care recipients. More specifically, care recipients with dementia whose primary caregivers were non-spousal caregivers exhibited decreased memory and behavior problems as a result of improved caregiver response to problem behaviors commonly displayed by people with dementia. Spousal caregivers in the treatment group displayed more positive responses to problems with activities of daily living in the PLST treatment group.

Other researchers have explored the effect of an environmental skill-building program on caregiver well-being and care recipient

TABLE 1. Review of Interventions for Individual Caregivers

Author	Population	N	Intervention	Outcomes
Buckwalter et al. (1999)	Dementia	245	Psychoeducation	Decreased depression, fatigue & tension.
Burns et al. (2003)	Dementia	167	Stress Reduction & Disease Ed.	More positive general well-being.
Gerdner et al. (2002)	Dementia	237	Psychoeducation	More positive caregiver response to behavior problems. Decreased memory & behavior problems among care recipients.
Gitlin et al. (2003)	Dementia	190	Skill Building	Improved caregiver affect & ability to manage responsibilities.

functioning (Gitlin et al., 2003). Over a six-month period of time, caregivers received five home visits and one phone call from an occupational therapist. The occupational therapist provided caregivers with information about dementia, the effect of the environment on people with dementia, problem-solving techniques, and ways to modify the home environment to minimize memory related behavior problems. The sample included 190 caregivers, 89 in the treatment group and 101 in the usual care comparison group. Results indicated that caregivers in the treatment group reported an improved affect and an improved ability to manage caregiving tasks with less assistance from family and friends when compared to the comparison group. More specifically, male caregivers in the treatment group reported a reduction in the amount of time necessary to complete their caregiving responsibilities compared to those in the comparison group. While there was no change for non-spousal caregivers, spouses in the treatment group were not as bothered by disruptive behaviors as were those in the comparison group.

Finally, a study conducted by Burns, Nichols, Martindale-Adams, Graney, and Lummus (2003) examined the effects of brief interventions delivered in conjunction with quarterly primary care physician visits to care recipients diagnosed with Alzheimer's disease or a related dementia. Participants (N = 167) were randomly assigned into one of two groups. One group, referred to as the Behavior Care group (n = 85), received an average of three hours of education regarding the management of problem behaviors during the 24-month study period. The other group, referred to as the Enhanced Care group (n = 82), received an average of four hours of education regarding the management of behaviors, as well as education regarding stress reduction measures during the 24-month intervention. The results of the study suggest that caregivers who received instructions regarding the management of problem behaviors and stress reported a more positive general well-being than those who only received instructions regarding managing behavior problems in the care recipient. In addition, the researchers found that those in the Behavior Care group were at a greater risk for depression than caregivers in the Enhanced Care group. The results suggest that interventions focused on the management of problem behaviors among care recipients without attention to caregiver stress may not be as effective as interventions that address both areas.

Group Interventions

In contrast to individual interventions, group interventions are therapeutic interventions that occur between one or more practitioners and a
group of multiple family caregivers. Support groups and educational
groups are common interventions that tend to be administered at
agency-based locations. Several researchers, as outlined in Table 2,
have studied the effectiveness of group interventions among family
caregivers.

To begin, Greene and Monahan (1989) studied the effects of support
groups among 289 caregivers of frail elders. Participants (n = 208) in
treatment groups met for two hours weekly over an eight-week period.
Opportunities for discussion, problem-solving, education, and relaxation training were available at each group meeting. Findings revealed
that caregivers participating in the support groups reported decreased
anxiety and depression when compared to the comparison group (n =
81) that did not participate in a support group. In 1987, Greene and
Monahan found in a similar study that participation in support groups
resulted in a decreased rate of institutionalization for care recipients.

Toseland, Rossiter, and Labrecque (1989) conducted a study in
which 56 adult daughters and daughters-in-law caring for aged parents
were randomly assigned into one of three groups: a professionally led
support group (n = 18); a peer led support group (n = 18); and a respite
only comparison group (n = 20). Professionally led groups were facilitated by master's prepared social workers while peer led groups were
facilitated by individuals with personal experience as caregivers. Professionally led groups utilized a two-part structured model of education
and problem-solving, while peer facilitated groups relied on a model of
mutual support and self-help. Each group met weekly for eight weeks,
with each session lasting approximately two hours. Findings revealed
that the primary difference between peer led and professionally led support groups could be found in social support and psychological outcomes for caregivers. Individuals in professionally led support groups
experienced a statistically significant improvement in psychological
functioning as measured by the Brief Symptom Inventory, while those
in peer-led groups developed more informal support in their social environment. More specifically, individuals in professionally-led support
groups experienced less perceived distress, obsessive compulsiveness, anxiety, and irrational fears. Individuals in both treatment
groups increased their knowledge of community resources and exhibited an improved ability to manage caregiving and other responsibili-

TABLE 2. Review of Group Interventions for Family Caregivers

Author	Population	N	Intervention	Outcomes
Greene & Monahan (1987)	Frail Elders	289	Support Group	Decreased rate of institutionalization among care recipients.
Greene & Monahan (1989)	Frail Elders	289	Support Group	Decreased caregiver anxiety & depression.
Kaasalainen et al. (2000)	Female caregivers	46	Education & Support Group	Increased knowledge of community resources & caregiving.
Toseland et al. (1989)	Dtrs & Dtrs-in-law of aged	56	Support Group	Professionally led support groups resulted in increased psychological functioning. Peer led support groups resulted in increased informal support. Both resulted in increased knowledge of community resources & improved caregiver well-being.

ties compared with the respite comparison group. The professionally led and the peer led support groups also experienced an increase in well-being compared to the respite comparison group that experienced a decrease in well-being.

Finally, Kaasalainen, Craig, and Wells (2000) conducted a study to assess the effectiveness of the community-based Caring for Aging Relative Group (CARG) on a sample of 46 female caregivers. Twenty-three caregivers participated in the group intervention. The usual care comparison group that consisted of 23 female caregivers were matched to treatment group participants by caregiver age, length of time as a caregiver, and relationship. The intervention consisted of weekly two-hour sessions over an eight-week period of time. During the weekly sessions participants were educated about a variety of caregiving issues including, but not limited to, the aging process, stress management and community resources. The groups were facilitated by bachelor-level public health nurses and included elements of education and social support. Social support was also provided by program facilitators who were nurses, and by other group members. Findings indicated that individuals in the CARG treatment group experienced a statistically significant increase in knowledge about caregiving based on pretest and posttest scores indicating the program was successful at educating participants about the caregiving process.

Multi-Modal Interventions and Meta-Analyses

Deciding which type of intervention to use with various types of caregivers can be a daunting task. To better understand the effectiveness of various interventions, it is helpful to review the effects of multi-modal interventions that involve a combination of both individual and group interventions, and meta-analyses that have explored the effectiveness of individual, group, and multi-modal interventions. An outline of multi-modal interventions and meta-analyses is provided in Tables 3 and 4. The first two studies discussed below, conducted by Mittleman and colleagues (1993) and Burgio, Stevens, Guy, Roth, and Haley (2003) respectively, report the findings of multi-modal interventions. The study by Toseland, Rossiter, Peak, and Smith (1990) and the final three meta-analyses provide a comparison of the effectiveness of individual, group, and multi-modal interventions.

To begin, Mittleman and colleagues (1993) assessed the impact of counseling, support groups, and consultations on caregiver outcomes and on care recipient placement in residential care settings among a

TABLE 3. Review of Multi-Modal Interventions for Family Caregivers

Author	Population	N	Intervention	Outcomes
Burgio et al. (2003)	Dementia	118	Ed. workshop, in-home consults, & phone calls	Most effective among African Americans. Decreased bother among caregivers and decreased behavior problems.
Mittleman et al. (1993)	Spouse caring for spouse with dementia	206	Ind. & fmly. counseling, support groups & consultations	Decreased likelihood of institutionalization among care recipients.
Toseland et al. (1990)	Dtrs. & Dtrs-in-law caring for frail elders	154	Support group, ind. counseling, or respite	Increased knowledge & improved attitudes toward caregiving among support groups & ind. counseling. Support group participants reported increased social support. Ind. counseling participants reported improved psychosocial symptoms.

TABLE 4. Review of Meta-Analyses

Author	Population	N	Intervention	Outcomes
Brodaty et al. (2003)	Dementia	30	Ind. & fmly. counseling, education, support groups, stress management, & others	Decreased caregiver burden with skill training. Interventions involving care recipient and caregiver more effective than interventions involving caregiver alone.
Forster et al. (2003)	Stroke	9	Educational interventions	Lectures may be more effective than the distribution of information pamphlets alone.
Sorenson et al. (2002)	Dementia, cancer, stroke, other	78	Psychoeducation, supportive, respite, psychotherapy, & multi-modal	Decreased caregiver burden with psychoeducation, psychotherapy & respite. Improved caregiver well-being with psychoeducation, psychotherapy, respite, care recipient training & multi-modal interventions. Improved caregiver knowledge & ability with psychoeducation, supportive interventions, psychotherapy, and multimodal interventions. Group interventions less effective than individual and mixed modality interventions.

sample of 206 spouses caring for a spouse with dementia at home. Participants were randomly assigned into a treatment group and a usual care comparison group. The treatment group received two individual counseling sessions and four family counseling sessions, during the first four months of the intervention. Following the counseling sessions, caregivers were required to participate in support groups and could access a counselor for consultations at any time over the next eight months. Researchers found that caregivers in the comparison group were twice as likely to place care recipients in a residential care facility compared to those in the treatment group. In addition, researchers identified a number of factors that predicted nursing home placement. Among the predictive factors were low income, severe dementia, younger caregivers, older care recipients, and excessive caregiver burden.

Burgio and colleagues (2003) evaluated the effectiveness of two psychosocial interventions for African American and Caucasian caregivers of people with dementia in Alabama. Participants (N = 118) were randomly assigned into two groups. One group (n = 61) received skills training that included problem-solving, cognitive restructuring, and education regarding the management of difficult behaviors. Skills training was administered over one year through a three-hour group workshop followed by 11 in-home sessions, and five supportive phone calls. The other group (n = 57) received only minimal support over the phone and written information. Researchers found a significant decrease in the average number of behavior problems experienced in both groups after six months. In addition, caregivers in both groups also reported less bother because of problematic behaviors in their care recipient. Skills training, however, appeared to be more effective among African American caregivers. When African American caregivers in the skills training group were compared to Caucasians in the skills training group, the African American caregivers reported less bother related to their caregiving activities than did Caucasian care providers. Within racial categories, African American caregivers in the skills training group reported less bother than their counterparts in the minimal support group as well. On the other hand, the provision of minimal support appeared to be more effective among Caucasian caregivers. When relationship to the care recipient was also considered, African American spousal caregivers in the skills training group and Caucasian spousal caregivers in the minimal support group reported the largest decline in behavior problems among their care recipients.

Researchers have also explored the effects of individual and group interventions facilitated by peers and professionals on caregiver well-being among adult daughters and daughters-in-law caring for frail older adults (Toseland et al., 1990). Participants (N = 154) were randomly assigned into one of three groups: a treatment group participating in group interventions; a treatment group receiving individual counseling; or a respite only comparison group. The group interventions met weekly for eight weeks with each session lasting approximately two hours. Participants receiving individual counseling met with the professional or peer counselor for about an hour a week for eight weeks. The comparison group received funds to employ 1-2 hours of respite care each week for eight weeks. Researchers explored the effects of participation in a group intervention and an individual intervention compared to a respite only comparison group. The study suggested that participants receiving individual and group interventions reported improved knowledge of and improved attitudes toward caregiving responsibilities. Participants receiving individual counseling reported a statistically significant improvement in the severity of psychiatric symptoms, including obsessive compulsiveness, depression, anxiety, hostility, phobic anxiety, and psychotic episodes. Those receiving group interventions reported greater social support than the other groups. Interestingly, those in the group intervention reported a greater knowledge of community-based resources, but increased knowledge did not translate into increased usage. These findings suggest that group interventions among adult daughters and daughters-in-law would be more effective at increasing the caregiver's knowledge of community resources and expanding their social support network, while individual interventions would be more effective at treating psychosocial issues among the caregivers.

Perhaps one of the most extensive studies was a meta-analysis of 78 studies conducted by Sorensen, Pinquart, and Duberstein (2002). Caregivers provided assistance to persons suffering from a variety of conditions including dementia, cancer, stroke, and other physical and mental conditions. Among the many interventions were psychoeducational interventions, supportive interventions, respite services, psychotherapy (primarily cognitive behavior treatments), and multi-modal interventions. The results of the meta-analysis revealed that psychoeducation, psychotherapy, and respite were effective at decreasing caregiver burden, while psychoeducation, psychotherapy, respite, care recipient training and multimodal interventions were effective at improving caregiver well-being. Improvements in caregiver knowledge and ability regarding the provision of their caregiving responsibilities were found with the use of psychoeducation, supportive interventions, psychotherapy, and multimodal interventions. Overall, group interventions were found to be less effective at addressing caregiver burden, depression, and well-being than were individual and mixed modality interventions.

Brodaty and colleagues (2003) conducted a meta-analysis of 30 studies exploring the effectiveness of interventions among 2,040 caregivers of people with dementia. Among the many interventions in the studies were caregiver counseling, education, family counseling, support groups, stress management, and training, to name a few. Researchers reported that only one intervention, a social skills training program, resulted in a statistically significant decrease in caregiver burden. Furthermore, interventions that involved both the care recipient and the caregiver were more effective at improving psychosocial outcomes among caregivers than interventions that involved the caregiver alone. The researchers also found that interventions involving more frequent contact resulted in a statistically significant decrease in caregiver physiological distress.

Forster and colleagues (2003) conducted a meta-analysis of nine studies to assess the effectiveness of educational strategies at increasing stroke patients' and caregivers' knowledge about strokes and stroke related services. Interventions included the provision of information and educational materials in the form of pamphlets, manuals, and lectures. The analysis revealed that the provision of information and educational materials, such as pamphlets, resulted in a minimal level of statistical significance. The findings from this meta-analysis suggest that two individual studies reported an increase in caregiver knowledge following educational sessions. Researchers reported weaker improvements in caregiver knowledge after caregivers were only provided with informational pamphlets. Researchers suggested that educational materials provided in a learning environment, such as lectures or discussions, might be more effective at statistically increasing the understanding of stroke related issues than providing informational pamphlets alone.

Technology-Based Interventions

More recently, researchers have explored the effectiveness of technology-based interventions among caregivers. Technology-based interventions involve the use of telephone and computer services to provide education and support to family caregivers. A distinct advantage of technology-based interventions is the ability of caregivers to access support and education 24 hours a day from their homes. Studies of the effectiveness of technology-based interventions are outlined in Table 5.

Eisdorfer and colleagues (2003) looked at the effects of interventions delivered through modern technology to caregivers of people with dementia in Florida. Caregivers (N = 225) were stratified by ethnicity (Cuban American or Caucasian American) and randomly assigned into two treatment groups and one comparison group. One treatment group (n = 75) received Structural Ecosystems Therapy (SET) over the course of one year. SET was used to identify interactions that contributed to caregiver burden and to develop individualized interventions to address maladaptive interactions. Participants in the SET group received weekly in-home visits for the first month, biweekly visits for the next two months, and monthly visits for the last six months. The second treatment group (n = 77) received SET and a Computer Telephone Integrated System (SET + CTIS). The first six months of the intervention were identical to the SET intervention, but in the last six months participants had access to CTIS. Caregivers could use CTIS to place conference calls to other family members, participate in online discussion groups, voice message, utilize reminder services, and access community resources. The minimal support comparison (MCS) group (n = 73) received minimally supportive phone calls and educational materials. Both white Americans and Cuban Americans in the SET + CTIS group reported a decrease in depression at six and 18 months compared to the other groups. The intervention appeared to be most effective at reducing depression among daughters of both ethnicities and Cuban American husbands.

Mahoney, Tarlow and Jones (2003) conducted a study to assess the effects of a computerized telephone voice response program among in-home caregivers of persons with dementia within the northeastern United States. The intervention provided caregivers with weekly conversations designed to monitor stress and provide caregivers with information to assist in managing problem behaviors. The system also provided caregivers with a personal voice mailbox that could be used to communicate with other caregivers and a clinical nurse. A bulletin board feature on the telephone system was used as a support group where caregivers communicated with one another via voice mail. The system could also be used to distract care recipients with phone calls. The study involved 100 caregivers, 49 of whom were randomly assigned to the treatment group, while 51 were in the usual care comparison group. The intervention resulted in minimal results. However, the findings did indicate that the intervention was most effective among

TABLE 5. Review of Technology-Based Interventions for Family Caregivers

Author	Population	N	Intervention	Outcomes
Eisdorfer et al. (2003)	Dementia Cuban & Caucasian Americans	225	SET* & CTIS**	Decreased caregiver depression at 6 & 18 mos. Most effective among dtrs. of both ethnicities & Cuban American husbands.
Mahoney et al. (2003)	Dementia	100	Computerized telephone voice response program	Decreased depression, anxiety & bother. Most effective among wives caring for husbands & those with low to mid levels of mastery.

*Structural Ecosystems Therapy **Computer Telephone Integrated System caregivers who initially exhibited a minimal to moderate level of comfort with caregiving activities rather than those who initially reported a high level of mastery over their caregiving responsibilities. Those with low to mid levels of mastery exhibited decreased depression, anxiety, and bother compared to those in the comparison group. The intervention was also noted to be more effective among wives caring for their husbands than among husbands caring for their wives.

TREATMENT SUMMARY

In summary, a variety of psychosocial treatment interventions have been used to assist caregivers in managing the effects that their caregiving responsibilities have on their physical and mental health. Individual psychoeducational interventions have been associated with decreased caregiver depression, fatigue and tension, as well as improved management of behavior problems among people with dementia. Group interventions have been effective at decreasing caregiver anxiety and depression, and giving an increased knowledge of community resources as well as increased social support. Multi-modal interventions have been successful at decreasing caregiver stress and burden, increasing caregiver knowledge, improving caregiver attitudes, and decreasing the likelihood of care recipient institutionalization. Other interventions, such as technology-based interventions, using computer and telephone-generated support, may be the key to assisting certain types or subpopulations of caregivers in our modern, computer-driven culture. Technology-based interventions have been shown to be effective at reducing caregiver burden, depression, anxiety, and bother.

Competent practitioners will want to use interventions that have been shown to be effective at treating the specific needs of their clients. Research has demonstrated that clients presenting with complaints of compromised well-being could benefit from stress reduction and disease education, support groups, psychoeducation, psychotherapy, respite, care recipient training, and multi-modal interventions. Psychoeducational interventions, support groups, and technology-based interventions have resulted in decreased caregiver depression. Caregiver anxiety has been reduced through participation in support groups and technology-based interventions. Decreased caregiver burden was observed after participation in skill training programs, psychoeducation, psychotherapy and respite. Caregiver knowledge and ability to manage caregiving responsibilities were improved as a result of skill-building, group interventions, psychoeducation, psychotherapy, respite, and multi-modal interventions. By matching caregiver needs with evidenced-based treatments that have been effective at treating those specific caregiver needs, practitioners will be better able to serve family caregivers and their care recipients.

CONCLUSION

Unlike other areas, research on caregivers has been explored in the gerontological literature for the past 25 years and has received a good deal of clinical attention. Despite this history, the emphasis on examining evidence-based treatments for caregivers is creating a need for more complex research methodologies, sophisticated sampling strategies, and analytical methods. With the expected growth of older adults, the demand for increased treatment strategies to support caregivers continues. Several steps should be taken to strengthen the evidence-based psychosocial treatments for caregivers of older adults.

First, the majority of the research on caregivers has used predominately Caucasian samples (Aranda & Knight, 1997; Dillworth-Anderson, Williams, & Gibson, 2002; Roff et al., 2004). Given the diversity that exists within the older adult community, it is necessary to examine how caregivers from different racial or cultural groups respond to various psychosocial interventions. Additionally, it is critical not to assume that intervention modalities that have been appropriate for Caucasian populations will be appropriate for other groups of caregivers. Thus, modifications may need to be made in many psychosocial interventions to ensure that they are culturally sensitive. Similarly, it is necessary to examine how issues such as geographic location, length of time in the United States, and overall cultural norms about caregiving impact the effectiveness of the intervention.

Second, while several of the reviewed studies used longitudinal designs (Buckwalter et al., 1999; Burns et al., 2003; Gerdner et al., 2002; Gitlin et al., 1999), additional future research should employ this methodological strategy to better account for changes in the overall caregiving experience, due to disease progression, placement in long-term care facilities, and changes in the physical and mental health of the caregiver. The majority of studies that used longitudinal designs were individual-based treatments. Greater attention needs to be given to the long-term benefits of group-based and technologically-based interventions as well. The use of longitudinal designs will better assist agency-based practitioners in determining the efficacy of treatments and their overall effectiveness with caregivers.

Third, research on caregivers of individuals with Alzheimer's disease and other forms of dementia has been the primary focal point in caregiving research. As seen in the review of literature, the majority of caregivers sampled were providing care to individuals with some form of progressive dementia. Even though dementia is one of the greatest concerns for older adults and places a great deal of physical and mental stress on caregivers, there are other chronic and non-chronic health conditions that impact older adults and, thereby, require the assistance of a familial caregiver. It should not be assumed that an intervention for a caregiver of an older adult with one type of health condition will be appropriate for a caregiver of an older adult with another type of health condition. Thus, research is needed that assists in differentiating what specific types of interventions are beneficial for individuals with different health conditions.

Finally, the use of interdisciplinary teams and collaborations may help expand the type of treatment strategies that are available to caregivers. Campbell and colleagues (1992) argued that interdisciplinary teams help facilitate a more holistic form of treatment and an overall higher quality of care. Unfortunately, interdisciplinary conflict within the health-care environment sometimes supersedes the goal of providing the best care to the client. Future research should focus on the impact of interdisciplinary interventions on caregivers.

In summary, a variety of evidence-based psychosocial treatment options exists for caregivers of older adults, but additional work is needed to ensure that caregivers receive the assistance, support, and services they need. The scholarly community active in gerontological research must expand their efforts to bring research and practice together in order to make certain that the needs of family caregivers are met. Caregivers play a vital role in the health and well-being of many frail older adults in America. As the number of caregivers in America continues to grow it is critical that research in this area also increases so practitioners and policy makers can formulate solutions to reduce the growing demands on those who willingly take on the role of caregiver.

TREATMENT RESOURCE APPENDIX

Alzheimer's Association National Office
www.alz.org
24/7 Nationwide Contact Center: 1-800-272-3900

The Alzheimer's Association is the first non-profit organization dedicated to finding suitable treatment strategies and an eventual cure for Alzheimer's disease. Chapters of the Alzheimer's Association are located throughout the United States and provide services to individuals with the disease and their familial caregivers. Included on this site is content related to family care provision, as well as ways to become more involved in advocacy efforts through contacting elected officials, and learning more about ways to serve in an advocacy role.

Alzheimer's Disease Education and Referral Center (ADEAR)
www.alzheimers.org
1-800-438-4380 (8:30 a.m. to 5:00 p.m. Eastern Time, Monday-Friday)

Created in 1990 by the U.S. Congress, ADEAR distributes education and research about Alzheimer's disease to health professionals, people with the disease, and familial caregivers. One section specifically lists resources for family care providers. The topics available to families are:

- Dealing with the Diagnosis
- Communication
- Bathing
- Dressing
- Eating
- Activities
- Exercise
- Incontinence
- Sleep Problems
- Hallucinations and Delusions
- Wandering
- Home Safety
- Driving
- Visiting the Doctor
- Coping with Holidays
- Visiting a Person with AD
- Choosing a Nursing Home

Coon, D. W., Gallagher-Thompson, D., & Thompson, L.W. (2003). Innovative interventions to reduce dementia caregiver distress: A clinical guide. This collection of 14 essays provides an overview of emerging themes in dementia research and a broad array of practical strategies for reducing caregiver distress. Individual contributions focus on family caregivers and distress; monitoring and evaluating interventions; interventions for a multicultural society; specific stressors of spousal caregivers (difficult behaviors, loss of sexual intimacy, and incontinence); family interventions to address the needs of the caregiving system; psychoeducational strategies; in-home interventions; partnering with primary care providers; capitalizing on technological advances; anticipatory grief and loss; ethnic minority caregivers; male caregivers; lesbian, gay, bisexual, and transgender caregivers; and future directions in dementia caregiving intervention research and practice.

Family Caregiver Alliance
www.caregiver.org
1-800-445-8106 (9:00am to 5:00pm, Monday-Friday)

The Family Caregiver Alliance was founded in 1977 to provide education and support to families who were providing care in the home. Programs and education are offered at the national, regional, and local level to support the daily work of familial caregivers. Several good resources are available on the site, for example:

- Caregiving across the states–which is a "clickable" map that is a data base of programs established for family caregivers in different locations.
- A TeleCaregiving site that has streaming audio programs for care providers. Topics include communicating with someone who has dementia, keeping away the blues, tips for sharing caregiving responsibilities among family members, among other topics.
- Information about upcoming workshops for family care providers.

National Family Caregiver Association
www.thefamilycaregiver.org
1-800-896-3650 (9:00am to 5:00pm, Monday-Friday)

The National Family Caregiver Association is dedicated to educating, supporting, and empowering familial caregivers. This organization is not disease-specific and instead focuses on the unique needs of each caregiver and the steps that need to be taken to reduce the disparities between caregivers and non-caregivers.

National Family Caregiver Support Program
http://www.aoa.gov/prof/aoaprog/caregiver/caregiver.asp
202-619-0724 (8:00am to 5:00pm, Monday-Friday)

The NFCSP provides information to health providers and familial caregivers about the location of caregiving services and current legislative initiatives that will impact caregivers. Available nationally, the NFCSP is administered through local Areas Agencies on Aging and state Departments on Aging.

Virtual Communities/Web Pages for Care Providers

Many virtual communities have started to develop web sites that allow care providers to establish a network with others. Some examples are:

CarePages
http://www.carepages.com/

CarePages are free, personal, private Web pages that help family and friends communicate when someone is receiving care. It takes just a few minutes to create a CarePage, share it with friends and family, and build a community of support.
CarePages help families:

- Create a virtual meeting place on the web
- Share news and photos as often as needed
- Receive emotional support during a time of need

Strength for Caring
http://www.strengthforcaring.com/

Strength for Caring is an online resource and community for family caregivers. Strength for Caring helps family caregivers take care of their loved ones and themselves. Strength for Caring is part of The Caregiver Initiative, created by Johnson & Johnson Consumer Products Company, Division of Johnson & Johnson Consumer Companies, Inc. Six sections are contained:

- *Caregiver Manual.* Within Caregiver Manual, the Strength for Caring Website visitors will find articles and content devoted to their needs–helping caregivers deal with stress, diet, managing work, spouses or partners, and siblings. In addition, the Caregiver Manual section helps caregivers relax and take time off.

- *Community.* The goal of the Community area is to empower and inform caregivers with a powerful and active online community. Strength for Caring provides 24/7 messageboards and a place where caregivers can tell their personal story to the world. Receive help and tips from other caregivers any time of the day or night in our Community.
- *Health Conditions.* The goal of this section is to help caregivers understand the main ailments that care recipients suffer from. The information on Strength for Caring is not meant as medical advice, but merely an overview. Please check with your doctor or your loved one's doctor for more information on any health condition.
- *Daily Care.* In our Daily Care section, we offer the practical, day-to-day information and advice from brushing someone's teeth and hair, to proper cleansing and bathing, to taking the keys away.
- *Housing.* This section contains information about the different types of housing options, and a friendly comparison chart. It contains practical tips and advice including "What to Look For" when choosing any type of home or housing situation.
- *Money & Insurance.* This section contains practical information, written in a simple and friendly way, about insurance, budgeting, eldercare law, and other topics related to Caregiving. This section will help caregivers understand what Power of Attorney or Guardianship mean; will explain Medicare Part D and the different types of supplemental insurance. This section will host experts in the financial, legal, insurance, and government arenas.

REFERENCES

Adkins, V. K. (1999). Treatment of depressive disorders of spousal caregivers of persons with Alzheimer's disease: A review. *American Journal of Alzheimer's Disease,* 14, 289-293.

Administration on Aging (2003a). A Profile of Older Americans. Retrieved February 25, 2005 from http://www.aoa.gov/prof/Statistics/profile/2003/2.asp

Administration on Aging (2003b). What we do makes a difference. Fact Sheet: Family Caregiving. Retrieved February 25, 2005 from http://www.aoa.gov/press/nfc_month/2003/nfcm_factsheets/8FamilyCaregiver.pdf

Aranda, M. P. & Knight, B. G. (1997). The influence of ethnicity and culture on the caregiver stress and coping process: A sociocultural review and analysis. *The Gerontologist,* 17, 342-354.

Arno, P. S., Levine, C., & Memmot, M. M. (1999). The economic value of informal care giving. *Health Affairs,* 18(2), 182-188.

Beach, S., Schulz, R., Williamson, G. M., Miller, L. S., Weiner, M. F., & Lance, C. E. (2005). Risk factors for potentially harmful informal caregiver behavior. *Journal of the American Geriatrics Society,* 53, 255-262.

Brodaty, H., Green, A., & Koschera, A. (2003). Meta-analysis of psychosocial interventions for caregivers of people with dementia. *JAGS,* 51(5), 657-664.

Buckwalter, K. C., Gerdner, L., Kohout, F., Hall, G. R., Kelly, A., Richards, B., & Sime, M. (1999). A nursing intervention to decrease depression in family caregivers of persons with dementia. *Archives of Psychiatric Nursing,* 13(2), 80-88.

Bullock, K., Crawford, S., & Tennstedt, S. L. (2003). Employment and caregiving: Exploration of African American caregivers. *Social Work,* 48, 150-162.

Burgio, L., Stevens, A., Guy, D., Roth, D. L., & Haley, W. E. (2003). Impact of two psychosocial interventions on white and African American family caregivers of individuals with dementia. *The Gerontologist,* 43(4), 568-579.

Burns, R., Nichols, L. O., Martindale-Adams, J., Graney, M. J., & Lummus, A. (2003). Primary care interventions for dementia caregivers: 2-year outcomes from the REACH study. *The Gerontologist,* 43(4), 547-555.

Butler, H. K., Holkup, P. A., & Buckwalter, K. C. (2001). The experience of caring for a family member with Alzheimer's disease. *Western Journal of Nursing Research,* 23, 33-55.

Campbell, L., Eisenburg, M., Elliott, T., Frank, R., Gardner, D., Garner, H., McClane, W., Patterson, D., Rothberg, J., & Saltz, C. (1992). *Guide to interdisciplinary practice in rehabilitation settings.* Glenview, IL: American Congress of Rehabilitation Medicine.

Cohen, C. A., Gold, D. P., Shulman, K. I., & Zucchero, C. A. (1994). Positive aspects in caregiving: An overlooked variable in research. *Canadian Journal on Aging,* 13, 378-391.

Dillworth-Anderson, P., Williams, I. C., & Gibson, B. E. (2002). Issues of race, ethnicity, and culture in caregiving research: A 20 year review (1980-2000). *The Gerontologist,* 42, 237-272.

Eisdorfer, C., Czaja, S. J., Loewenstein, D. A., Rubert, M. P., Arguelles, S., Mitrani, V. B., & Szapocznik, J. (2003). The effect of a family therapy and technology-based intervention on caregiver depression. *The Gerontologist,* 43(4), 521-531.

Farran, C. J. (1997). Positive aspects of caring for elderly persons with dementia: A theoretical examination. *The Gerontologist,* 37, 250-256.

Forster, A., Smith, J., Young, J., Knapp, P., House, A., & Wright, J. (2003). Information provision for stroke patients and their caregivers. *The Cochrane Library,* Issue 3, 2003. Oxford: Update Software.

Fredriksen-Goldsen, K., & Farwell, N. (2004). Dual responsibilities among black, Hispanic, Asian, and white employed caregivers. *Journal of Gerontological Social Work,* 43, 25-44.

Gallant, M. P. & Connell, C. M. (1998). The stress process among dementia spouse caregivers: Are caregivers at risk for negative health behavior change? *Research on Aging,* 20(3), 267-297.

Gerdner, L. A., Buckwalter, K. C., & Reed, D. (2002). Impact of a psychoeducational intervention on caregiver response to behavioral problems. *Nursing Research,* 51(6), 363-374.

Gitlin, L. N., Winter, L., Corcoran, M., Dennis, M. P., Schinfeld, S., & Hauck, W. W. (2003). Effects of the home environmental skill-building program on the caregiver-care recipient dyad: 6-month outcomes from the Philadelphia REACH initiative. *The Gerontologist,* 43(4), 532-546.

Greene, V. L. & Monahan, D. J. (1989). The effect of a support and education program on stress and burden among family caregivers to frail elderly persons. *The Gerontologist,* 29 (4), 472-477.

Greene, V. L. & Monahan, D. J. (1987). The effect of a professionally guided caregiver support and education group on institutionalization of care receivers. *The Gerontologist,* 27 (6), 716-721.

Kaasalainen, S., Craig, D., & Wells, D. (2000). Impact of the caring for aging relatives group program: An evaluation. *Public Health Nursing,* 17(3), 169-177.

Mahoney, D. F., Tarlow, B. J., & Jones, R. N. (2003). Effects of an automated telephone support system on caregiver burden and anxiety: Findings from the REACH for TLC intervention study. *The Gerontologist,* 43(4), 556-567.

MetLife (1999). The MetLife Juggling Act Study: Balancing caregiving with work and the costs involved. Westport, CT: Metropolitan Life Insurance Company.

MetLife (1997). The MetLife Study of Employer Costs for Working Caregivers. Westport, CT: Metropolitan Life Insurance Company.

Mittleman, M. S., Ferris, S. H., Steinberg, G., Shulman, E., Mackell, J. A., Ambinder, A., & Cohen, J. (1993). An intervention that delays institutionalization of Alzheimer's disease patients: Treatment of spouse-caregivers. *The Gerontologist,* 33(6), 730-740.

National Alliance for Caregiving and AARP (2004). Caregiving in the U.S. Retrieved February 25, 2005 from http://research.aarp.org/il/us_caregiving.pdf

National Alliance for Caregiving and AARP (1997). Family caregiving in the U.S.: Findings from a national study. National Alliance for Caregiving, Bethesda, MD.

National Family Caregiver Association (2000). NFCA Caregiver survey. Retrieved May 31, 2005 from http://www.thefamilycaregiver.org/who/2000_survey.cfm

Roff, L. L., Burgio, L. D., Gitlen, L., Nicols, L., Chaplin, W., & Hardin, M. (2004). Positive aspects of Alzheimer's caregiving: The role of race. *Journal of Gerontology, Psychological Sciences,* 59B, 185-190.

Sherwood, P. R., Given, C. W., Given, B. A., & Von Eye, A. (2005). Caregiver burden and depressive symptoms: Analysis of common outcomes in caregivers of elderly patients. *Journal of Aging and Health,* 17, 125-147.

Sorensen, S., Pinquart, M., & Duberstein, P. (2002). How effective are interventions with caregivers? An updated meta-analysis. *The Gerontologist,* 42 (3), 356-375.

Toseland, R. W., Rossiter, C. M., & Labrecque, M. S. (1989). The effectiveness of peer led and professionally led groups to support family caregivers. *The Gerontologist,* 29(4), 465-471.

Toseland, R. W., Rossiter, C. M., Peak, T., & Smith, G. C. (1990). Comparative effectiveness of individual and group interventions to support family caregivers. *Social Work,* 35, 209-217.

U.S. Bureau of the Census Statistical Brief (1995). Sixty-Five Plus in the United States. Retrieved May 31, 2005 from http://www.census.gov/apsd/www/statbrief/sb95_8.pdf

Chapter 13

Grandparent Caregivers

Stacey Kolomer

Caregiving is a natural occurrence within families. At some point in a person's life, one can expect to provide care to a loved one or to receive care from a family member. Unexpected caregiving relationships may occur within families as well. In some families, grandparents (and even great-grandparents) become primary caregivers to their grandchildren. Many of these care providers are older and feel somewhat unprepared to raise a new generation of children. The following chapter will summarize characteristics of grandparent caregivers in our society, the challenges that they face, and how organizations are attempting to help with their care provision responsibilities. Recommendations for future research and intervention design will also be discussed.

DEMOGRAPHICS AND PREVALENCE

In the United States, it is estimated that one in 10 grandparents will be the primary caregiver for at least six months for a grandchild(ren) before the child(ren)'s 18th birthday (Burnette, 1999; Silverstein & Vehvilainen, 1998). Five percent of all children are living in grandparent-headed households which represents approximately five to six million children (Generations United, 2003). Casper and Bryson (1998) found that in 40% of grandparent-headed households, the child(ren)'s parent was not living in the home.

Although grandparent caregiving is not a new phenomenon in the United States, there has been a dramatic increase in grandparent-headed households in the last two decades (Burnette, 1997; Emick & Hayslip, 1999; Minkler, 1994; Mullen, 1996). The factors that account for this increase vary and include parental addiction, abuse and neglect, incarceration, decrease in foster home availability, teenage mother/fatherhood, divorce, illness, death, military deployment, unemployment, and homelessness (Burton, 1992; Dressel & Barnhill, 1994; Emick & Hayslip, 1999; Fuller-Thomson, Minkler, & Driver, 1997; Jendrek, 1994; Kelley, Yorker, & Whitley, 1997; Minkler, 1994; Minkler & Roe, 1993; Silverstein & Vehvilainen, 1997; Smith & Beltran, 2000). For the purposes of this chapter *grandparent caregiver* will be defined as an individual who has assumed primary care for a child, is at least one generation removed from the child's own parent, and perceives her/ himself in a grandparenting relationship with the child (Janicki, McCallion, Grant-Griffen, & Kolomer, 2000).

Similar to other late life caregiving roles, most grandparent caregivers are grandmothers (Burnette, 1997; Dressel & Barnhill, 1994). In the 2004 U.S. Census, 62% of all grandparents who were responsible for children under age 18 were female (U.S. Census, 2004). This percentage is consistent with several studies of grandparent caregivers. In a profile of 173 grandparents, Fuller-Thomson and colleagues (1997) found that 77% of the participants were grandmothers. In Hayslip and colleagues' (1998) study of 193 grandparents, 80% of the custodial grandparents were women. A telephone survey of 134 grandparent caregivers conducted by the University of Massachusetts-Boston found 86% of the caregivers to be women (Silverstein & Vehvilainen, 1997). Clearly, women are the predominant care providers for their grandchildren.

Though data are limited, available studies indicate that grandparent caregivers are also more likely to be married (Burnette, 1997; Fuller-Thomson et al., 1997; Hayslip et al., 1998; Silverstein & Vehvilainen, 1997). Based on Census (2004) data, 71% of all grandparent households report being headed by a married couple. However, insufficient data exists to determine if this is true across all racial/ethnic groups.

While the grandparent role may be assumed by individuals across a substantial age range, most grandparent caregivers are in late mid-life. In a review of studies of grandparent caregivers, Kelley and colleagues (1997) found that the mean age of caregivers ranged from 52 to 57 years. Burnette (1997) noted that the age range of grandparent caregivers in the studies she reviewed was from 45 to 64 years of age. A significant percentage of grandmothers are reported to be older than age 60, however (Dubowitz, Feigelman, & Zuravin, 1993; Minkler, Roe, & Price, 1992). In 1996, the U.S. Bureau of the Census estimated that 19% of grandparent caregivers were over age 65 and 48% were between ages 50 and 64 years (Generations United, 1999). In their study of 101 grandmothers raising grandchildren, Burton and De Vries (1992) found grandmother caregivers as young as 29 years old, and great-grandmother caregivers as young as 56 years old. The 2000 Census reported that 2.3 million co-resident grandparents were aged 60 or over as compared to 3.5 million who were younger than 60 (U.S. Department of Commerce, 2003).

Grandparent care providers are represented in all racial and ethnic categories. The breakdown of grandparent-headed households by ethnicity/race is reported to be: 43.6%, Caucasian; 35.9%, Black; and 18%, Hispanic/Latino (Generations United, 1999). As reported by Minkler and colleagues (1992), these data indicate that a disproportionate number of the families are African American in comparison to their overall population in the United States. Jendrek (1994) also reported that African American and Latino/Hispanic grandparents are more likely to be the primary caretakers of a grandchild than are Caucasian grandparents. However, assumptions should be avoided about these households. A higher incidence of grandparent caregiving in African American households does not mean that grandparent caregiving is a common experience for African Americans (Minkler, 1999).

Grandparent caregiving disproportionately affects lower-income households (Minkler, 1999). The 2004 U.S. Census estimated that 19.5% of all grandparent-headed households were living in poverty (U.S. Census, 2004). Whether providing formal or informal care, grandmother caregivers most frequently live in inner cities, have less than a high school education, and are poor (Minkler et al., 1992; Woodworth, 1996). An estimated 59% of grandparent caregivers are currently in the labor force (U.S. Census, 2004).

NATURE OF PROBLEM

There are several different legal issues which impact grandparent-headed households. Children who are removed from their parents' home and taken into the legal custody of the state either because of parental abuse or neglect can be placed in the physical custody of a grandparent caregiver. The family member in whose care the child is placed must meet licensing requirements to be approved as an appropriate formal kinship foster care placement (Child Welfare League of America, 1994). Yet the formal caregiver in this situation has limited rights, and the state is considered the legal guardian of the child. In an informal caregiving situation, the decision that the child will live with a grandparent or another family member is made within the family system and the state is neither involved nor aware of the change in the child's primary caregiver (Child Welfare League of America, 1994). While challenges are different depending on the type of caregiving role, both formal and informal grandparent caregivers confront significant legal challenges in raising grandchildren.

As the availability of traditional foster care households has dwindled due to the increases of women in the work force, grandparents and other relatives have assumed roles of kinship care providers. The passage of the Adoption Assistance and Child Welfare Act of 1980 and later the Adoption and Safe Families Act of 1997 both pushed the agenda that children who are removed from their parents' care should be placed with family, if possible. This legislation made kin caregivers eligible for foster care stipends in some states (Burnette, 1997; Genty, 1998). By 1993, one-half of the children removed by states from their parents' custody were reported to be formally placed by foster care agencies with their grandmother (Dubowitz et al., 1993). These households typically receive much less financial support than traditional foster care homes (Hegar & Scannapieco, 1998; Smith & Beltran, 2000). Children in kinship foster homes are twice as likely to be living in poverty than children in non-kinship foster homes (Macomber, Genn, & Main, 2003). Families who have gained temporary guardianship of grand-child(ren) may experience insecurities for both generations due to the vagueness of the relationship (Waldrop & Weber, 2001).

Those families who do not have a formal caregiving relationship have a variety of problems in accessing education and medical services for the grandchildren in their care (Smith & Beltran, 2000). With the ex-ception of vaccinations, proper consents are needed for the children to receive medical treatment and often informal caregivers do not have these consents in place. Enrollment in school may also be challenging as school districts each have unique policies about what documentation is needed to register. In response to this problem, individual states have been developing policies to assist grandparent families with custody programs such as subsidized guardianship and education and medical consent laws (Smith & Beltran, 2000).

Becoming a caregiver has been reported to cause changes in employ-ment and retirement statuses (Phillips & Bloom, 1998). Those who were not working prior to becoming a grandparent caregiver also report finan-cial stressors. Limited income needs to be stretched further, and there is a fear of being stigmatized if public assistance is needed (Minkler, 1999). Previously, grandmothers who were not working frequently relied on AFDC, which provided support for an eligible child. The introduction of the Personal Responsibility and Work Opportunity Reconciliation Act of 1996 (P.L. 104-193) created additional stress for these grandparent-headed families. Some of the issues with which they are contending in-clude the fear of having to return to work following retirement, the bur-den of providing proof of citizenship, and the requirement of providing personal information about the grandchild's parent (Mandelbaum, 1995; Mullen, 1996; Robinson-Dooley & Kropf, in press).

Housing is another challenging issue for grandparent caregivers. Fuller-Thomson and Minkler (2003) reported that one quarter of the 2,350,000 grandparent caregivers in the United States were renting their homes. In addition, approximately one-third of renters were paying more than 30% of their earnings on housing. Fourteen percent of grand-parent-headed housholds families lived in public housing and three out of 10 of the grandparent-headed households were living in overcrowded conditions.

Grandparent-headed households also experience difficulties when grandparents are living in housing specifically designed for older adults, as senior housing occupants are required to be over age 55. Grandparents living in senior housing must forfeit their apartment, negotiate with the housing managers, or conceal their grandchildren. Public housing causes similar problems for these families. Tenants living in public housing are required to change the lease to reflect the actual composition of the household. Frequently, grandparent families are reluctant to take this course of action as a large household size creates risk for an eviction (Flint & Perez-Porter, 1997).

An additional housing problem may be that a grandparent's home is too small to accommodate additional tenants (Generations United, 1999). Grandparents who had scaled down their living arrangements now are cramped with added family members. For many grandparent families, however, moving is not an option due to limited finances and poor health (Generations United, 1999). Grandparents may also not want to move from their residence for other reasons such as proximity to their support network, attachment to their home, or familiarity with the neighborhood.

When a grandparent is part of the foster care system, there is pressure to move to housing that has ample space. The foster care system also has strict safety requirements. If a grandparent's home is found to be out of compliance with the regulations the grandparent is at risk for either losing funding or having the grandchild removed from the home. Frequently, the foster care agency involved with the family does not assist the grandparent with moving or in making adaptations to the home, adding to the stressfulness of these concerns (Kolomer, 2000).

CONSEQUENCES OF CAREGIVING FOR GRANDPARENTS

Grandparent caregivers are at risk for multiple physical, mental, and emotional problems due to the stresses and strains of care provision. In Minkler and Roe's (1993) study of grandmothers, 37% reported that their health had deteriorated since becoming a caregiver. Several factors place this population of caregivers at risk for health problems including, but not limited to, the stress of the new caretaking role, aging, lack of insurance, and socioeconomic status (Kelley et al., 1997). Common physical health problems reported by grandparent caregivers include arthritis, hypertension, insomnia, pain, stiffness, headaches, and hearing problems (Emick & Hayslip, 1999; Kelley et al., 1997; Silverstein & Vehvilainen, 1998).

Many grandparents report that they are concerned about their health, but lack time to take care of themselves (Emick & Hayslip, 1999). A possible explanation is that grandmothers tend to deny their health problems for fear that their grandchildren may be taken away (Minkler & Roe, 1996). Frequently, grandparent caregivers will ignore their symptoms or diminish the severity of illnesses. Grandparent caregivers may feel the need to cover up health problems for fear that their ability to care for grandchildren will be questioned.

As a way to cope, some grandparents report increased drinking and smoking since becoming caregivers to their grandchildren (Burton, 1992; Emick & Hayslip, 1999; Minkler et al., 1992). These addictions may further contribute to a compromised health status. In their study of 52 grandparent caregivers, Kolomer and colleagues found that 17 of the grandparents were misusing and/or under-using pain medication (Kolomer, McCallion, Dugan, & Robinson, in preparation). Abuse of prescription medication can have serious consequences for these caregivers.

Acquiring a new role in life can be both a welcomed, and a dreaded, event. When asked to raise their grandchildren, grandparents are often caught off guard by the change in the meaning of grandparenthood. For both the grandparent and grandchild, there is role confusion about who they are to one another (Emick & Hayslip, 1999; Kropf & Robinson, 2004). This is true even for grandparents who have raised their grandchildren since infancy.

Many grandparent caregivers have feelings of loss or shame for their own children. Whether living or deceased, the son or daughter has often become "lost" to the parent, and the grandparent mourns for the relationship. The grieving process may never be acknowledged because caregiving for the grandchildren takes priority over experiencing their loss (Woodworth, 1996). Grandparents may also experience feelings of anger, shame, and hurt because of their children's irresponsibility and inability to care for their own children (Roe et al., 1996). They may feel embarrassed due to their own children's alcohol and substance abuse problems (Minkler & Roe, 1996). There may be shame about how they became the primary caregivers of their grandchildren if substance abuse, HIV or incarceration were involved (Roe, Minkler, Saunders, & Thomson, 1996; Phillips & Bloom, 1998; Poindexter & Linsk, 1999). In addition, some are fearful of their children because of violent behaviors brought on by substance abuse (Roe et al., 1996).

Another psychosocial struggle of grandparents is a feeling of divided loyalty between their own children and the grandchildren in their care. Although they are responsible for the well-being of their grandchildren, they may continue to feel an allegiance to their children. While the child welfare system might define the best interest of the child as severing ties with an addicted or violent parent, grandparents may also be concerned about the impact of this action on any remaining hope for improvement in the child's parent.

Many grandparents experience exhaustion from caregiving, especially if they have not had child-rearing responsibilities for numerous years. New children in the house may disrupt the family's routine and new ways of relating to one another may have to be developed. Partners who are unrelated to the child may feel resentment toward the addition to the household and choose to withdraw from the relationship. Other grandparent care providers are also caring for other family members (e.g., their older parent or a disabled spouse) in addition to their grandchildren (Burton, 1992). Other family members usually offer limited support to the care provider which contributes to the fears grandparent caregivers have about who will care for their grandchildren if something were to happen to them (Roe et al., 1996). Additional stressors experienced by grandparent care providers are dangers in their neighborhoods, a lack of understanding about "this generation" of children, problems with the school system their grandchildren attend, and the impact of public policies and provisions for caregivers (Burton, 1992).

Depression and anxiety are concerns when working with grandparent caregivers. Grandmothers report feeling cheated, a loss of freedom, and increased social isolation (Kelley et al., 1997; Roe et al., 1994). Increased symptoms of anxiety have been found (Sands & Goldberg-Glen, 1998), but the most common concern is heightened symptoms of depression (Burnette, 2000; Janicki et al., 2000). In a study by Minkler and colleagues (1997), 25.1% of the caregiving grandparents were experiencing depression as compared to 14.5% for the non-caregiving grandparents. In Janicki and colleagues' (2000) sample of inner city African American grandparents caring for at least one child with a developmental disability, more than 50% reported experiencing symptoms of depression. High rates of depressive symptoms in Latino grandparents caring for child(ren) with disabilities have also been reported (Burnette, 2000; Kolomer, McCallion, & Janicki, 2002). Many grandparents lack support to provide temporary respite from their care responsibilities (Minkler & Roe, 1996)

EMPIRICAL LITERATURE

Within the literature on grandparent caregivers, several interventions and programs have been reported. Yet, unfortunately, very few interventions include evaluative data. This gap may be due to lack of staff support, unwillingness from the grandparents to participate in evaluation processes, or limited agency time and finances. Databases that were used to locate interventions included Ageline, Social Work Abstracts and PsychInfo, and articles were included from 1995 through 2005. Key search terms were *grandparent caregivers, grandparents as parents,* and *skipped generation households.* The interventions sought were ones that were designed to improve grandparents' health, mental health or quality of life. Table 1 outlines nine intervention studies for grandparent caregivers and their families.

Case Management Approaches

An intervention methodology that has been employed with grandparents who are raising grandchildren is case management. Using an exploratory study design, Kelley and colleagues (1997, 2001) developed a strength-based case management intervention titled Project Healthy Grandparents™ (PHG). The intervention was designed to reduce psychological stress, improve mental and physical health, strengthen support systems and increase resources. The six-month intervention included home visits by registered nurses, social workers, and legal assistants. Social workers and nurses administered psychosocial assessments and gathered information regarding health status. Social workers visited monthly and maintained regular telephone contact. Along with the grandparent, the social worker identified problems and designed an action plan to resolve the identified problems. Nurses monitored the health status of all family members on a monthly basis and made appropriate referrals when needed. Third-year law students, who were under the supervision of an attorney, screened and provided legal assistance in custody issues. Grandparents also participated in monthly support group meetings.

The participants of PHG were recruited from health-care and community sites. Grandparents were eligible if they had full-time responsibility for at least one grandchild and resided in one of two Atlanta counties. If there were multiple grandparents in the household, the

TABLE 1. Interventions with Grandparent Caregivers

RESEARCHERS	SAMPLE	INTERVENTION	OUTCOMES
Kelley, Yorker, Whitley, & Sipe, 2001	24 grandparent caregiving families	Home-based case management intervention	Improved hostility, interpersonal sensitivity, mental health
Robinson, Kropf, & Myers, 2000	25 rural grandparent families	Case management and support groups	Improved mental health & increased resources
McCallion, Janicki, Grant-Griffin, & Kolomer, 2000	103 grandparents and great grandparents caring for children with developmental disabilities	Case management and support groups	Improved depression, mastery, & empowerment
Cohon, Hines, Cooper, Packman, & Siggins, 2003	424 African American families	Case management services	Program satisfaction
Burnette, 1998	11 grandparent caregivers	School-based small group intervention	Decreased depression and improved coping
Grant, Gordon, & Cohen, 1997	23 grandparent-headed households	Comprehensive school-based medical and social service care program	Increase in accessing support services
Smith & Dannison, 2002	33 grandparent caregivers 41 preschool grandchildren 71 education professionals	School-based intervention	Reduced loneliness and isolation
Cox, 2002	15 African American grandmothers	Group intervention for empowerment training	Satisfaction with program; increased leadership behaviors
Strozier, Elrod, Beiler, Smith & Carter, 2004	46 Kinship caregivers	8 week computer training course	Increased technology skills and social support

grandparent who provided most of the care was considered the participant. Twenty-five grandparents initially approached agreed to participate in the evaluation of the intervention. Data that includes pre- and
post-test scores at six months were reported on the initial 25 participants. The final sample consisted of 24 grandparents after six months of
receiving the intervention. The mean age of the grandparents who
participated was 55.7 years old (s.d. 10.46, range 39-78).

Data collected included the Brief Symptom Inventory, Family Resource Scale, Grandparent Interview form, Short form-36 and the General health survey (SF 36). Information about legal relationships was also
collected. All measures were found to have strong internal and external
validity. Caregivers were found to have improved scores on hostility and
interpersonal sensitivity following the sixth month intervention. There
was also improvement in mental health, perception of social support,
enhanced resources and services, and increases in the establishment of
legal relationships with the grandchildren in their care.

PHG was replicated in a three-county rural area with 25 families
(Robinson, Kropf, & Myers, 2000). Although 25% of grandparents
raising grandchildren reside in non-urban areas (Casper & Bryson,
1998), this program was an initial one to provide service to rural grandparents. The goals for this intervention were to mobilize a family's
strengths, marshal resources, and maximize family functional capacity
(Myers, Kropf, & Robinson, 2002). As in the original PHG model, social work students, nursing students and lawyers provided the services
to families. In addition to monthly support groups for grandparent caregivers, the grandchildren were provided with their own support groups
as well as tutoring, recreation, and mentoring.

Grandparents were recruited via the media, schools, social service
agencies, and churches. The grandparent was determined eligible if he
or she had the primary responsibility for at least one grandchild and no
parent was living in the home. Data was completed on 22 grandparents
with the average age of the participants being 58.9 years old (s.d. 7.4,
range 46-71). All grandparents completed questionnaires before participating and following one year of being in the program. The following
measures were used: Brief Symptom Inventory, Parental Locus of Control, Child Neglect Inventory, Self-Esteem Index, Family Resource
Scale, Family Social Support Scale, Family Empowerment Scale,
Child's Attitude toward mother/father/grandmother/ grandfather, Short
Form-36 Health Survey, and Child Behavior Checklist. The pre- and
post-test scores (at entry to the program and one year later) showed a

significant increase in family support and family resources, and significant decreases in somatization, interpersonal sensitivity, and paranoia.

A somewhat different case management intervention using a quasi-experimental design was developed by McCallion and colleagues (2000) specifically for grandparents caring for a grandchild with a developmental disability. Three community agencies were provided with funding for one year to provide case management and support group services to grandparent-headed households that were caring for at least one grandchild with a developmental disability. Each agency appointed a staff person to provide intensive case management and counseling. The case managers provided the families with benefits counseling, education assistance, advocacy, housing, respite, summer camp, and assessment and treatment for both the grandchildren and grandparents. Services were provided in the home and within the agency. Grandparent caregivers also participated in a six to eight week education/support group which covered topics such as how to get services, caring for a child with a developmental disability, planning for the future, and custody and guardianship. In addition to the specialized topics, grandparents were provided with relaxation and stress-reducing activities at the end of every support group meeting.

Each agency was required to recruit at least 30 participants with one agency providing services to a total of 43. Schools, churches, current clients, newspapers and the radio were all utilized to sign up grandparent caregivers. At least one child in care had to have some type of disability. The criteria for a disability were loosely defined, however, since a significant part of the intervention was getting the child in care a correct diagnosis. A total of 103 grandparent caregivers were recruited for this intervention. The mean age of the grandparents was 60 years (s.d. 8.94).

Using a quasi-experimental design, every grandparent was provided with case management services following the initial assessment; however, only 10 grandparents could participate in each support group meeting during the six to eight week period, thus constituting a treatment and control group. By the end of the year all grandparents had participated in the support group intervention. Pre- and post-tests indicated that both the treatment and control groups had decreased depression scores after participating in the intervention, although statistical significance was only reached for the control group. In addition, the control group had increased scores on mastery. These findings might indicate that the later participation in the support group within the overall program protocol may have been a more effective strategy.

Cohon and colleagues (2003) provided case management services to kinship caregivers in the foster care system, the majority of whom were skipped generation households. The researchers described the evaluation as a descriptive evaluative study. The case management services were focused on filling the gaps and reducing barriers to public services. A community worker was assigned to each family and constructed an assessment and case plan. In addition, the worker provided monthly home visits, weekly phone calls, linkage to support groups, recreation, respite, trainings, tutoring, mentoring, and transportation services. The sample consisted of kinship caregivers and relatives who received the case management services over a period of almost six years. All those referred to the program were enrolled and the researchers reported that a very small number declined to participate. Of the 424 families who received services, 266 were headed by grandparents and 25 were great-grandparent caregivers. The mean age of the grandparents was 55 years old, and 69 years old for great-grandparents.

The data collected on the families included a family assessment of needs, caregiver's physical and mental health, caregiver's satisfaction with social support network, and client satisfaction. The initial intake found that grandparents and great grandparents had significantly worse health than other types of caregivers. A total 122 participants graduated from the program. Comparing the T1 (intake) and T2 (graduation) measures, kin caregivers' resource needs (e.g., connection to available services) diminished following participation in the program. Overall, participants reported satisfaction and increased social support and competence in caregiving abilities.

Group Interventions

While case management has been used in a variety of contexts for grandparents, group interventions are more frequently employed with this population of care providers. In an early evaluation of a grandparent group, Burnette (1998) conducted a small exploratory intervention with 11 grandparent caregivers in a public elementary school. The intervention consisted of eight weekly 90-minute education/support group meetings. Each week consisted of a specialized topic followed by support and problem-solving techniques. The educational component focused on social supports, behavioral coping, managing interpersonal conflict, parenting skills, legal options, and community-based initiatives. The participants were recruited in a school-based mental health program using posters, school staff, and word of mouth. A pre-test was administered before the start of the first session and a post-test following the final session. The scales included the general health questionnaire, ways of coping scale, social support behaviors, short version of the social desirability scale, and knowledge of formal services. Prior to the start of the group, these grandparent caregivers were found to have high overall well-being. Following participation in the group, there was a slight improvement in participants' depression and coping scores.

Grant and colleagues (1997) also designed a weekly education/support group for grandparent caregivers within four public schools. Grandparent caregivers (N = 23) participated in weekly health education/support groups. The sessions focused on information, skill development, and self-advocacy training. The participants completed pre-tests about health-care usage, health status, and insurance. Prior to participation, many grandparents indicated that they did not use health-care resources due to problems with access and poor quality services. Grandparents reported that their phone calls were not returned, follow-up appointments were delayed and the doctors did not adequately explain health issues. At six months post-intervention, most caregivers had reengaged with health resources. In addition, emergency room visits for this group also decreased following their participation in the intervention.

Dannison and Smith (2003) developed a unique multidimensional intervention to address the needs of grandparent caregivers, their grandchildren, and educators. The program was designed for the grandparents to improve their social and emotional functioning. Participants were recruited through the school system. A total of 33 grandparent caregivers, and 41 grandchildren participated. There were eight support group meetings for grandparents and eight support group meetings for grandchildren. Pre- and post-tests were administered. At post-intervention, grandparents reported decreased loneliness, and increased social support.

Educators were also involved in the intervention, and participated in service professional trainings (Smith & Dannison, 2002). A total of eight hours of training focused on teaching the educators to recognize the strengths of the grandparent-headed household, increase their awareness of legal issues, and enhance knowledge of available resources and services. In addition, the training also planned ways to modify curriculum and adapt classroom techniques to better serve grandparent-headed families. After the in-service, participants had increased knowledge about the needs of grandparent care providers and greater knowledge of ways to modify the curriculum to provide grandparent caregivers with needed information, positive feedback, and referrals to existing services.

Cox (2002) developed an empowerment training specifically for grandparent caregivers. The training consisted of 12 group sessions with topics that included an introduction to empowerment; building self-esteem; communicating with grandchildren; dealing with loss, grief, and behavior problems; legal and entitlement issues; talking to grandchildren about sex, drugs and HIV/AIDS; developing advocacy skills and negotiating systems. The group sessions used a variety of methodologies including didactic content, hand-outs, homework assignments, and role plays. Participants were selected from an ongoing support group for grandparent caregivers in Harlem that had been initially established in 1994.

For this intervention, 15 African American grandparent caregivers participated (mean age = 64 years) and were selected based upon their commitment to attend classes, length of time in the support group, and interest in the project. Fourteen grandparents completed the session, as one grandmother had to stop due to health problems. The grandparents met twice a week and transportation was provided. Following every training session, the caregivers completed a brief evaluation of the training to assess what they had learned, what was helpful and what was not helpful. In evaluating the ratings of each session, the grandparents scored several sessions very highly. The content on self-esteem, grief and loss, and communicating with children received the highest ratings. An additional outcome of this intervention was the expectation that grandparents would share their new knowledge with other grandparents within the community. Specifically, grandparents who finished the group gave presentations to other grandparents in the community on content that had been covered within the group sessions. This behavioral outcome demonstrated increased empowerment and self-efficacy.

Strozier and colleagues (2004) employed a different type of group experience for caregivers to enhance computer skill development. Caregivers were drawn from area kinship support groups (N = 46) to participate in a computer-based intervention to promote technology-based skill attainment and support for care providers. The intervention consisted of an eight-week computer training course provided in a group format. The caregivers completed pre- and post-tests measuring the caregivers' computer efficacy, using the Caregiver Computer Efficacy

Scale (CCES) which was designed by the researchers. The CCES measured level of computer skills to improve employability, increase social supports, and increase access to information via the internet and world wide web. At post intervention, one-half of the participants had significant increases in all areas of the CCES. In addition, commentary from all caregivers indicated that their ease in using technology and pride in their advanced skills in this area was markedly more positive after completing the intervention.

TREATMENT SUMMARY

Based upon the available outcome literature, the most common intervention with grandparent caregivers is delivered in a group format. While it is difficult to accurately estimate the number of support groups for grandparent caregivers currently available, in 2003 AARP estimated that over 800 registered support groups existed nationally (Davies & Williams, 2003). This estimate is probably low, however, as many groups that are in existence may not register with AARP. Even using a higher number, it is questionable whether support and educational groups are available in all communities to serve as a resource for grandparents who are care providers to their grandchildren.

Group formats offer many resources to grandparents. The educational component provides grandparent caregivers with information about medical, legal, educational, and financial issues. Group formats provide a way to sort through this complex and confusing content with others in care provision roles. Participants in support groups also report that they are less isolated and lonely, which are two of the biggest challenges for these families. Grandparent caregivers have the opportunity to meet other caregivers who share their experiences at these meetings.

The second intervention that appears to be promising for grandparent-headed households is the interdisciplinary case management model. Although this model takes significant human and financial support, it also provides a holistic approach to meeting the biopsychosocial needs of a family. In conjunction with a support group intervention, grandparent families who received services from an interdisciplinary case management team showed improvement in their physical, mental, and emotional health. By including social workers, nurses, educators, and legal professionals in case management services, the critical needs of these families can be addressed. The outcome of McCallion and colleagues' (2000) intervention would indicate that including support groups with the case management component is essential for a successful program.

CONCLUSION

Despite the number of support groups and pilot programs available for grandparent caregivers, very few have been systematically evaluated. The interventions presented in this chapter include a small number of innovative programs designed for grandparents raising their grandchildren. The level of research design used in these studies, however, is a limitation. The majority of studies were pre-experimental, and all used small convenience samples. The addition of control or comparison groups would increase the rigor, and add to the knowledge about the efficacy of the various interventions. Also, the studies cited above measure a variety of outcomes. Unfortunately, there is a lack of consistency in measured outcomes and a lack of standardized measurement. For all of these reasons, it seems external validity is greatly compromised.

More research is needed to better understand what elements are necessary for a successful intervention with this population. There are significant gaps in the literature as many articles outline what components would be helpful to include in designing interventions for this population, but few report the results of actual intervention studies. In addition, the cross-sectional nature of the research is problematic as this research design does not provide information concerning whether the intervention approaches promote lasting change for the grandparents.

There are some indicators of factors that increase support group participation for all caregivers. For support groups to be successful there are three components which are necessary. The first is child care. Support groups need to occur when children are in school or daycare, or the agency must provide child care on site for grandparents to participate. Another important component is transportation/location of the meeting. For caregivers to participate they need to be able to get to the meeting. Therefore, the meeting either has to be held at an easy-to-access location or transportation for the caregivers should be provided. Support groups that provide transportation are more likely to be successful. The last component that is essential to the success of a support group is flexibility. Meeting at times that suit the needs of the caregivers rather than the agency is necessary for participation and building the credibility of the organization (Kolomer, McCallion, & Overendyer, 2003)

At this point, most interventions focus on the grandparent or the family unit. Evidence-based treatment for the grandchildren within these families would also be a useful addition to the literature. Programs for children in the care of their grandparents need to be constructed and evaluated. Child-focused support groups or recreational programs that bring together children in grandparent care are a method to create relationships among these children. In addition, school-based curricula can include examples of diverse family forms to create a sense of normalcy for children who are part of non-traditional family structures. An excellent example is the film "That's a Family" (Chasnoff & Cohen, 2000) in which children discuss growing up in grandparent-headed families, same-sex households, blended, interracial, and single parent families. This type of curriculum-based intervention would also benefit from evaluation to see if education about diverse family systems creates a greater tolerance and acceptance for children who are raised within grandparent households by classmates and peers.

In conclusion, the number of grandparent caregivers has increased due to some of the social conditions that are being experienced within society. Factors associated with an increase in this family structure include the rising rate of drugs (e.g., crack cocaine and methamphetamines), a growth in the incarceration rates of women with children, the ongoing HIV/AIDS epidemic, and related social challenges. Since the majority of grandparents who are in care provision roles are in mid- to later-life, these caregivers are experiencing the concomitant challenges of performing child-rearing tasks and coping with their own health, economic and social changes. As a result, grandparents are often involved with diverse formal services systems including health care, school systems, child welfare agencies, and even aging services. Additional evidence-based research is warranted to gain additional knowledge about how to effectively intervene within and across these multiple contexts where social workers and other practitioners work with grandparents who are in caregiving roles.

TREATMENT RESOURCE APPENDIX

AARP Grandparent Information Center
www.aarp.org

This information, located under the menu "Grandparenting," offers help for grandparents who are raising grandchildren. Information contained on the site includes ways to find local support groups, information about legal, financial, education, health, and other sources of support.

The Brookdale Center on Aging
www.brookdale.org/fh2h/index.html

From Hardship to Hope Project. This unique curriculum is for support groups or special one-time groups who want to focus particularly on the feelings and struggles of the grandparent caregiver. While the sessions certainly presuppose that children bring their own needs to the family situation, this curriculum encourages caregivers to allow themselves to concentrate on their own needs–a challenging task for many caregivers. It is not a parenting course, nor is it a course about resources, advocacy, and the child welfare system. The six modules are:

* MODULE 1–Living in Two Worlds: Bridging the Gap
* MODULE 2–It's Getting to Me: Dealing with Stress and Anger
* MODULE 3–I'm Too Depressed to Think: When the Sadness Never Leaves
* MODULE 4–How Did This Happen: Am I at Fault?
* MODULE 5–I'm Too Old for This: Aging and Health Issues
* MODULE 6–Living the Good Life: Simple Strategies for a Long and Healthy Life

Tools for Working with Grandparent Caregivers
http://www.hunter.cuny.edu/socwork/nrcfcpp/downloads/Tools-for-working-with-kinship-caregivers.pdf

Provides information about where to get toolkits and curriculum to help grandparent caregivers. Provides a number of links to various resources that are available at different sites. The following information is included:

Training Materials:

* *Tradition of Caring Curriculum*: Six-session curriculum that provides kinship care providers with resources and materials. During the course of this experience, care providers develop an individualized action plan to meet family and resource needs. *http://www.cwla.org/pubs/*

- Two programs on kinship care have been developed by the Center for Child and Family Programs at Eastern Michigan University:
  - *Kinship Training Program* provides factual information to sensitize workers to the strengths and needs of kinship family. It consists of four three-hour modules.
  - *The Kinship Caregiver Forums* provide guidelines for presentation to caregivers. Each of the nine forums provides participants with an opportunity to discuss issues, exchange ideas, and develop support networks.

  Materials for both are available at: *www.iscfc.emich.edu.*
- *Empowering Grandparents Raising Grandchildren: A Training Manual for Group Leaders.* Developed by Carol Cox (2000), this manual provides training sessions focused on communicating with children; dealing with problematic behaviors; teaching grandchildren about drugs, sex, HIV; helping children cope with grief and loss; developing advocacy skills; and helping children develop self-esteem. *www.springerpub.com*
- *Assessing Adult Relatives as Preferred Caregivers in Permanency Planning: A Competency-Based Curriculum.* This curriculum was developed by the National Resource Center for Family-Centered Practice and Permanency Planning and is intended to be used in coordination with existing state laws and practices regarding family studies and assessments. Available at: *www.hunter.cuny. edu/socwork/nrcfcpp/info_services/kinship-relative-care.html.*
- *Grandparents' and Other Relative Caregivers' Guides.* Written by the Children's Defense Fund, these guides provide information about health care and insurance, raising children with disabilities, child care and early education programs, and food and nutrition programs. The guides answer questions, provide information about federal programs and eligibility requirements, and how to enroll children. Available at: *www.childrensdefense.org/childwelfare/ kinshipcare/guides.asp.*

Grandsplace
www.grandsplace.org

This website has been specifically developed for grandparents who are raising grandchildren. The site has a chatroom, and provides FAQs on various caregiving issues, message boards, and numerous other resources.

Generations United
www.gu.org

This is the only national organization advocating for the mutual well-being of children, youth, and older adults. GU provides information about national and state programs and policies affecting grandparent caregivers.

REFERENCES

Burnette, D. (1997). Grandparents raising grandchildren in the inner city. *Families in Society, 78* (5), 489-501.

Burnette, D. (1998). Grandparents raising grandchildren: A school-based small group intervention. *Research on Social Work Practice, 8* (1), 10-27.

Burnette, D. (1999). Custodial grandparents in Latino families: Patterns of service use and predictors of unmet needs. *Social Work, 44* (1), 22-34.

Burnette, D. (2000). Latino grandparents rearing grandchildren with special needs: Effects on depressive symptomatology. *Journal of Gerontological Social Work, 33*(3), 1-16.

Burton, L. (1992). Black grandparents rearing children of drug addicted parents: Stressors, outcomes, & social services needs. *The Gerontologist, 32* (6), 744-751.

Burton, L. & DeVries, C. (1992). Challenges and rewards: African American grandparents as surrogate parents. *Generations, 16* (3), 51-54.

Casper, L.M. & Bryson, K.R. (1998). *Grandparents and Their Grandchildren: Grandparent Maintained Families.* Washington, DC; U.S. Bureau of the Census.

Chasnoff, D. (Director) & Cohen, H.S. (Executive Producer) (2000). *That's a Family!* [Videotape]. (Available from Women's Educational Media, 2180 Bryant Street, Suite #203, San Francisco, CA 94110).

Child Welfare League of America (1994). *Kinship Care: A Natural Bridge.* Washington, DC: Child Welfare League of America.

Cohon, D., Hines, L., Cooper, B.A., Packman, W., & Siggins, E. (2003). Preliminary study of an intervention with kin caregivers. *Journal of Intergenerational Relationships, 1* (3): 49-72.

Cox, C.B. (2002). Empowering African American grandparents. *Social Work, 47*(1), 45-54.

Dannison, L.L. & Smith, A.B. (2002). (2003). Custodial Grandparents Community Support Program: Lessons learned. *Children and Schools, 25* (2), 87-95.

Davies, C. & Williams, D. (2003). Lean on Me: Support and Minority Outreach for Grandparents Raising Grandchildren. *Research Report.* Retrieved December 7, 2005. http://www.aarp.org/research/reference/minorities/aresearch-import-483.html

Dressel, P.L. & Barnhill, S. (1994). Reframing gerontological thought and practice: The case of grandmothers with daughters in prison. *The Gerontologist, 34* (5), 685-691.

Dubowitz, H., Feigelman, S., & Zuravin, S. (1993). Children in kinship care. *Child Welfare, 72* (2),153-169.

Emick, M.A. & Hayslip, B. (1999). Custodial grandparenting: Stresses, coping skills, and relationships with grandchildren. *International Journal of Aging and Human Development, 48* (1), 35-61.

Flint, M. & Perez-Porter, M. (1997). Grandparent caregivers: Legal and economic issues. *Journal of Gerontological Social Work, 28* (1/2), 63-76.

Fuller-Thomson, E. & Minkler, M. (2003). Housing issues and realities facing grandparent caregivers who are renters. *The Gerontologist, 43* (1), 92-98.

Fuller-Thomson, E., Minkler, M., & Driver, D. (1997). A profile of grandparents raising grandchildren in the United States. *The Gerontologist, 37* (3), 406-411.

Generations United (2003). *Fact Sheet: Grandparents and Other Relatives Raising Children: Their Inclusion in the National Family Caregiver Support Program.*

Generations United (1999). *Fact Sheet: Grandparents and Other Relatives Raising Children: Challenges of Caring for the Second Family.*

Genty, P. (1998). Permanency planning in the context of parental incarceration: Legal issues and recommendations. *Child Welfare, 77* (5), 543-559.

Grant, R., Gordon, S.G., & Cohen, S.T. (1997). An innovative school-based intergenerational model to serve grandparent caregivers. *Journal of Gerontological Social Work, 28* (1/2), 47-61.

Hayslip, B., Jr., Shore, J., Henderson, C.E., & Lambert, P.R. (1998). Custodial grandparenting and the impact of grandchildren with problems on role satisfaction and role meaning. *Journals of Gerontology: Series B: Psychological Sciences and Social Sciences, 53B* (3), s164-s173.

Hegar, R.L. & Scannapieco, M. (Eds.) (1998). *Kinship Foster Care: Policy, Practice, and Research.* New York : Oxford University Press.

Janicki, M.P., McCallion, P., Grant-Griffin, L., & Kolomer, S.R. (2000). Grandparent caregivers I: Characteristics of the grandparents and the children with disabilities they care for. *Journal of Gerontological Social Work. 33* (3), 35-55.

Jendrek, M.P. (1994). Grandparents who parent their grandchildren: Circumstances and decisions. *The Gerontologist, 34*(2), 206-216.

Kelley, S.J., Yorker, B.C., & Whitley, D. (1997). To grandma's house we go . . . and stay. *Journal of Gerontological Nursing, 23* (9), 12-20.

Kelley, S.J., Yorker, B.C., Whitley, D, & Sipe, T. (2001). A multimodal intervention for grandparents raising grandchildren: Results of an exploratory study. *Child Welfare, 80* (1), 27-50.

Kolomer, S.R. (2000). Kinship foster care and its impact on grandmother caregivers. *Journal of Gerontological Social Work, 33* (3), 85-102.

Kolomer, S.R., McCallion, P., Dugan, S., & Robinson, M.M. (in preparation). Grandparent caregivers use of prescription medication: A pilot study.

Kolomer, S.R., McCallion, P., & Janicki, M. (2002). African-American grandmother carers of children with disabilities: Predictors of depressive symptoms. *Journal of Georntological Social Work, 37* (3/4), 45-63.

Kolomer, S.R., McCallion, P., & Overendyer, J. (2003). Why support groups help: Successful interventions for grandparent caregivers of children with developmental disabilities. In Eds. B. Hayslip, Jr. & J.H. Patrick. *Working with Custodial Grand-parents.* 111-126. New York, NY: Springer Publishing.

Kropf, N.P. & Robinson, M.M. (2004). Pathways into caregiving for rural custodial grandparents. *Journal of Intergenerational Relationships, 2* (1), 63-77.

Macomber, J.E., Geen, R., & Main, R. (2003). Custody, Hardships, and Services. Retrieved November 7, 2005. http://www.urban.org/url.cfm?ID=310893

Mandelbaum, R. (1995). Trying to fit square pegs into round holes: The need for new funding scheme for kinship caregivers. *Fordham Urban Law Journal, 22,* 907-936.

McCallion, P., Janicki, M.P., Grant-Griffin, L., & Kolomer, S.R. (2000). Grandparent caregivers II: Service needs and service provision issues. *Journal of Gerontological Social Work, 33* (3), 57-84.

Minkler, M. (1994). Grandparents as parents: The American experience. *Aging International, 21* (1), 24-28.

Minkler, M. (1999). Intergenerational households headed by grandparents: Contexts, realities, and implications for policy. *Journal of Aging Studies, 13* (2), 199-218.

Minkler, M. & Roe, K.M. (1993). *Grandmothers as Caregivers: Raising Children of the Crack Cocaine Epidemic.* Newbury Park: Sage Publications.

Minkler, M. & Roe, K.M. (1996). Grandparents as surrogate parents. *Generations, 20* (1), 34-38.

Minkler, M., Fuller-Thomson, E., Miller, E., & Driver, D. (1997). Depression in grandparents raising grandchildren. *Archives of Family Medicine, 6,* 445-452.

Minkler, M., Roe, K.M., & Price, M. (1992). The physical and emotional health of grandmothers raising grandchildren in the crack cocaine epidemic. *The Gerontologist, 32* (6), 752-761.

Mullen, F. (1996). Welcome to Procrustes' house: Welfare reform and grandparents raising grandchildren. *Clearinghouse Review, 30* (5), 511-520.

Myers, L., Kropf, N.P. & Robinson, M.M. (2002). Grandparents raising grandchildren: Case management in a rural setting. *Journal of Human Behavior in the Social Environment, 5* (1), 53-71.

Phillips, S. & Bloom, B. (1998). In whose best interest? The impact of changing public policy on relatives caring for children with incarcerated parents. *Child Welfare.* 77(5), 531-541.

Poindexter, C.P. & Linsk, N.L. (1999). "I'm just glad that I'm here": Stories of seven African American HIV-affected grandmothers. *Journal of Gerontological Social Work, 32(1),* 63-81.

Robinson, M.M., Kropf, N.P., & Myers, L. (2000). Grandparents raising grandchildren in rural communities. *Journal of Aging and Mental Health, 6,* 353-365.

Robinson-Dooley, V. & Kropf, N.P. (In Press). Second generation parenting: Grandparents who receive TANF. *Journal of Intergenerational Relationships.*

Roe, K.M. & Minkler, M. (1998/9). Grandparents raising grandchildren: Challenges and responses. *Generations, 22* (4), 1-9.

Roe, K.M., Minkler, M., & Barnwell, R.S. & (1994). The assumption of caregiving: Grandmothers raising the children of the crack-cocaine epidemic. *Qualitative Health Research, 4* (3), 281-303.

Roe, K.M., Minkler, M., Saunders, F. & Thomson, G.E. (1996). Health and grand-mothers raising children of the crack cocaine epidemic. *Medical Care, 34* (11), 1072-1084.

Sands, R.G. & Goldberg-Glen, R.S. (1998). Impact of employment and serious illness on grandmothers who are raising their grandchildren. *Journal of Women & Aging, 10* (3), 41-58.

Silverstein, N.M. & Vehvilainen, L. (1998). *Raising Awareness About Grandparents Raising Grandchildren in Massachusetts.* University of Massachusetts-Boston, MA: Gerontology Institute.

Smith, A.B. & Dannison, L.L. (2002). Educating educators: Programming to support grandparent-headed families. *Contemporary Education, 72* (2), 47-51.

Smith, C.J. & Beltran, A. (2000). Grandparents raising grandchildren: Challenges faced by these growing numbers of families and effective policy solutions. *Journal of Aging & Social Policy, 12* (1), 7-16.

Smith, G. (2003). How caregiving grandparents view support groups: An exploratory study. In Eds. B. Hayslip, Jr. & J.H. Patrick. *Working with Custodial Grandparents.* 69-91. New York, NY: Springer Publishing.

Strozier, A.L., Elrod, B., Beiler, P., Smith, A., & Carter, K. (2004). Developing a net-work of support for relative caregivers. *Children and Youth Services Review, 26,* 641-656.

United States Census Bureau (2004). Selected Social Characteristics: 2004. Data Set: 2004 American Community. Retrieved January 4, 2005. http://factfinder.census.gov/servlet/ADPTable

Waldrop, D.P. & Weber, J.A. (2001). From grandparent to caregiver: The stress and satisfaction of raising grandchildren. *Families in Society: The Journal for Contemporary Human Services, 82* (5), 461-472.

Woodworth, R.S. (1996). You're not alone . . . You are one in a million. *Child Welfare, 75* (5), 619-635.

Chapter 14

Evidence-Based Interventions with Older Adults: Concluding Thoughts

Nancy P. Kropf, PhD
Sherry M. Cummings, PhD

Within this volume, the chapter authors have done a remarkable job summarizing and critiquing the available outcome literature for the older population. In some topical areas, the literature is robust such as the outcome studies on caregiving and depression. Other areas, however, have relatively scant literatures (e.g., HIV/AIDS, grandparents raising grandchildren, and DD) which signify these areas as emerging foci for research energies. Taken collectively, the status of social work intervention research with the older population is uneven at best.

In spite of this fact, there is appreciation in social work for conducting outcome and evaluative research. As Padgett (2005) argues, social work research has progressed over the past decade with a number of efforts to strengthen the research base in the profession. Through initiatives such as the annual Society for Research on Social Work conference, and additional workshops on and applications for NIH funding and other non-traditional sources of funding (e.g., NSF funding opportunities [Jasykyte, 2005]), social work researchers have become more prominent in adding additional knowledge to the outcome literature on psychosocial interventions.

Specifically in aging, progress has been made in constructing a research agenda. In an important study on the current status and future directions for gerontological social work research, the top priority reported by gerontological social workers and researchers was the development and testing of psychosocial interventions for older adults and their families (Morrow-Howell & Burnette, 2001). Clearly, researchers acknowledge that greater understanding about how different intervention approaches promote beneficial outcomes within the diversity of the older adult population is required. Since limited evidence exists in many areas of practice with older adults, researchers have abundant opportunities to conduct research that will add to the knowledge base about effective intervention approaches.

Unfortunately, the profession of social work did little to heed early warnings that additional understanding of aging was necessary to work with an increasingly older population. Back in 1970, Elaine Brody chastised the social work profession for the lack of attention to the older population, yet limited change occurred until the late 1990s when greater resources were devoted to capacity-building in gerontological social work. In particular, the John A. Hartford Foundation must be credited for supporting many initiatives to enhance faculty, student, and curricular enhancements in aging (Rosen & Zlotnik, 2001). For example, many of the authors in this volume have received generous support from the Hartford Foundation as Doctoral Fellows, Faculty Scholars, or through the Geriatric Enrichment Program. In addition, organizations such as the Association for Gerontological Education in Social Work (AGE-SW) and the Baccalaureate Program Directors (BPD) Gerontology Committee support networking and development for faculty in aging. As a greater number of social work researchers are conducting studies in aging, additional knowledge about effective interventions in late life should increase significantly.

STATE OF INTERVENTION RESEARCH

Taken collectively, the articles in this volume provide a beginning method to assess outcome research in aging. A heartening finding is that treatment efficacy has been the focus of various sub-populations within the older population including people with developmental disabilities, terminal illness, and various health conditions (e.g., diabetes, arthritis, cancer, HIV), and grandparents who are raising their grandchildren. These efforts begin the process of contextualizing treatment protocols across various later life issues. Interventions that are appropriate and helpful for those with one specific chronic health condition may be ineffective with another patient population, for example. In addition, relieving caregiving stress for care providers of older adults is quite different from stress experienced by grandparents who are raising grandchildren. Evaluation of approaches that are effective across various health conditions or caregiving roles is an effort to differentiate practice with diverse client populations.

In addition, the literature includes meta-analyses or consensus reports for several of the topical areas contained with this volume. This finding suggests that the state of the psychosocial literature in several areas is at the point of drawing conclusions about treatment efficacy across multiple intervention approaches. Specifically, outcomes for increasing competence and decreasing stress for care providers of older adults, psychosocial interventions in geriatric depression and anxiety, managing arthritis pain, and cardiac wellness have been analyzed through meta-analyses or consensus reports. The outcome of most of this research indicates that interventions often produce moderate success at best, if a clear indication of efficacious treatment can be determined at all. As additional analyses are conducted across treatment studies, a clearer picture of effective interventions will add clarity about useful practice approaches.

One interesting finding across chapters is the introduction of innovative treatment within various areas of practice. Several articles, for example, include studies that employed technology-based interventions and have produced positive impacts for the participants of the studies.

Some interventions were structured to provide information or support, such as telephone and internet support groups for care providers of older adults, grandparents who are raising their grandchildren, and cancer patients. Other technological interventions have monitored risk situations such as blood sugar levels of diabetics and pain status of those with arthritis. Telemedicine is an area that has vast potential to provide services to traditionally underserved populations of older adults (Buckwalter, Davis, Wakefield, Kienzle, & Murray, 2002; Kropf & Grigsby, 1999; Mahoney, Tarlow, & Jones, 2003). Within this volume, it is heartening to learn that technology is providing innovative ways to expand psychosocial and support services to older individuals.

In spite of the gains that have been made in determining effective psychosocial treatment for older adults, certain research areas need to be more robust. One is the strength of the studies' research design, as currently, the majority of psychosocial intervention research uses pre-experimental or quasi-experimental designs. Many researchers use naturalistic settings to conduct outcome research, such as agencies where a treatment situation can be compared to a wait list or usual care procedure. This demonstrates the creativity of the researchers who seize opportunities to evaluate their practice, as well as the challenges in conducting psychosocial evaluations. Yet, more rigorous designs would allow for additional control over interventions and data collection.

Many authors in this volume provide commentary on the lack of consensus over outcomes within their area of focus. Waldrop, for example, reports that in end-of-life care a debate continues concerning the issue of appropriate "outcome." As medical interventions create greater fluidity between chronic and terminal conditions, what are appropriate outcomes for end-of-life researchers to measure? Adamek and Slater discuss treatment resistance in the areas of depression and anxiety which creates complications in determining efficacy. They describe the possibility of including treatment initiation techniques to enhance clients' motivation and decrease resistance to participate in intervention protocols. These types of debates create both empirical and methodological issues that are captured in many of the articles in this volume.

Another challenge is the lack of specificity about treatment interventions in many of the studies reviewed. As the outcomes of interventions require operationalization, the treatment or practice approach also requires definition. In numerous outcome studies cited in this volume, there is a lack of specificity about the intervention or treatment provided. Gaps in knowledge about *how much* treatment was provided (e.g., three months of weekly group sessions), or *service context* (e.g., sessions within the home or a clinician's office) are critical. In medicine, dosage is an important component of evaluating whether a medication regime is effective. Having an older patient ingest three pills at once, for example, is quite different from taking one pill three times per day. Similarly, psychosocial interventions also require specific information about amount and timing of treatment. In order to replicate studies, understanding about what, how, and when treatment was provided is vitally important.

EFFECTIVE INTERVENTION APPROACHES IN LATER LIFE

Although the outcome literature on effective interventions with older adults is uneven across condition and treatment approaches, there are some particular intervention methods that are common across various late life issues. In an effort to analyze outcomes by type of treatment and client condition, three tables are presented that condense the rich analyses presented by the volume authors. Each table presents various treatment types that are associated with important functional domains (health, mental health/cognitive status, and social role functioning) identified by the authors. Outcomes are then summarized within the various treatment protocols (e.g., case management, support groups, etc.) to present an overview of the conditions that have been achieved through these various intervention methods.

Several chapters reported on psychosocial treatment approaches for older adults experiencing various health conditions (see Table 1). Within this body of literature, education, training, and support interventions have numerous effective outcomes. In particular, education and training interventions tend to focus on skill attainment for the management of chronic health conditions. These protocols also enhance coping strategies that can alleviate or reduce stress or discomfort that accompany some of these conditions. Support groups, either face-to-face or via technology, motivate patients to manage tasks and health behaviors to maintain or preserve functioning. These groups also connect patients to others with similar conditions, and potentially decrease stress on family members and care providers. CBT treatments have also been successfully used to manage the psychosocial aspects of chronic conditions.

For later life cognitive and mental health issues (see Table 2), psychotherapy is a primary method of treatment. Across various conditions, CBT and other forms of therapy have promoted social participa-

TABLE 1. Effective Interventions with Late Life Health Conditions

Chapter	Case Management	Education/ Training	CBT Protocols	Support Group	Technological Interventions
Cancer		Journaling increased emotional expression and decreased risk of PTSD, exercise group had improved body image and fitness, lowered depression when paired with peer counselor, audio tapes increased self-efficacy, meditation/wellness increased relaxation and decreased stress	Group decreased depression and increased optimism, improved family functioning	Partners had less stress, enhanced marital quality, patients had decreased negative affect, enhanced social support network	Phone group had positive experience with care providers, phone education intervention lead to greater knowledge of disease
Cardiac Conditions		Increased sexual functioning, lowered health care costs, increased quality of life, decreased chest pain	Decreased re-hospitalization, decreased additional cardiac events, decreased depression and isolation	Especially for me, increased quality of life	
Diabetes	Increased independence, ADLs, knowledge of condition, overall functioning	Increased self-efficacy, self-care behaviors, diet adherence, exercise, weight management		Increased self-care behaviors, social support network, weight maintenance and adherence to diet	Increased diet knowledge, diet adherence, independence
Pain		Decreased experience of pain and physician visits, improved self-efficacy behaviors	Enhanced functioning, pain tolerance, self-efficacy for patient and family members, decreased depression	Improved self-efficacy behaviors, enhanced coping behaviors	Improves pain and disability status, reduced doctor visits
HIV/AIDS				Increased social support, coping, well-being, quality of life	Increased support and health-related knowledge

tion and decreased isolation. In addition, therapy also seems to assist with enhancing functioning such as remaining abstinent from alcohol and increasing memory recall. Therapeutic interventions are delivered within a group format, as well as individually or within a family system.

In Table 3, interventions that promote social role functioning are presented. The various chapters confirm that support and psychoeducational groups are effective approaches to facilitate role transitions and performance. Outcome data indicate that individuals, care providers, and family members who participated in such groups experienced decreased grief and loss issues, decreased feelings of isolation and alienation, and enhanced coping ability and skill performance. Case management has also been used in the area of social role performance, and is effective in enhancing participants' ability to gain access to needed services and in promoting functioning. Psychotherapy approaches also effectively increase individuals', families', and groups' well-being and future planning ability, and improve role functioning. Taken collectively, there are some intervention approaches that are gaining credibility as effective treatments for social issues and role transitions with older adults and their care providers.

FUTURE RESEARCH EFFORTS

The limitations of the current status of the literature point to areas for future research endeavors. One is the strength of the design that is employed. Researchers can seek ways to improve external validity of intervention studies, even if the most stringent designs (e.g., randomized control trials) are impossible. Studies that include multiple research sites, control or comparison groups such as waiting lists, are encouraged. In addition, the inclusion of data about non-completing participants is also critical to determine if mortality or attrition is present and skews results and conclusions.

Outcome studies also need to provide additional data on the persistent impact of the intervention on functioning. Unfortunately, numerous studies cited in this volume collect post-intervention data immediately following the intervention (e.g., at the end of the last group session). This design does not answer the question about whether change has a lasting impact. At minimum, an additional data collection period after the conclusion of an intervention is necessary to determine lasting change.

TABLE 2. Effective Treatments with Late Life Cognitive and Mental Health Issues

Chapter	Social Support/Psycho-Educational Groups	Psychotherapy or Wellness Groups	Individual/Family Psychotherapy	CBT
Dementia		Decreased anxiety and depression, improved reminiscence, decreased depression and agitation, enhanced communication	Memory training improved recognition and recall, improved well-being, improved quality of life, life review enhanced social interaction and decreased isolation	Improved relaxation and social participation
Depression & Anxiety	Social support interventions decreased depression	Reminiscence decreased depression, relaxation decreases anxiety	Behavioral, reminiscence, life review, bibliotherapy, problem-solving approaches and psychodynamic therapies decreased depressive symptoms	Individual and group interventions decreased depression and anxiety
Substance Abuse	Age specific groups enhanced treatment completion		Problem-solving increased abstinence, enhanced community adjustment, elder specific treatment enhanced abstinence and increased overall health status	Increases abstinence, increased treatment adherence

TABLE 3. Effective Interventions with Late Life Social Roles

Chapter	Social Support/Psycho-Educational Grps	Psychotherapy or Wellness Grps	Individual/Family Psychotherapy	Case Management/ Interdisciplinary Team
End of Life	Enhanced social adjustment of bereaved spouses, reduced depression, helped with coping	Increased engagement of bereaved spouses, improved role function and mental health		Improved satisfaction and symptom management
Family Caregivers	Decreased depression and anxiety for caregivers, decreased behavior problems for care recipients, improved caregiver affect, increased caregiver knowledge of resources	Increased general well-being	Decreased/delayed institutionalization of care recipient	
Grandparent Caregivers	Reduced loneliness and isolation, increased access to services, increased grandparent skills, enhanced technology proficiency			Improved grandparent functioning, mental health, access to resources, satisfaction with services
People with DD and Caregivers	Increased future planning, increased caregiver skills, increased knowledge for people with DD, increased leisure choices and life satisfaction		Increased family ability to plan for future care issues	Increased future planning efforts and access to services

As the older population diversifies, additional research on sub-populations must be increased. While there has been substantial attention and acknowledgement that older adults of color are increasing at significant rates (c.f. Cummings, 2004), this understanding has not translated into studies that identify effective interventions with this segment of the older population. Other diverse sub-populations, such as those living in rural areas and people who are gay, lesbian or bisexual, are not present in most of the studies discussed within this volume.

Additionally, a greater array of practice modalities need to be evaluated with the older population. Except in the areas of caregiving, dementia, and end-of-life topics, family interventions are relatively scarce. In addition, these interventions cluster around older adults' functional declines and the families' ability to cope with these losses. These are vital parts of family life and should continue to command research and practice efforts. Yet, extended life expectancies produce other transitions in later life that also require support and practice knowledge. As older adults are living longer, social work practitioners are dealing with families in which an older adult has remarried or re-partnered. Other older adults are outliving their adult children who experience death through significant health problems (e.g., cancer, HIV/AIDS) or through violence or other tragic occurrences (e.g., accidents, suicides). Family intervention modalities that progress beyond care provision and functional decline need to be employed and evaluated to address the social and structural diversity in later life families.

In conclusion, this volume provides an important contribution to the outcome literature. With a focus on psychosocial interventions across physical, emotional and social issues of late life, practice approaches that have empirical support are highlighted. In addition, authors provide treatment resources that can be reviewed for more in-depth information about the nature and consequences of various topics as well as treatment approaches. Hopefully, these beginning efforts will provide a foundation for additional outcome studies that focus on older adults and their families.

REFERENCES

Brody, E. M. (1970). Serving the aged: Educational needs as viewed by practice. *Social Work, 15*, 42-51.

Buckwalter, K. C., Davis, L. L., Wakefield, B. J., Kienzle, M. G., & Murray, M. A. (2002). Telehealth for elders and their caregivers in rural communities. *Family & Community Health, 25*(3), 10-41.

Cummings, S. M. (ed.) (2004). Diversity and aging in the social environment. *Journal of Human Behavior in the Social Environment* (entire-issue), *9*(4).

Jaskyte, K. (2005). The National Science Foundation: Funding opportunities for social workers. *Research on Social Work Practice, 15*, 47-51.

Kropf, N. P. & Grigsby, R. K. (1999). Telemedicine for older adults. *Home Health Care Services Quarterly, 17*(4), 1-11.

Mahoney, D. F., Tarlow, B., & Jones, R. (2003). Effects of an automated telephone support system on caregiver burden and anxiety: Findings from the REACH for TLC intervention study. *The Gerontologist, 43*, 556-567.

Morrow-Howell, N. & Burnette, D. (2001). Gerontological social work research: Current status and future directions. *Journal of Gerontological Social Work.* 36(3/4): 63-79.

Padgett, D. K. (2005). The Society for Social Work and Research at 10 years of age and counting: An idea whose time had come. *Research on Social Work Practice, 15*, 3-7.

Rosen, A. L. & Zlotnik, J. L. (2001). Demographics and reality: The "disconnect" in social work education. *Journal of Gerontological Social Work, 36*(3/4): 81-9.

Index